Allergopedia
Clinical Protocols in Pediatric Allergy

Equipping the Next Gen in Allergy Care

Allergopedia
Clinical Protocols in Pediatric Allergy

Equipping the Next Gen in Allergy Care

Editors

Neeraj Gupta
MBBS DCH DNB FRCPCH DAA FAAAAI IDPCCM DPSM
Allergist, Pediatric Intensivist, and Sleep Medicine Specialist
Department of Pediatrics
Sir Ganga Ram Hospital
New Delhi, India

Krishna Mohan R
DNB DAA MNAMS ICPP
Consultant Pediatrician and Pediatric Allergist
Department of Health Services
Malappuram, Kerala, India

Foreword

Ruchi Gupta

JAYPEE BROTHERS MEDICAL PUBLISHERS
The Health Sciences Publisher
New Delhi | London

Jaypee Brothers Medical Publishers (P) Ltd

Headquarters
EMCA House, 23/23-B
Ansari Road, Daryaganj
New Delhi 110 002, India
Landline: +91-11-23272143, +91-11-23272703
+91-11-23282021, +91-11-23245672
e-mail: jaypee@jaypeebrothers.com

Corporate Office
4838/24, Ansari Road, Daryaganj
New Delhi 110 002, India
Phone: +91-11-43574357
Fax: +91-11-43574314
e-mail: jaypee@jaypeebrothers.com

Overseas Office
JP Medical Ltd.
83, Victoria Street, London
SW1H 0HW (UK)
Phone: +44-20 3170 8910
e-mail: info@jpmedpub.com

EU GPSR Authorised Representative
Logos Europe, 9 rue Nicolas Poussin
17000, La Rochelle, France
Phone: +33 (0) 6 67 93 73 78
e-mail: contact@logoseurope.eu

Website: www.jaypeebrothers.com
Website: www.jaypeedigital.com

Inquiries for bulk sales may be solicited at: jaypee@jaypeebrothers.com

Allergopedia: Clinical Protocols in Pediatric Allergy

First Edition: **2026**

ISBN: 978-93-7202-212-4

Printed at: Samrat Offset Pvt. Ltd.

Dedication

To our patients and their families—
whose courage, resilience, and trust inspire us every day
To our teachers and mentors—
who ignited in us the passion for learning and the commitment to excellence
To our colleagues and friends—
who walk with us in the shared mission of advancing pediatric allergy care
And to our families—
whose unwavering love, support, and understanding have been our greatest strength

Neeraj Gupta
Krishna Mohan R

Contributors

Afaq Jalali
Consultant
Jawahar Lal Nehru Memorial Hospital
Srinagar, Jammu and Kashmir, India

Areeba Shaan
Medical Officer
Jawahar Lal Nehru Memorial Hospital
Srinagar, Jammu and Kashmir, India

D Rama Rajyam
Associate Professor
Department of Pediatrics
Paderu Medical College
Alluri Sitharama Raju, Andhra Pradesh, India
Consultant, Swasa Allergy and Asthma Center
Visakhapatnam, Andhra Pradesh

Dhanesh Volvoikar
Consultant and Pediatric Allergist
Healthway Hospital
Panaji, Goa, India

Dipti Pujari
Consultant Allergist and Pediatrician
Head
Department of Allergy
Deenanath Mangeshkar Hospital and Research Center
Pujari Pediatric and Allergy Center
Pune, Maharashtra, India

Gayatri S Pandit
Consultant Allergist and ENT Specialist
Director
Samarth ENT and Allergy Centre
Manipal Hospital
Bengaluru, Karnataka, India

Hadeeqa Aijaz
Resident
Jawahar Lal Nehru Memorial Hospital
Srinagar, Jammu and Kashmir, India

Hima Mathews P
Consultant Allergist and Pediatrician
Ernakulam, Kerala, India

Kagithapu Surender
Professor and Head
Department of Pediatrics
Government Medical College
Jayashankar Bhupalpally, Telangana, India

Krishna Mohan R
Consultant Pediatrician and Pediatric Allergist
Department of Health Services
Malappuram, Kerala, India

Mahesh PA
Pulmonologist and Allergy Specialist
Professor
Department of Respiratory Medicine
JSS Medical College
JSS Academy of Higher Education and Research
Mysuru, Karnataka, India

MD Ziaul Haque
Pulmonologist
Apollo Multispecialty Hospital
Kolkata, West Bengal, India

Mitesh Kakkad
Consultant Pediatric Pediatrician and Allergist
Director
Neo Children Allergy and Asthma Centre
Ahmedabad, Gujarat, India

Mohammad Naveed
Medical Officer
Jawahar Lal Nehru Memorial Hospital
Srinagar, Jammu and Kashmir, India

Mohit Poddar
Consultant Pediatric Allergist
Medihub Multispecialty Clinic
Jaipur, Rajasthan, India

Muzima Jeelani
Allergy Asthma Counsellor
Jawahar Lal Nehru Memorial Hospital
Srinagar, Jammu and Kashmir, India

Nandana Bala
Consultant Pediatrician
Allergy and Asthma Specialist
Rainbow Children's Hospital
and Prudent Health Specialty Clinic
Bengaluru, Karnataka, India

Naresh Grover
Consultant Pediatrician and Allergy Specialist
Director
Dr Naresh Grover's Advanced Pediatric
and Allergy Management Centre
Amritsar, Punjab, India

Nayan Mani Deka
Consultant Pediatrician and Allergist
Pratiksha Rainbow Children's Hospital
Guwahati, Assam, India

Neeraj Gupta
Allergist, Pediatric Intensivist,
and Sleep Medicine Specialist
Department of Pediatrics
Sir Ganga Ram Hospital
New Delhi, India

Rachna Mehta Shroff
Pediatric Allergist
Devasya Clinic
Mumbai, Maharashtra, India

S Narmada Ashok
Consultant Pediatrician and Allergy Specialist
Director
Nalam Medical Centre and Hospital
Vellore, Tamil Nadu, India

Saibal Moitra
Adjunct Professor and Senior Consultant
Division of Allergy and Immunology
Department of Pulmonology
Apollo Multispecialty Hospitals
Kolkata, West Bengal, India

Sanjukta De
Consultant Allergist and Pediatrician
Clinical Director
Department of Pediatrics
Peerless Hospital
Kolkata, West Bengal, India

Shalini Tyagi
Consultant Allergist and Pediatrician
Asthma and Allergy Centre and
MCRD Allergy Centre
Metro Hospital
Noida, Uttar Pradesh, India

Shamsa Tariq
Resident
Department of Medicine
Hamdard Institute of Medical Sciences
and Research
New Delhi, India

Shebna A Khader
Pediatrician and Allergist
ALLERGO KIDZ Allergy clinic
Midtown Medical Centre
Kochi, Kerala, India

Sinchana Bhat
Consultant Pediatrician and Allergy Specialist
Dr Sinchana's Allergy and Asthma Clinic
Mangaluru, Karnataka, India

Soundarya M
Consultant Pediatrician and Allergist
Kasturba Medical College
Mangaluru, Karnataka, India

Sowmya Arudi Nagarajan
Consultant Allergist and Pediatrician
Sanjeevini Specialty Clinic and Mallige Hospitals
Bengaluru, Karnataka, India

Taha Ashraf Qureshi
Consultant Allergist
Jawahar Lal Nehru Memorial Hospital
Srinagar, Jammu and Kashmir, India

Uppin Narayan Reddy
Consultant Pediatrician and Allergy Specialist
Laxmi Child Clinic
Hyderabad, Telangana, India

Vikram Patra
Allergist and Pediatrician
Senior Consultant
Apollo Hospital
Navi Mumbai, Maharashtra, India

Vinay Mehta
Consultant Allergist
Allergy and Asthma Associates of Southern California
Irvine, CA, USA

Foreword

Allergies are no longer a niche concern. They are a global health challenge affecting every age group, specialty, and region. In recent decades, we have seen a troubling rise in allergic diseases, from asthma and allergic rhinitis to food allergies and anaphylaxis. This burden is especially pronounced in developing countries like India, where rapid urbanization, environmental changes, and evolving lifestyles have created a perfect storm for allergic conditions to thrive.

Allergopedia: Clinical Protocols in Pediatric Allergy is a timely and vital initiative that bridges cutting-edge global allergy science with the unique, context-specific needs of the Indian population. This book offers a comprehensive, evidence-based, and deeply practical roadmap for allergists, pediatricians, and frontline practitioners navigating the complexities of allergic diseases in everyday clinical settings.

What truly sets this book apart is its unapologetic focus on India's distinct challenges and opportunities. From the epidemiology of allergies across diverse Indian regions to the development of diagnostic and therapeutic protocols tailored to local constraints and allergens, each chapter reflects both scientific rigor and cultural relevance. The inclusion of practical algorithms, clinical flowcharts, and real-world scenarios makes this an indispensable resource for clinicians and academic centers training the next generation of allergy specialists.

As someone deeply engaged in allergy research and policy worldwide, I am especially inspired by the vision behind this book—to unify and elevate allergy care in India through collaboration, standardization, and education. Dr Neeraj Gupta and Dr Krishna Mohan R, along with their outstanding team of authors and reviewers, deserve immense credit for creating a high-quality, accessible reference that will have a lasting impact on allergic disease management in the region.

I am confident that *Allergopedia* will serve not only as a protocol guide but also as a cornerstone in the journey toward better allergy awareness, diagnosis, and care across India and beyond. It is a privilege to write this foreword, and I wholeheartedly commend this important contribution to all stakeholders in allergy care.

Ruchi Gupta MD MPH
Professor of Pediatrics and Medicine
Northwestern University Feinberg School of Medicine
Clinical Attending, Ann & Robert H Lurie Children's Hospital of Chicago
Director, Center for Food Allergy and Asthma Research (CFAAR)

Preface

Allergic diseases are no longer rare clinical curiosities—they have emerged as a significant public health challenge in India, affecting individuals across all ages and socioeconomic strata. Rapid urbanization, environmental changes, evolving dietary habits, and increasing pollution have contributed to an alarming rise in asthma, allergic rhinitis, food allergies, and other hypersensitivity disorders. Despite this growing burden, the availability of standardized, India-specific clinical protocols remains limited.

Allergopedia: Clinical Protocols in Pediatric Allergy was conceptualized to address this critical gap. This book brings together the expertise of leading allergists, pediatricians, pulmonologists, dermatologists, and other specialists from across the country to create a practical, evidence-based, and regionally relevant reference for clinicians. Each chapter blends the latest scientific knowledge with pragmatic approaches tailored to Indian realities—be it allergen profiles, diagnostic limitations, or therapeutic accessibility.

The aim is not merely to inform but to empower. From foundational immunology to advanced diagnostics, from pharmacotherapy to immunotherapy, and from environmental control to preventive strategies, *Allergopedia* offers step-by-step, ready-to-apply protocols that can enhance patient outcomes in everyday practice. Special attention has been given to pediatric care, seasonal variations, and culturally sensitive management plans, making this volume a valuable companion in both primary and specialty care settings.

This book is the result of collaborative effort, professional dedication, and a shared vision—to equip the next generation of clinicians with the tools, knowledge, and confidence to deliver optimal allergy care in India. It is our hope that *Allergopedia* will become a trusted, go-to resource in every clinic, hospital, and academic library, ultimately contributing to improved quality of life for patients and families living with allergic diseases.

Neeraj Gupta
Krishna Mohan R

Acknowledgments

The journey of creating *Allergopedia: Clinical Protocols in Pediatric Allergy* has been one of passion, learning, and shared commitment to improving allergy care for children in India. This work is deeply personal to us, yet it would not have been possible without the wisdom, encouragement, and generosity of so many friends and colleagues from across the country.

We are profoundly grateful to the many distinguished pediatricians, allergists, pulmonologists, dermatologists, ENT specialists, and other healthcare professionals who shared their experience, insights, and practical pearls with us during the development of this book. Their contributions—whether in the form of scientific input, clinical guidance, or thought-provoking discussions—have enriched these pages immeasurably.

We also wish to acknowledge the guidance and goodwill of our mentors, seniors, and peers who have inspired our academic journey and strengthened our resolve to pursue this work.

We are indebted to our families for their patience, understanding, and unwavering support during the many long hours of writing, revising, and refining. Their encouragement has been the quiet force that sustained us through this endeavor.

We also extend our sincere appreciation to the publishing team at M/s Jaypee Brothers Medical Publishers (P) Ltd, New Delhi, India, for their professionalism, meticulous attention to detail, and belief in the vision of this book.

Finally, we dedicate *Allergopedia* to every clinician striving to provide the best possible care to children with allergies. It is our hope that this work will serve as a practical companion, a trusted reference, and a small step toward raising the standard of pediatric allergy care in India.

Contents

Introduction

Neeraj Gupta

OVERVIEW OF THE ALLERGY LANDSCAPE IN INDIA

Allergic diseases have emerged as a significant public health challenge in India, paralleling global trends but with distinct regional and socio-environmental dimensions. Once perceived as diseases of affluence and industrialization, allergies are now omnipresent across rural and urban geographies in India, affecting both pediatric and adult populations. The increasing burden of asthma, allergic rhinitis, atopic dermatitis, urticaria, food allergies, and drug hypersensitivities signals a pressing need for comprehensive and culturally adapted clinical guidelines.

The allergy landscape in India is shaped by a confluence of *environmental*, *genetic*, and *lifestyle* factors. Rapid urbanization, climate change, vehicular and industrial pollution, dietary transitions, and changes in microbial exposures have disrupted the delicate immune balance in genetically susceptible individuals. These evolving exposures are believed to skew the immune system toward allergic phenotypes, often manifesting early in life and persisting chronically.

India's vast biodiversity, regional climate variations, and traditional dietary habits introduce a complex web of allergens—ranging from pollens, mites, fungi, and cockroach antigens to food and drug allergens. These require a nuanced approach to diagnosis and management, yet existing international protocols often lack relevance in our setting.

Despite this burden, allergy as a discipline remains under-recognized and under-resourced in India. There is a lack of formal training, limited availability of standardized allergen extracts, non-uniform diagnostic practices, and fragmented care pathways. It is in this context that *Allergopedia* is envisioned—as a timely and essential initiative to streamline and strengthen allergy care across the country.

THE RISING BURDEN OF ALLERGIC DISEASES IN THE INDIAN POPULATION

Epidemiological Trends

In recent years, multiple studies have highlighted a stark rise in the prevalence of allergic disorders in India. The *International Study of Asthma and Allergies in Childhood (ISAAC)* Phase III reported asthma prevalence of up to 20% in certain urban centers. Allergic rhinitis affects nearly 15–30% of school-aged children, with significant overlap with asthma. Atopic dermatitis, once considered rare, is now being reported in 10–15% of pediatric consultations in urban clinics.

Food allergies, though traditionally under-reported due to lack of awareness and diagnostic capacity, are emerging as a growing concern, particularly in children. Drug allergies and anaphylaxis are increasingly encountered in both outpatient and inpatient settings, often managed without standardized protocols.

Regional and Environmental Influences

India's climatic diversity and distinct ecosystems result in substantial *regional variation in allergen exposure*. For instance:

- *Northern India*, with its dry seasons and widespread poplar and parthenium weed exposure, sees high pollen-related respiratory allergies.
- *Southern India*, characterized by humidity and monsoonal patterns, fosters mold overgrowth, and dust mite proliferation.
- *Eastern and northeastern India*, with extensive vegetation and unique pollens such as Albizia and Acacia, reports seasonal flares.
- *Urban megacities*—Delhi, Mumbai, and Bengaluru—grapple with unprecedented levels of *PM2.5, nitrogen dioxide, and ozone*, significantly aggravating asthma and rhinitis.
- *Indoor allergens*, such as *Dermatophagoides* species, cockroach antigens, and mold spores, contribute to perennial symptoms, especially among children living in congested or poorly ventilated homes.

Influence of Urbanization and Lifestyle

Urban living has reshaped dietary patterns, hygiene practices, and environmental exposures in India. Children born and raised in cities are more likely to experience early-life antibiotic use, reduced microbial diversity, lack of breastfeeding, and diminished exposure to protective farm environments—factors contributing to allergic sensitization.

The *"hygiene hypothesis"* and more recently the *"microbiome hypothesis"* posit that reduced microbial stimulation in early life leads to immune dysregulation. In India, this immune dysregulation is compounded by malnutrition, parasitic load, and genetic predisposition in certain populations. Moreover, indoor pollutants from biomass fuels, incense sticks, mosquito coils, and damp housing conditions amplify the allergenic load.

THE NEED FOR TAILORED PROTOCOLS IN INDIAN HEALTHCARE SETTINGS

Diagnostic Gaps and Clinical Challenges

In the absence of national guidelines, clinicians in India often rely on Western protocols that may not align with local realities. Common challenges include:

- *Non-availability of region-specific allergen panels* for skin prick testing or serum-specific immunoglobulin E (IgE) assays
- *Over-diagnosis due to non-standardized testing*, poor interpretation, and lack of clinician training
- *Under-reporting of food and drug allergies* due to diagnostic limitations, societal perceptions, and labeling inadequacies
- *Lack of validated questionnaires* in regional languages, complicating history-taking and symptom scoring

While academic interest in allergy is increasing, there is still a *lack of structured postgraduate training*, and allergists remain a rarity in many regions. Pediatricians, pulmonologists, dermatologists, ENT specialists, and general practitioners form the frontline of allergy care—but often lack formal exposure to current best practices.

Challenges in Therapeutic Strategies

Allergen-specific immunotherapy (AIT), one of the only disease-modifying therapies in allergy, is grossly underutilized in India due to:

- Limited awareness and training
- High cost and import-dependence of allergen extracts
- Perceived risks of adverse reactions and medicolegal apprehensions

Similarly, *biologic therapies* for severe asthma and atopic dermatitis are scarcely prescribed due to cost, lack of protocols, and uncertainty about indications in Indian patients. Even basic pharmacotherapy is marred by over-the-counter misuse, steroid phobia, and non-adherence due to low health literacy.

Hence, there is an urgent need for *India-specific practice protocols*—grounded in evidence, yet adaptable to local resource constraints and sociocultural dynamics.

GOALS AND VISION OF ALLERGOPEDIA

Allergopedia is conceived as the first effort to curate *standardized, practical, and regionally contextualized protocols* for allergy diagnosis and management in India. This compendium is a milestone in India's journey toward rational, equitable, and science-based allergy care.

Key Objectives

- *To bridge the knowledge-practice gap* by equipping healthcare providers with user-friendly, evidence-informed, and India-relevant protocols.
- *To harmonize clinical practice* by minimizing variability in allergy diagnosis and treatment across regions and specialties.
- *To promote rational use of diagnostic tests* through standardized indications, interpretation guidelines, and allergen panel design.
- *To empower generalists and specialists alike*, enabling early recognition, appropriate referral, and safe in-office management of allergic conditions.
- *To advocate for structured allergy education and training*, encouraging inclusion in undergraduate, postgraduate, and CME curricula.
- *To stimulate policy conversations* around the inclusion of allergy services under national health programs and insurance coverage.

Structure and Content

Allergopedia is organized into 16 comprehensive chapters spanning:

- Basic science and immunology of allergy
- Regional epidemiology and burden
- Diagnostic strategies and novel technologies
- Disease-specific management (asthma, rhinitis, eczema, urticaria, food allergy, etc.)
- Pharmacotherapy and immunotherapy protocols
- Ethical and legal dimensions of allergy practice
- Environmental control, preventive strategies, and special population considerations
- Creation of an integrated allergy care network

Each chapter is authored by subject experts and peer-reviewed for scientific accuracy and clinical relevance. Chapters follow a uniform structure—*Introduction, Main Content, Summary, and Key Learning Points*—with emphasis on tables, flowcharts, algorithms, and real-world scenarios.

Appendices include *practical tools* such as region-wise pollen maps, patient history forms, consent templates, and referral protocols.

A CALL TO ACTION

Allergopedia is more than a protocol book—it is a *manifesto for the future of allergy care in India*. It calls upon healthcare providers, academic institutions, policymakers, and patient advocacy groups to:

- *Recognize allergy as a major public health challenge*, not a niche specialty.
- *Invest in capacity building*, including training of healthcare workers, laboratory standardization, and indigenous allergen extract development.
- *Integrate allergy services* into national programs addressing non-communicable diseases and environmental health.

- *Support research and surveillance* to build India-specific data on allergen prevalence, treatment outcomes, and economic burden.

CONCLUSION

The rising tide of allergic diseases in India is undeniable—and so is the urgency to respond with cohesive, contextual, and compassionate care models. *Allergopedia* represents a landmark step in this journey, uniting the expertise of clinicians, researchers, and educators to offer a *gold standard of allergy protocols tailored for India*.

As this book finds its way into clinics, hospitals, classrooms, and conference halls, we envision a ripple effect—*better diagnosis, safer treatment, fewer exacerbations, and ultimately improved quality of life for millions of allergy sufferers across India*.

CHAPTER

1

Immunology of Allergy

Taha Ashraf Qureshi, Muzima Jeelani, Mohammad Naveed, Afaq Jalali, Hadeeqa Aijaz, Areeba Shaan, Shamsa Tariq, MD Ziaul Haque

Reviewer: *Saibal Moitra*

INTRODUCTION

Allergy is an exaggerated immune response to normally harmless environmental substances known as allergens. This exaggerated immune response is classified under the broader category of hypersensitivity reactions. As was described by Gell and Coombs, these include type I (immediate), type II (cytotoxic), type III (immune complex-mediated), and type IV (delayed-type) hypersensitivities. Among these, type I hypersensitivity is mediated by immunoglobulin E (IgE) antibodies and involves rapid activation of mast cells and basophils, leading to symptoms ranging from mild allergic rhinitis to life-threatening anaphylaxis. This chapter will be delving upon the commonest mode of presentation of different clinical allergies which envisage the type I mechanism of hypersensitivity reaction.

TYPE I (IMMEDIATE OR IMMUNOGLOBULIN E-MEDIATED HYPERSENSITIVITY)

Type I hypersensitivity, or immediate or anaphylactic hypersensitivity, is mediated by IgE. During initial exposure to an allergen (e.g., pollen, dust mite, or food proteins), the immune system is sensitized and forms IgE antibodies.

The IgE antibodies attach to mast cell and basophil receptors. When exposed again later to the same allergen, it cross-links the IgE on these cells, leading to degranulation and release of histamine and other pro-inflammatory mediators. This results in symptoms such as sneezing, itching, wheezing, hives, and anaphylaxis in severe forms—a sudden, life-threatening event with airway constriction, blood pressure decrease, and shock.

THE ROLE OF IMMUNOGLOBULIN E IN ALLERGIC REACTIONS

Immunoglobulins are glycoproteins secreted by plasma cells in response to pathogens, with IgE among the five primary classes (IgA, IgD, IgE, IgG, and IgM) of antibodies. IgE, as opposed to IgG or IgA, is produced in small amounts and is mainly involved in allergic response and prevention of parasitic infections. Structurally, IgE consists of two heavy chains (epsilon) and two light chains **(Fig. 1)** and binds to receptors of high affinity to

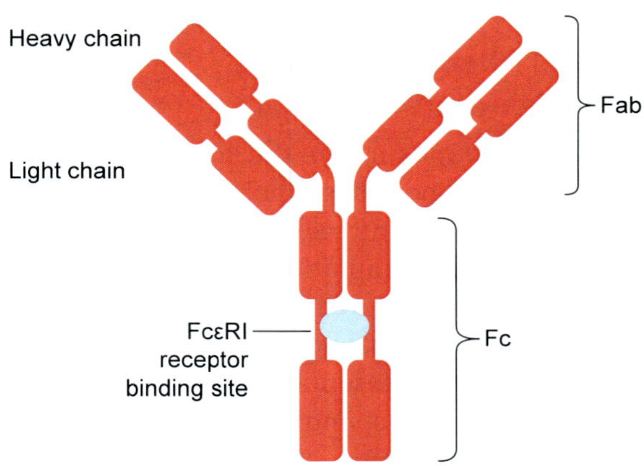

Fig. 1: Structure of immunoglobulin E (IgE) antibody.

IgE (FcεRI) which are present on the surface of various immune cells including mast cells and basophils.

MECHANISM OF HYPERSENSITIVITY REACTION

The IgE-mediated allergic response is a complex molecular process that involves a lot of cellular interactions and signaling pathways.

Immunoglobulin E Sensitization

The allergens' first interaction with an individual initiates the allergen-presenting cells such as dendritic cells to process and present the allergen to T-helper cells (Th2). The immune response in allergic individuals is typically a Th2-dominant immune response which further activates B cells to become plasma cells and produce allergen-specific IgE.

After allergens combine with specific IgE antibodies, they are released into the bloodstream. These allergen-specific IgE bind to a high-affinity receptor for IgE (FcεRI) on the surface of mast cells and basophils, which are distributed throughout tissues, particularly in the skin, lungs, and gastrointestinal (GI) tract. This sensitization process is crucial for the subsequent allergic reaction upon re-exposure to the same allergen.

Clinical Allergy and the Role of Various Cells

On second exposure to the allergen, cross-linking of FcεRI-bound IgE molecules by allergen triggers a series of intracellular signaling events that leads to degranulation of mast cells and basophils, releasing preformed mediators, such as histamine, heparin, and proteases. This results in varied clinical presentation of IgE-mediated allergic reactions depend on the organ system affected **(Fig. 2)**.

ROLE OF MAST CELLS IN ALLERGIC REACTIONS

Mast cells are known for their central role in allergic reactions. These immune cells are primarily located in connective tissues, particularly in the skin, lungs, gastrointestinal tract, and mucosal surfaces. Upon activation, mast cells release a broad array of inflammatory mediators, which can lead to a wide range of allergic symptoms, including inflammation, tissue damage, and hypersensitivity responses.

Mast Cell Development and Distribution

Originating from hematopoietic stem cells in the bone marrow, mast cells differentiate into progenitor cells that circulate before migrating to tissues where they mature. In the tissues, mast cells settle in areas exposed to the external environment including the skin, lung, and gut, making them ideally situated to respond to pathogens, allergens, and environmental insults.

Mast cells are characterized by large granules containing preformed mediators such as histamine, proteases (e.g., tryptase and chymase), heparin, and cytokines. These mediators are kept stored in a quiescent state within the granules and are released upon mast cell activation. Mast cells exhibit specific characteristics, which include multiple receptors and the ability to synthesize different effector molecules, allowing them to mediate complex immune responses.

Mast Cell Activation and Degranulation

The activation of mast cells begins when the allergen cross-links the IgE antibodies on the mast cell surface. This cross-linking leads to the aggregation of FcεRI receptors, activating intracellular signaling pathways, including the phosphorylation of Syk kinase, phospholipase C (PLC), and protein kinase C (PKC). The intracellular signaling pathways increase intracellular levels

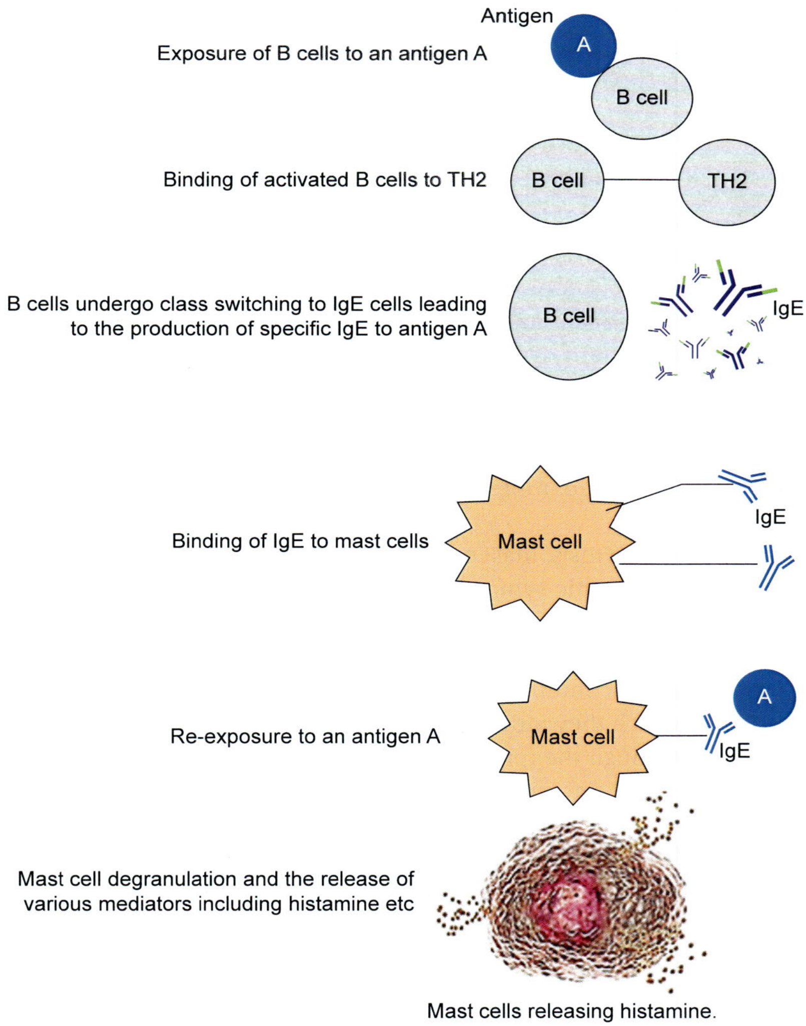

Fig. 2: Mechanism of hypersensitivity reaction.

of calcium, leading to the release of preformed granules containing histamine, cytokines, proteases, and other inflammatory mediators. Histamine, one of the most well-known released when mast cells are activated, is the major mediator of the pathophysiology of allergic reactions. Histamine causes contraction of smooth muscle, vasodilation, and increase in vascular permeability, and mucus secretion which are characteristic of allergic symptoms such as itching, swelling, and nasal congestion. Leukotrienes, prostaglandins, and platelet-activating factors (PAF) are also newly synthesized upon mast cell activation and are mediators of the late-phase inflammatory response. Mast cells also secrete pro-inflammatory cytokines like interleukin (IL)-4, IL-5, IL-6, and tumor necrosis factor (TNF)-α. These cytokines also enhance the allergic reactions by triggering the differentiation of Th2 cells and the recruitment of eosinophils and other immune cells. They are responsible for the chronic inflammation seen in allergic diseases, such as asthma and allergic rhinitis.

Mast Cells in Non-immunoglobulin E-Mediated Allergic Reactions

Although mast cells are classically associated with IgE-dependent reactions, they are also involved in non-IgE-dependent allergic reactions. In non-IgE-dependent allergic reactions, mast cells may be activated directly by certain drugs (e.g., opiates), physical stimuli (e.g., cold, exercise), or by activation by other receptors such as TLRs (toll-like receptors), which have the capacity to recognize pathogen-associated molecular patterns.

In conditions such as mastocytosis, mast cells are overactivated, leading to chronic symptoms such as flushing, diarrhea, and anaphylactoid-like manifestations even without IgE. Mast cells are also implicated in autoimmune conditions such as rheumatoid arthritis, in which they induce the inflammation of the joints through the release of pro-inflammatory mediators and cytokines.

THE ROLE OF BASOPHILS IN ALLERGIC REACTIONS

Basophils are a granulocyte, a white blood cell that plays important role in the immune response, especially in allergic reactions. Although the least common of the granulocytes (<1% of the circulating white blood cells), basophils are key mediators of both the early and late allergic reactions. Basophils are involved in allergic reactions by releasing several pro-inflammatory mediators and by modulating the function of other immune cells.

Basophils and Immunoglobulin E-Mediated Allergic Reactions

One of the most important roles of basophils in allergy is their involvement in the IgE-mediated immune response. The traditional allergic response is triggered when an allergen is identified by the immune system in a genetically predisposed host.

Sensitization and Activation of Basophils

Basophils, much like mast cells, play a critical role in the initiation and propagation of allergic and inflammatory responses. Their mechanism of activation parallels that of mast cells, particularly in their capacity to respond to IgE-mediated stimuli. Cross-linking of allergen-bound IgE on high-affinity FcεRI receptors on the surface of basophils with exposure to allergens initiates degranulation and histamine, leukotrienes, and cytokine release. Besides IgE-dependent mechanisms, basophils can also be triggered by IgG receptors, complement components (e.g., C5a), and other cytokines like IL-3. Basophils play roles in both immediate hypersensitivity responses and the regulation of adaptive immune responses, further establishing their functional similarity to mast cells while maintaining distinct characteristics regarding kinetics, localization, and regulatory interactions.

Promotion of Th2 Immune Response

Basophils play a pivotal role in the regulation of the Th2-predominant immune response that defines allergic disease, such as asthma, allergic rhinitis, and atopic dermatitis. Basophils are producers of IL-4 and IL-13, which are Th2-predominant cytokines. Basophils are of great importance in initiating production of IgE and in activating other inflammatory cells such as eosinophils, which perpetuate the cascade of inflammation.

Basophils in Chronic Allergic Inflammation

Basophils are not only involved in the immediate response (early-phase reactions such as pruritus, redness, swelling, and urticaria) but also contribute to the chronic phase of allergic inflammation (late-phase allergic responses, i.e., tissue inflammation) thereby serving to maintain the allergic response even after mast cells have been eliminated.

Basophil Contribution to Airway Remodeling and Allergic Asthma

In chronic allergic illnesses such as asthma, basophils contribute to airway remodeling through the induction of eosinophil and other inflammatory cell recruitment into the lung. This is facilitated by cytokines such as IL-4 and IL-13 secreted by basophils in the late-phase response. These cytokines help to coordinate tissue remodeling, fibrosis, and mucus hyperproduction that are pathogenic processes in the chronicity of conditions such as asthma.

THE ROLE OF EOSINOPHILS IN ALLERGIC REACTIONS

Eosinophils are white blood cells that play an important role in the immune response, particularly in allergic disease. Eosinophils have a central function in the inflammatory responses of asthma, allergic rhinitis, atopic dermatitis, and eosinophilic esophagitis. Eosinophils play a role in the acute and late allergic reactions, and their function is pivotal in tissue damage, chronic inflammation, and remodeling of most of the allergic diseases.

Eosinophil Recruitment and Activation in Allergic Reactions

Eosinophils are generally recruited to allergic inflammatory tissues by a variety of signals, mainly eotaxin, a chemokine that binds to eosinophil receptors. Mobilization is mainly induced by the presence of Th2 cytokines, mainly IL-4, IL-5, and IL-13, produced by Th2 cells, mast cells, and basophils in an allergic reaction.

Role of Interleukin-5 in Eosinophil Activation

Of the cytokines, IL-5 is the most crucial to eosinophil activation and development. IL-5 promotes eosinophil differentiation from bone marrow hematopoietic progenitors and survival and cell proliferation. IL-5 also stimulates eosinophil granule release in the form of toxic proteins and thus contributes to the inflammatory process. Indeed, IL-5 blockade has been noted to decrease blood and tissue eosinophils and also the symptoms of asthma.

Eosinophils in the Chronic Phase of Allergic Inflammation

Eosinophils are also important in the late-phase or chronic phase of the allergic response. After the first encounter with an allergen and acute immune response, eosinophils contribute to the chronic inflammation and tissue remodeling that are characteristic of chronic allergic diseases such as asthma and allergic rhinitis.

Eosinophil Contribution to Airway Remodeling in Asthma

Eosinophils also contribute to airway remodeling, a condition where the architecture of the airway is changed and permanent changes in lung function follow. Eosinophils also release transforming growth factor-beta (TGF-β), a cytokine that stimulates the production of extracellular matrix proteins such as collagen and fibronectin, leading to fibrosis and thickening of the airway wall. Airway remodeling leads to airway hyperresponsiveness and airway constriction, leading to chronic wheezing and breathlessness symptoms.

Besides fibrosis, eosinophils are also implicated in mucus hypersecretion by releasing IL-13 that stimulates mucus secretion in airway epithelial cells. Air flow obstruction and asthma exacerbation are a result of mucus deposition.

GENE AND ENVIRONMENTAL INFLUENCES

Gene-environment interactions and epigenetics are important elements in determining the etiology of allergies. Genetic susceptibility as well as environmental factors significantly contributes to regulating immune functions, possibly causing allergic conditions such as asthma, rhinitis, and atopic dermatitis. Gene-environment interaction and epigenetic research in allergy development has increased in the last few decades, and evidence for the Indian population has begun to be studied.

Gene-Environment Interactions in Allergy Development

Gene-environment interactions refer to the ways in which genetic predisposition interacts with environmental factors to influence the risk of developing allergic diseases. For example, individuals with specific genetic variants may be more susceptible to environmental triggers such as air pollution, dietary factors, or infections, which may in turn increase the likelihood of allergic diseases.

Genetic factors: Studies have identified several genes that are linked to the development of allergies. These include genes involved in immune responses, such as those coding for cytokines, immunoglobulins, and receptors for allergens. One of the most commonly studied genes is the *IL-4* gene, which plays a key role in the development of allergic reactions by promoting the differentiation of T-helper cells into Th2 cells. In Indian populations, polymorphisms in the *IL-4* gene have been associated with an increased risk of asthma and rhinitis.

Additionally, genes related to the *filaggrin* gene (*FLG*), which is crucial for maintaining the skin barrier, have been linked to atopic dermatitis. Mutations in *FLG* have been found to increase susceptibility to eczema and other allergic conditions. Studies have shown that Indian children with specific FLG mutations are more prone to developing skin-related allergic reactions, though these genetic variations are not as prevalent in the Indian population as in Western cohorts.

Environmental factors: Environmental influences such as air pollution, allergen exposure (pollen, dust mites, etc.), hygiene habits, and diet are imperative in the development of allergies. In India, urbanization and exposure to elevated levels of air pollution have been found to aggravate asthma and other allergic diseases among children. For example, exposure to particulate matter (PM2.5) has been highly linked to asthma attacks among children in cities such as Delhi. Likewise, the greater adoption of modern cleansing products and decreasing exposure to pathogenic agents in early childhood (hygiene hypothesis) are suspected to be contributing to the growth in allergic illness.

EPIGENETICS IN ALLERGY DEVELOPMENT

Epigenetics is the process of gene expression changes that are not accompanied by alterations in the base deoxyribonucleic acid (DNA) sequence but remain heritable. Epigenetic changes, including DNA methylation, histone modification, and regulation by non-coding ribonucleic acid (RNA), can affect the immune response to environmental stimuli and consequently affect allergy formation. Epigenetic changes can be affected by exposures during early life, such as diet, pollution, infections, and lifestyle **(Table 1)**.

- *Deoxyribonucleic acid methylation and allergies:* DNA methylation, or the deposition of methyl groups onto the DNA molecule, is one of the most important epigenetic pathways to influence gene expression. When it comes to allergies, epigenetic DNA

TABLE 1: Epigenetic modification in allergy.

Epigenetic mechanism	*Role in allergy development*	*Key findings/examples*	*Relevance to Indian studies*
Deoxyribonucleic acid (DNA) methylation	Alters gene expression by adding methyl groups to DNA, influencing immune function	Hypomethylation of the *IL-4* gene promoter is associated with increased asthma susceptibility	Indian study showed children from polluted areas had altered DNA methylation in inflammation-related genes
Histone modifications	Affects chromatin structure through acetylation/ methylation, modulating gene accessibility and immune responses	Histone modifications regulate genes involved in allergic inflammation pathways	*Sundararajan et al. (2020)* found urban air pollution triggered histone changes increasing allergic sensitization
MicroRNA (miRNA) regulation	Post-transcriptional gene silencing of immune-related genes, influencing allergy development	Dysregulation of miRNAs affects *Th2 pathway*, a key player in allergic diseases such as asthma	*Pillai et al. (2018)* identified specific dysregulated miRNAs in Indian children with asthma
Environmental exposures	Early-life exposures (e.g., air pollution, maternal diet, infections) induce lasting epigenetic modifications	Air pollution during pregnancy alters DNA methylation in offspring, raising future allergy risk	Environmental factors common in India (e.g., poor air quality, infections) shown to influence epigenetic programming

methylation modification can impact the functioning of the immune system, which in turn may trigger allergic reactions. An example is that hypomethylation of the *IL-4* gene promoter correlates with higher susceptibility to asthma among children. Researchers in an Indian study discovered children growing up in polluted communities had different DNA methylation patterns in inflammatory-related genes, suggesting a possible connection between environmental pollution and epigenetic alterations leading to asthma.

- *Histone modifications and immune response:* Histone modification, in turn, impacting gene expression and chromatin structure is also responsible for the formation of allergy. Experiments revealed that histone methylation and acetylation could modulate immune pathway activation involved in the central allergic inflammation. A research conducted by Sundararajan et al. (2020) found that exposure to particulate matter in urban settings may cause histone modifications leading to increased allergic sensitization in children, especially in Indian cities with high air pollution levels.
- *MicroRNA regulation in allergies:* MicroRNAs (miRNAs), small non-coding RNAs, can also modulate immune responses and have been found to be involved in the pathogenesis of allergy. Pillai et al. (2018) investigated the function of miRNAs in the regulation of immune responses in Indian children with asthma. They found certain miRNAs that were dysregulated in patients with asthma, which could be responsible for the development and worsening of allergic diseases. These miRNAs were identified to target genes that play a role in the Th2 immune response, which is the key to allergy development.
- *Environmental exposures and epigenetic modifications:* In Indian children, environmental

exposures such as nutrition, air pollution, and infections have been found to affect epigenetic changes. As an instance, exposure to air pollution during pregnancy has been found to change DNA methylation profiles, elevating the risk of allergic conditions in adulthood.

Three Signal Paradigm in Development of Allergy Phenotype

The interactions between antigen-presenting cells (APCs) and T cell are a cornerstone of the adaptive immune response. This interaction is governed by a well-established "three signal paradigm" which is essential for the activation, differentiation, and functions of T cells.

The three signal incudes:

1. Antigen-specific recognition
2. Co-stimulatory interactions
3. Cytokine-mediated polarization

Signal 1 involves antigen specific recognition, where a T cell receptor (TCR) binds to a peptide-MHC (major histocompatibility complex) complex displayed on the surfaces of the APC. CD4+ T cells recognize antigenic peptides presented by MHC class II molecules (on dendritic cells, macrophages, and B cells). Although this signal provides antigen specificity, it is insufficient alone for full T cell activation and may instead lead to T cell anergy or tolerance if not accompanied by co-stimulatory signals.

Signal 2 consists of co-stimulatory interactions that amplify the TCR signals and are crucial for full T cell activations, survival, and proliferations. One major co-stimulatory pathway involves the binding of CD28 on T cells with B7-1 (CD80) or B7-2 (CD86) on APCs. Other important pathways include the ICOS-ICOSL (inducible T cell co-stimulator and its ligand) interaction, which modulates the function of follicular helper T cells (Tfh), and the CD40-CD40L interactions, which enhances antigen presentation, antibody production by B cells and cytokine production. The absence of co-stimulatory signals causes T cell to enter a state of anergy there by preserving self-tolerance and preventing autoimmunity.

Signal 3 is characterized by the release of cytokines from APCs and the surrounding immune environment, directing the functional specialization of activated T cells. For instance, IL-4 drives Th2 cell development (important for defense against extracellular bacterial defense), and IL-10 along with TGF-beta help generate regulatory T cells (Tregs), which suppress immune overactivity and maintain tolerance. Cytokine signaling is primarily mediated via the JAK-STAT pathway, facilitating the plasticity and adaptability of the immune response to various pathogens.

Together these three signals ensure precise control of T cell activation, preventing harmful immune responses while enabling robust defense mechanisms.

SUMMARY

This foundational chapter delves into the immunological underpinnings of allergic diseases, with a primary focus on type I (IgE-mediated) hypersensitivity reactions. It outlines the complex interplay of immune cells—mast cells, basophils, eosinophils—and molecular mediators such as histamine and cytokines that culminate in allergic inflammation. The chapter describes how allergen exposure leads to sensitization, IgE production, and subsequent allergic reactions upon re-exposure. It further explores the unique roles of mast cells in both IgE and non-IgE-mediated allergies, the contribution of basophils to both early and late-phase allergic responses, and the pivotal function of eosinophils in chronic allergic inflammation and airway remodeling. Additionally, the influence of genetic and environmental factors, particularly in the Indian context, and emerging insights into epigenetics are discussed. The three-signal paradigm of T-cell activation provides a conceptual framework for understanding immune polarization in allergy development.

Key Learning Points

- *Immunoglobulin E-mediated reactions (type I hypersensitivity):*
    - Allergens induce IgE production, which sensitizes mast cells and basophils. Re-exposure leads to degranulation and release of inflammatory mediators causing immediate allergic symptoms such as asthma, rhinitis, or anaphylaxis.
- *Role of effector cells in allergy:*
    - Mast cells and basophils mediate early-phase allergic responses through histamine and cytokine release; eosinophils drive chronic inflammation and tissue remodeling, particularly in conditions such as asthma and atopic dermatitis.
- *Molecular signaling pathways:*
    - Activation of FcεRI on mast cells initiates signaling cascades (e.g., MAPK, NF-κB) leading to mediator release. Cytokines such as IL-4, IL-5, and IL-13 amplify allergic responses and immune cell recruitment.
- *Gene-environment-epigenetic interactions:*
    - Genetic predisposition (e.g., *IL-4*, *FLG* mutations) interacts with environmental exposures (e.g., pollution, hygiene) to influence allergy risk. Epigenetic modifications such as DNA methylation and microRNA dysregulation are increasingly recognized in allergy pathogenesis, with Indian studies highlighting regional relevance.
- *Three-signal paradigm in T-cell activation:*
    - *Allergic sensitization involves three essential signals:* Antigen recognition (TCR-MHC interaction), co-stimulatory signals (e.g., CD28-CD80/86), and cytokine-mediated polarization (e.g., IL-4 for Th2 bias), facilitating T-cell activation and differentiation central to allergic disease progression.

SUGGESTED READING

1. Bloom BR, Bennett B. Mechanism of a reaction in vitro associated with delayed-type hypersensitivity. Science. 1966;153(3731):80-2.
2. Dispenza MC. Classification of hypersensitivity reactions. Allergy Asthma Proc. 2019;40(6): 470-473.
3. Dixon FJ. The Pathogenesis of Serum Sickness. N Eng J Med. 1969;280(24):1295-1300.
4. Galli SJ. The mast cell as a critical effector in allergic inflammation. Clin Immunol Immunopathol. 2000;95(2):88-97.
5. Gell PGH, Coombs RRA. The classification of allergic reactions underlying disease. In: Clinical Aspects of Immunology. 1963.
6. Gould HJ, Sutton BJ. IgE in allergy and asthma today. Nat Rev Immunol. 2008;8(3):205-17.
7. Irani C, Hallit S, Mouzannar M, Salameh P. Aeroallergen sensitization and upper respiratory allergies among patients living in rural and urban areas: Real-life exploration of the hygiene hypothesis. World Allergy Organ J. 2019;12(9): 100059.
8. Iype J, Fux M. Basophils Orchestrating Eosinophils' Chemotaxis and Function in Allergic Inflammation. Cells. 2021;10(4):895.
9. Kashiwakura J, Yokoi H, Saito H, Okayama Y. T cell–mediated selective activation of basophils in chronic allergic inflammation. J Immunol. 2004;173(1):769-75.
10. Kemp SF, Lockey RF. Anaphylaxis: a review of causes and mechanisms. J Allergy Clin Immunol. 2002;110(3):348-58.
11. Kousha A, Mahdavi Gorabi A, Forouzesh M, Hosseini M, Alexander M, Imani D, Razi B, Mousavi MJ, Aslani S, Mikaeili H. Interleukin 4 gene polymorphism (-589C/T) and the risk of asthma: a meta-analysis and met-regression based on 55 studies. BMC Immunol. 2020; 21(1):55.
12. Kumar A, Choudhary R. Immunology of asthma. Allergy Rhinolog. 2014;5(2):67-74.
13. Lambrecht BN, Hammad H. The role of dendritic cells and eosinophils in allergic disease. Nature Immunology, 2010;11(4):244-50.
14. Metcalfe DD, Baram D, Mekori YA. Mast cells. Physiol Rev. 1997;77(4):1033-79.
15. Miyake K, Karasuyama H. Emerging roles of basophils in allergic inflammation. Allergol Int. 2017;66(3):382-391.

16. Morita H, Saito H, Matsumoto K, Nakae S. Regulatory roles of mast cells in immune responses. Semin Immunopathol. 2016;38(5):623-9.
17. Nagase H, Ueki S, Fujieda S. The roles of IL-5 and anti-IL-5 treatment in eosinophilic diseases: Asthma, eosinophilic granulomatosis with polyangiitis, and eosinophilic chronic rhinosinusitis. Allergol Int. 2020;69(2):178-186.
18. Perera F, Herbstman J. Prenatal environmental exposures, epigenetics, and disease. Reprod Toxicol. 2011;31(3):363-73.
19. Rathi A, Sharma S. Changing Allergy Patterns in India. M J Immu. 2017;1(1):003.
20. Reddy KRBK, Gupta N, Bhattacharya BG, Deka NM, Chandane P, Kapoor R, Gupta S, Nagarajan SA, Basavaraja GV, Parekh BJ. Impact of Air Pollution on Allergic Rhinitis and Asthma: Consensus Statement by Indian Academy of Pediatrics. Indian Pediatr. 2021;58(8):765-70.
21. Rothenberg ME. Eosinophilic gastrointestinal disorders (EGID). J Allergy Clin Immunol. 2009; 124(3):615-20.
22. Samuels J. Immunoglobulin E (IgE) and allergy: An overview. Ann Allergy Asthma Immunol. 2019;123(1):10-8.
23. Sicherer SH, Sampson HA. Food allergy. J Allergy Clin Immunol. 2014;134(5):983-91.
24. van de Veen W, Akdis M. Mechanisms of immune regulation in allergy. In: Akdis CA, Agache I (Eds). EAACI Global Atlas of Allergy. Zurich: European Academy of Allergy and Clinical Immunology. 2015. pp. 90-1.
25. Weller PF, Spencer LA. Functions of tissue-resident eosinophils. Nat Rev Immunol. 2017; 17(12):746-60.
26. Wernersson S, Pejler G. Mast cell secretory granules: Armed for battle. Nat Rev Immunol. 2014;14(7):478-94.

CHAPTER

2

Epidemiology of Allergic Diseases in India

Soundarya M
Reviewer: *Kagithapu Surender*

INTRODUCTION

As we advance further into the 21st century, the trend toward an increasing burden of allergic diseases has been noted. With the advent of potent antibiotics, better methods of sanitation and control of infections, there is a steady rise in non-communicable diseases including allergies. This rise was first noted in the Western countries and is now being noted in India as we have begun to adopt urbanization and westernization; and allergies have a complex interaction between the genetic make-up of an individual and the environment. Recent epidemiological studies done also report an increasing incidence of allergic diseases in India across the last 20–25 years. This has been in all types of allergies—asthma, allergic rhinitis, atopic dermatitis, and even food allergies. Numerous studies have been done on the incidence and prevalence of asthma and its changing trends. The ISAAC study done early this century in 2009, showed that wide variations existed in the prevalence of childhood asthma symptoms and even though these were more prevalent in the developed nations, they were found to be more severe in the developing nations. These changes are due to global climatic changes as a result of pollution, deforestation and urbanization. And as India is now stepping into the urbanization, that the world moved into the last century, the allergy epidemic is now marching forward in India.

PREVALENCE STATISTICS IN ALLERGIES

Across the world almost 30–35% children have an allergic disorder. Studies regarding the prevalence of allergies have been done in western countries but not much literature is available from India. With a large population of 1.45 billion and contributing to 17.78% of the world's population, the studies done from India reflect mainly the urban population and a large number in rural population have not been represented in the scientific literature. Studies done at multiple centers all over the world have shown a reduction in the incidence and prevalence of allergies however, studies in India have reported an increase in the same.

Allergic rhinitis (AR): It impacts quality of life and causes substantial morbidity. It impacts a significant proportion of the population and has been reported in a recent study done by Sundaraman in 2023 to be as high as 30–40% which means it affects nearly one in six people. According to the ISAAC Phase I study, nasal symptoms are the primary complaints in 12.5% of 6–7-year-old and 18.6% of 13–14-year-old children which increased to 12.9% in the 6–7-year-group and to 23.6% in 13–14-year-group by ISAAC phase-III studies. Chandrika et al. in 2017 has also reported an increase in the rhinoconjunctivitis over the last decade. Recent studies such as the Global Asthma Network phase I in India reported a prevalence of 7.7% among 6–7 years old, 23.5% among adolescents and 9.8% in adults. In 2018, Singh S had reported similarly with a prevalence of 11.3% in 6–7 years old and 24.4% in adolescents. Similar statistics have been reported among adolescents in another study done by Moitra et al. in 2023.

Asthma: It has become one of the very common diseases impacting both children and adults. The popular ISAAC phase III study also reported in 2009 that the prevalence ranged from 7 to 20% in various areas with an important aspect being that nearly 50% of these were poorly controlled asthma. Since then, the prevalence of asthma has been studied as self-reported asthma in adults and as objective physician diagnosed asthma. The self-reported asthma prevalence is 1.8% in adult men and 1.9% among women. And once known risk factors were adjusted for, the risk for women was 1.2 times higher than men. Among children the prevalence of childhood asthma was reported to range from 2% in some states to 18.2% in some other states and was an average of 7.9%. Over the last decade asthma prevalence in adults in India was studied in the Global Burden of Diseases (GBD), Injuries and Risk Factors Study Indian cohort analysis (Salvi et al.) to be 37.9 million cases in 2016 with a disability adjusted life years being 2.4 times higher than the world average. Between the Indian states, North Indian states had a higher prevalence as was seen in states which are low socioeconomic status. Systematic reviews and meta-analysis done by Daniel AR in 2022 showed that the prevalence varied based upon the type of study done. It was 7.6% in school-based studies and 8.7% in community-based studies, perhaps because of the types of methodology used in school based as compared to community-based studies. Another aspect studied was the prevalence with respect to gender which differed between boys and girls i.e., 8% and 5.9%, respectively.

There have been studies to analyze the comorbidity of AR with asthma and this prevalence was as high as 65.4%; more in males than females. This shows the association where the allergic rhinitis is a part of the unified airway and is not a separate entity than asthma rather a part of it.

According to the global Asthma network phase I study done in 2022, 35% of India's population suffers from asthma. Upon comparison of the prevalence of asthma, the GAN study showed a lower prevalence of asthma as reported by the ISAAC Phase III study. This conflicts other reports as it does not take into consideration the inadequate representation in rural areas, the under diagnosis and the inability to control causal factors especially in poor homes.

Food allergies: Among all the facets of allergic disease, food allergy prevalence has not been studied as much as the others. This is because the difficulty in exactly making a diagnosis of food allergy is the main challenge, unlike in allergic rhinitis, asthma, or atopic dermatitis. Despite this, the prevalence of true food allergy is much lesser than the others. The connection between allergy and foods is made in many ways and can be patient perceived as well and not true food allergy. This also can be difficult as food allergy is not only the typical immunoglobulin E (IgE) reaction but also the non-IgE reaction. In 2015, studies done by Turnbull showed that the prevalence of self-reported adverse food reaction was as high as 20% however true food allergies in the population were only 4%. In the west, the prevalence of food allergies has been increasing, due to multiple epigenetic, environmental, and parenting reasons and in the United States alone, the incidence is nearly 8%. In India however, the prevalence of true food allergies has always been low probably due to the cultural practices of food and influences over the gut microbiome. Mahesh et al. studied the prevalence of food allergies in South India using the EuroPrevall model and found the prevalence of self-reported food reactions as 26% and that of true food allergy to be a lot lesser at 1.2%. The recent EuroPrevall-INCO study in 2019 reported a prevalence of food allergy in India to be as low as 0.14% though the sensitization to foods was as high as 19%. PA Mahesh reported in 2023 in a study done on food allergy and sensitization in low income countries that the overall prevalence of allergic sensitization to "any" food among children was 0.11–16.8% when tested with serum-specific IgE and 0.14–9.6% when analyzed with skin test.

In infancy, mainly milk and egg allergy is reported and nearly half of them outgrow this allergy by 1 year of age and this reduces even more by the end of their second year. The prevalence of milk allergy in infancy was around 1.5–3% which reduces to <1% by 6 years. Allergies to nuts and seafood tend to persist throughout life with the prevalence being as high as 2.7% to peanuts and 1.7% to tree nuts.

Atopic dermatitis: Atopic dermatitis is one of the common inflammatory conditions of the skin in children with an early onset of 3–6 months of age and nearly 60% manifesting symptoms in infancy. The varied prevalence of atopic dermatitis is due to regional, cultural, and epidemiological differences and ranges from 0.2 to 36% in children. Studies in India done by De A in 2023 stated that the prevalence of AD as 3.1–7.21% among the pediatric population (up to 16 years of age) with a mean age of onset at 5.2 months to 3.63 years. The prevalence of AD ranged from 0.98 to 9.2% in studies including pediatric and adult patients. This prevalence varies based upon the criteria used either the Hannifin and Rajka or William's criteria. In Asia, the prevalence of AD was 0.96–22.6% at 1 year of age. These statistics increased in Europe and America to 13.5–20%, however the prevalence of severe AD was <15%. When the global prevalence of AD was researched, the prevalence was reported as 2.0% in adults and 4.0% among children. There was a female preponderance noted with the global prevalence of AD among females being 2.8%, while among males it was 2.4%.

IMPACT OF URBANIZATION AND CLIMATE CHANGE ON THE PREVALENCE OF ALLERGIES

While delving into the epidemiology of allergy, the study implies research into all the factors that determine the presence or absence of diseases and disorders. These in allergy are essentially implied the interactions between the individual and their genetic composition, the allergens in the environment and the factors that worsen allergies such as pollution, climate change, etc.

POLLUTION, CLIMATE CHANGE, AND ALLERGIES

The increasing prevalence of allergies over the last few decades in India has been attributed to westernization and the increase in pollution in the bargain. Air pollution implies an increase in the toxic compounds, volatile substances, and particulate matter in the inhaled air. With asthma and allergic rhinitis being inflammatory conditions in the airway, increase in airway irritants and inflammatory substances in the air, worsen the asthma and allergic rhinitis. Studies have shown a positive correlation between air pollution and airway allergies wherein the airway epithelial inflammatory cells degranulate, releasing inflammatory mediators and further damaging the epithelium in response to pollutants (both indoor and outdoor). Particulate matter has been accepted as one of the indicators of air quality and children are the maximally susceptible population to the changes in air quality. The Indian subcontinent has one of the highest air pollution statistics due to use of biomass fuel, mosquito coils and incense sticks which contribute to the large amounts of particulate matter (PM2.5, PM5, and PM10) in the air. This results in a very poor air quality index in many urban and rural areas. The National air quality standards has mentioned that the maximum allowed particulate matter in the air must be 40 μg/m^3. However nearly 77% of the population is exposed to PM levels more than this which impacts the airway and increases the prevalence of asthma. The 11 most polluted cities of South Asia are in India, accounting for the increasing occurrence of airway allergies due to indoor and outdoor pollution with primary pollutant being PM2.5.

Air pollution causes increase in greenhouse gases and increases the overall temperature variations in any place. This results in climate change where the seasons are offset, there are longer warmer periods which result in longer pollination seasons. This exposes the populations to longer durations of pollen shedding and subsequent increasing prevalence in pollen allergies. Scoping review done by Verscheure reported that increase in atmospheric nitrogen pollution results in increasing atmospheric pollen levels causing alterations in pollen structure and increasing the allergenicity. The impact of nitrogen pollution causing allergies is still to be determined in controlled studies. The national consensus statement on air pollution and allergies in India by Reddy B et al. detailed the ambient air pollution, traffic related air pollution, and the effects of these on the increasing prevalence of asthma and allergic rhinitis.

Along with outdoor air pollution, a significant contribution to the airway allergies is due to the indoor air pollution. This is due to the burning of biomass fuels, use of chemical sprays, disinfectants, mosquito repellents, use of air conditioning in urban households, and exposure to environmental tobacco smoke. When this is combined with sedentary activities, easy availability of ready-to-eat foods, the rise in obesity/overweight occurs which acts as an independent risk factor increasing the allergy severity and prevalence.

With the change in air quality and particulate matter, there are also changes in the meteorological conditions and this in turn can affect the airway responsiveness. Studies on the meteorological conditions and particulate matter showed that there is an inverse relation between temperature and particulate matter in the outdoor air. As the temperature rises, so does the particulate matter and hence the air quality becomes poor. With poor air quality, there is an increase in allergic rhinitis and asthma, however with humidity, there exists an inverse relation between these two parameters. As humidity rises, there is a fall in the particulate matter and vice versa. Hence in dry less humid areas, there is more air pollution and more allergies/asthma. Increased humidity causes increased precipitation which reduces pollen concentrations.

Another aspect of environmental pollution is the effect it has over plant physiology. Due to increased warming due to the greenhouse gases CO_2, photosynthesis is augmented and there are extended pollination seasons. Other factors, such as changes in temperature of air, humidity, precipitation, and wind speed, together affect the pollen production as well. The allergenicity of the pollens also varies greatly with pollution as the pollen counts, pollen morphology, immunogenicity, pollen dispersal, and immunomodulatory effects of the allergenic proteins increase. In areas where diesel is used, the diesel exhaust particles act as carriers for the pollens and increase the allergenicity of the pollen thereby worsening asthma and allergic rhinitis.

EMERGING TRENDS

Over the last few decades, apart from the respiratory allergies that have shown an increase in food allergies, drug allergies, and occupational allergies.

Increasing trends in food allergies: Food allergies have shown a significant increasing trend, only next to respiratory allergies. This increase has been primarily attributed to the changing environment, changing dietary habits and changes in parenting of children. Studies done in Western countries show that there is an increased incidence of food allergies in children born to non-local population but brought up in the migrant country. Similar findings were found in local children who adopted a westernized lifestyle. These changes were found to be more in the migrant population and explained as due to gene environment interactions and epigenetics.

Increasing trends in drug allergies: The prevalence of drug allergies is very difficult to estimate as the drug reactions are very unpredictable, and reporting systems are very tedious and not complete in most countries. Studies have shown that nearly 10% of the population who are in the healthcare profession claim to have an allergy to a drug with the most common being penicillin allergy. The emergency room visits due to anaphylaxis are common and nearly 20% of them are due to drug allergies. In hospitalized patients, this becomes around 15–20%. There is also rise in the adverse drug reactions by almost 2.6 times, reported nearly a decade back. The reasons for this were given as higher usage of antibiotics, interactions between the antibiotics and viral infections such as EBV and CMV and newer classes of drugs being available.

Increasing trends of occupational allergies: There has also been an increasing report of occupational allergies over the last two decades. This has been attributed to the changes in the workplace environment, the emergence of newer occupations and newer allergens, the excessive use of chemicals in today's industries, increasing pollution which acts as an additive factor, epigenetics, and the individual predisposition. Condition such as the Baker's asthma has been described in the latter part of the 20th century and this has been changed to grain-induced asthma in this century with the changing pattern of the disease. Occupational rhinitis has been detailed as any rhinitis that occurs due to exposure to certain substances in the workplace environment. This has been further divided as work-related rhinitis and work-exacerbated rhinitis, based on whether the symptoms occur only at the workplace or are pre-existent with worsening at the workplace.

SUMMARY

This chapter highlights the increasing burden of allergic diseases in India, reflecting global trends influenced by urbanization, pollution, climate change, and lifestyle shifts. While data from India remain limited in scope—particularly from rural areas—available evidence shows rising rates of asthma, allergic rhinitis, atopic dermatitis, and food allergies. Air quality deterioration, westernized living, and epigenetic changes further exacerbate this health challenge. Better surveillance, public awareness, and preventive strategies are urgently needed.

Key Learning Points

- *Rising trend in allergic diseases:* Asthma, allergic rhinitis, atopic dermatitis, and food allergies are increasing in India, mirroring global trends.
- *Environmental contributors:* Pollution, urbanization, and climate change significantly influence allergy prevalence, particularly through particulate matter and prolonged pollen seasons.
- *Regional and socioeconomic disparities:* Prevalence varies widely between regions and socioeconomic strata, with underdiagnoses common in rural populations.
- *Emerging allergy patterns:* Food, drug, and occupational allergies are emerging concerns, driven by environmental, lifestyle, and workplace factors.
- *Need for comprehensive data:* Robust, nationwide epidemiological studies are needed to accurately capture and address the burden of allergic diseases in India.

SUGGESTED READING

1. Barne M, Singh S, Mangal DK, Singh M, Awasthi S, Mahesh PA, et al. Global Asthma Network Phase I, India: Results for allergic rhinitis and eczema in 127,309 children and adults. J Allergy Clin Immunol Glob. 2022;1(2):51-60.
2. Daniel RA, Aggarwal P, Kalaivani M, Gupta SK. Prevalence of asthma among children in India: A systematic review and meta-analysis. Lung India. 2022;39(4):357-67.
3. Jagpal PK, Alshareef S, Marriott JF, Krishna MT. Characterization, epidemiology and risk factors of multiple drug allergy syndrome and multiple drug intolerance syndrome: A systematic review. Clin Transl Allergy. 2022;12(8):e12190.
4. Kotz S, Pechtold L, Jörres RA, Nowak D, Chaker AM. Occupational rhinitis. Allergol Select. 2021;5:51-6.
5. Krishna MT, Mahesh PA, Vedanthan PK, Mehta V, Moitra S, Christopher DJ. The burden of allergic diseases in the Indian subcontinent: barriers and challenges. Lancet Glob Health. 2020;8(4):e478-9.
6. Lai CKW, Beasley R, Crane J, Foliaki S, Shah J, Weiland S, et al. Global variation in the prevalence and severity of asthma symptoms: Phase Three of the International Study of Asthma and Allergies in Childhood (ISAAC) Thorax. 2009;64:476-83.
7. Mahesh PA, Moitra S, Mabalirajan U, Garg M, Malamardi S, Vedanthan PK, et al. Allergic diseases in India - Prevalence, risk factors and current challenges. Clin Exp Allergy. 2023;53(3):276-94.
8. Matthai J, Sathiasekharan M, Poddar U, Sibal A, Srivastava A, Waikar Y, et al. Guidelines on Diagnosis and Management of Cow's Milk Protein Allergy. Indian Pediatr. 2020;57:723-9.
9. Moitra S, Mahesh PA, Moitra S. Allergic rhinitis in India. Clin Exp Allergy. 2023;53(7):765-76.
10. Rosario CS, Urrutia-Pereira M, Murrieta-Aguttes M, D'Amato G, Chong-Silva DC, Godoi RHM, et al. Air pollution and rhinitis. Front Allergy. 2024;5:1387525.
11. Silverberg JI, Barbarot S, Gadkari A, Simpson EL, Weidinger S, Mina-Osorio P, et al. Atopic dermatitis in the pediatric population: A cross-sectional, International Epidemiologic Study. Ann Allergy Asthma Immunol. 2021;126(4):417-28.e2.
12. Silverberg JI, Barbarot S, Gadkari A, Simpson EL, Weidinger S, Mina-Osorio P, et al. Atopic dermatitis in the pediatric population: A cross-sectional, international epidemiologic study. Ann Allergy Asthma Immunol. 2021;126(4):417-28.e2.
13. Singh D, Gupta I, Roy A. The association of asthma and air pollution: Evidence from India. Econ Hum Biol. 2023;51:101278.
14. Tang ML, Mullins RJ. Food allergy: is prevalence increasing? Intern Med J. 2017;47(3):256-61.
15. Tian J, Zhang D, Yang Y, Huang Y, Wang L, Yao X, et al. Global epidemiology of atopic dermatitis: a comprehensive systematic analysis and modelling study. Br J Dermatol. 2023;190(1):55-61.
16. Turnbull JL, Adams HN, Gorard DA. Review article: the diagnosis and management of food allergy and food intolerances. Aliment Pharmacol Ther. 2015;41(1):3-25.
17. Verscheure P, Honnay O, Speybroeck N, Daelemans R, Bruffaerts N, Devleesschauwer B, et al. Impact of environmental nitrogen pollution on pollen allergy: A scoping review. Sci Total Environ. 2023;893:164801.
18. Warren CM, Jiang J, Gupta RS. Epidemiology and Burden of Food Allergy. Curr Allergy Asthma Rep. 2020;20(2):6.
19. Zender-Świercz E, Galiszewska B, Telejko M, Starzomska M. The effect of temperature and humidity of air on the concentration of particulate matter - PM2.5 and PM10. Atmos Res. 2024;312:107733.

CHAPTER

3

Diagnosis of Allergic Diseases

Shalini Tyagi
Reviewer: *Naresh Grover*

INTRODUCTION

Recent years have seen significant advancements in identifying the prevalence of allergic diseases and developing diagnostic modalities. Diagnosing allergic diseases involves two main steps: Diagnosing the condition and identifying the underlying allergens and irritants. Diagnosis of allergy to certain external substance usually commands the identification of inciting allergens and irritants for precision of treatment and planning of symptom control medications. The clinical diagnosis of allergic disorders in practice is often done accurately in specialist doctor's office based on history and symptoms of patient, but to figure out what is the underlying relevant allergen is not always easy and possible. This chapter will look at the rational approach to diagnosis of allergies.

Diagnosing allergies is not a linear process, unlike other diseases. Instead, it is shaped like a U-pattern, where doctors review the patient's history and correlate with their symptoms and tests repeatedly **(Fig. 1)**.

The diagnosis of allergic diseases does not follow a linear progression; rather, it necessitates repeated correlation of symptoms, examination findings, and the patient's response to interventions such as avoidance and challenges to allergens based on their medical history **(Flowchart 1)**.

Diagnosis of allergic diseases will require following steps:

1. History-taking
2. Physical examination
3. *Investigations:*
   a. Investigations to establish diagnosis of allergy
   b. Investigations to identify the inciting allergen

HISTORY-TAKING

Eliciting the clinical history is the most important tool in diagnosing allergic diseases. Physicians should spend adequate time taking and documenting every detail of the patient's history. The physician should keep in mind following questions while extracting information from patient:

- History-taking to establish clinical disease are the symptoms of patients suggesting toward allergic rhinitis (AR) or asthma.
- *History of personal atopy:* The history of atopic dermatitis (AD) in early infancy, coupled with repeated coughs in a preschooler, strongly suggest an atopic cause for his symptoms.
- *Family history of atopy:* The positive history of atopic diseases in family members increases the probability of diagnosis because of the well-documented strong genetic association between them.

Step 1
History
Step 2
Examination
Step 3
Investigation
Step 4
Revisit history
Step 5
Final diagnosis

Fig. 1: Sequence in the diagnosis of allergic diseases.

Flowchart 1: Sequence of the diagnosis of allergic diseases.

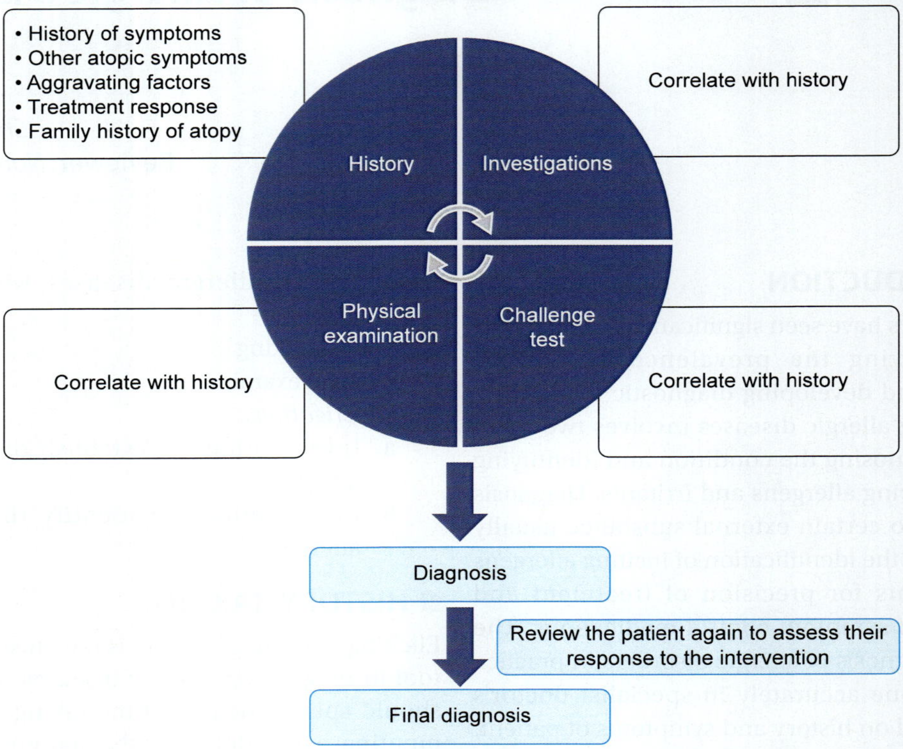

- *History of associated comorbid conditions and complications:* Allergic diseases like asthma and AR are often complicated by sinusitis, adenoids GERD, allergic conjunctivitis, and secondary infections. These complications are often the presenting complaints and require proper understanding to manage the underlying allergic diseases in a better way.
- History suggestive of inciting allergens and irritants

Various allergens exist, including house dust mites, indoor/outdoor molds, tree, grass, and weed pollen, animal dander, food, insect venom, drugs, etc. Their prevalence fluctuates based on weather conditions, indoor or outdoor exposure, temperature, humidity, and numerous other environmental factors. A comprehensive history of the onset of symptoms, triggers, seasonal patterns, exposure to pets, farm animals, damp walls, and molds in homes and schools can aid in identifying the specific responsible allergens.

History-taking to establish clinical disease:

- AR
- Asthma
- AD
- Food allergies
- Anaphylaxis

Allergic Rhinitis

Symptoms in favor of AR:

- *Persistent runny nose:* Children are prone to frequent viral infections in early childhood. However, underlying allergies can be suspected if the runny nose persists beyond the usual duration or occurs with frequent watery nasal discharge without fever and infections.

- *Frequent sneezing:* Excessive sneezing, particularly in the early mornings, during seasonal changes, or in response to cold air or strong odors, suggests nasal allergy.
- *Nasal itching:* Children with rhinitis often sniff and rub their noses multiple times a day to alleviate the itch. This frequent rubbing is often referred to as the "*allergic salute*".
- *Nasal obstruction:* Most children complain of nasal obstruction, especially when lying down, and require nasal drops for comfortable breathing during sleep.
- *Mouth breathing and snoring:* This question is typically raised by the attending clinician and is not explicitly expressed by the patient or caregiver.

Symptoms against AR:

- *Sinusitis:* Persistent thick mucosal discharge accompanied by headache, facial pain, and fever
- *Onset of symptoms at an early age:* This may favor congenital anomalies and gastroesophageal reflux disease (GERD).
- *Growth failure:* From early childhood can indicate underlying diseases such as cystic fibrosis (CF), primary ciliary dyskinesia (PCD), and growth loss later on may be suggestive of Koch's disease
- *Unilateral nasal discharge and foul odor:* May be due to the presence of a long-standing foreign body

Asthma

Symptoms in favor of asthma:

- *Dry, recurrent, and prolonged cough:* Asthma coughs are characterized by dryness, recurrence, and typically prolonged duration. They are more prevalent during the night and early mornings when natural steroid levels are at their lowest. Coughing intensity increases with exertion, such as running, crying, playing, or during exercise.
- *Rapid breathing:* Breathlessness or breathing faster than usual is a hallmark of asthma. It can be triggered by viral infections, exercise, exposure to allergens or triggers, such as viral infections, smoke exposure (incense sticks, tobacco, etc.), strong smells, or even cold drafts of air.

Symptoms of asthma in children:

- *Wheezing:* Wheezing is a whistling sound produced by air flowing through narrowed windpipes. It typically begins as an expiratory wheeze and worsens as the windpipes tighten further. Asthma wheezing is a generalized sound that resonates throughout both lungs, exhibiting a diverse range of notes and a polyphonic quality. This phenomenon arises from the vibration of windpipes of varying calibers.
- *Chest tightness:* Older children, adolescents, and adults may experience chest tightness, often accompanied by feeling of suffocation.
- *Shortness of breath:* Occasionally, older children may express concerns about having difficulty inhaling deeply during inspiration, resulting in a sensation of chest tightness.
- Cough bouts on running, cycling, climbing stairs, and playing physical games in younger children also point toward asthma.

Symptoms against asthma:

- *Early onset:* Wheezing from the first year of life can be a sign of anatomical malformation or GERD.
- *Failure to thrive:* Children with asthma may experience difficulty in gaining weight and growing adequately.
- *Persistent wet cough:* Children with mucociliary dyskinesia may have a persistent wet cough, which can be bothersome for both the child and their caregivers.

- *Unilateral or monophonic wheeze:* Children with a foreign body may experience unilateral or monophonic wheezing, which can be challenging to diagnose.

Atopic Dermatitis

Atopic dermatitis is a chronic and relapsing inflammation of the skin that typically affects the extensor areas of the skin in infancy and the flexural areas in later childhood. It is often associated with itching, scaling, and lichenification of the skin. AD is a clinical diagnosis, and there are no definitive laboratory tests for its identification.

Some severe cases of AD may be due to food or even dust mite allergy for which allergists might prove very helpful **(Fig. 2)**.

History Directed at Food Allergy

Food allergies can cause immunoglobulin E (IgE)-mediated allergies such as anaphylaxis and urticaria, as well as non-IgE-mediated reactions like FPIES (food protein-induced enterocolitis syndrome), FPIAP (food protein-induced allergic proctocolitis), FPE (food protein-induced enteropathy), and mixed allergies like AD.

Taking a detailed history is essential for establishing a diagnosis of food allergy with certainty and identifying the offending allergens.

Drug Allergy

Drug reactions are uncommon, yet they can cause substantial morbidity and mortality. Drug reactions are influenced by both the chemical structure of the drug and the host's immune responses. Certain drugs cause significant non-IgE-mediated reactions by virtue of mast cells degranulation. Such reactions do not have any immunological memory. Intradermal testing for assessing allergic reactions is validated for penicillin allergy. Negative intradermal test followed by negative oral challenge helps to rule out false labels of penicillin allergy. Employing

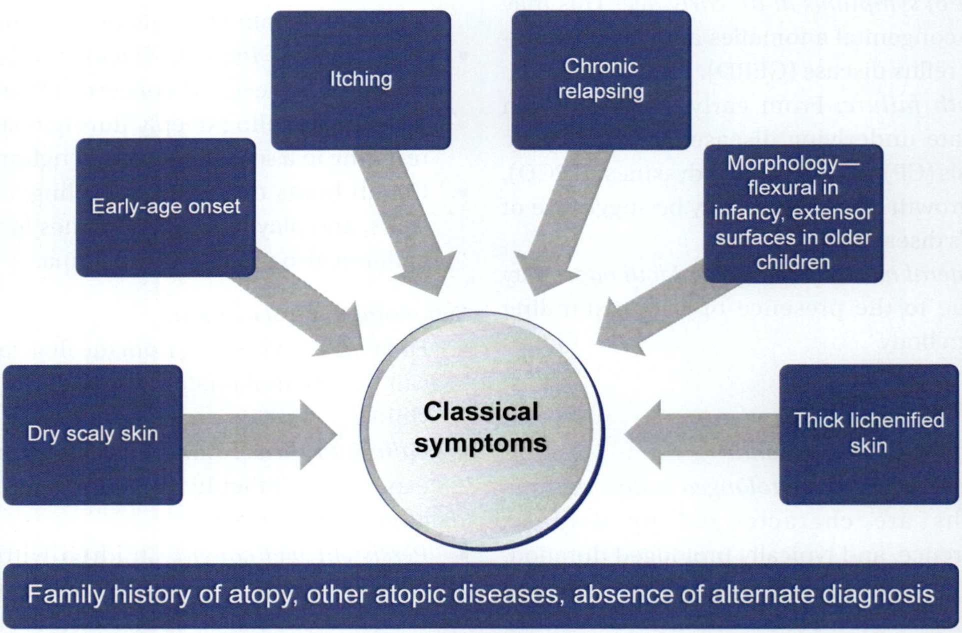

Fig. 2: Various symptoms of allergy.

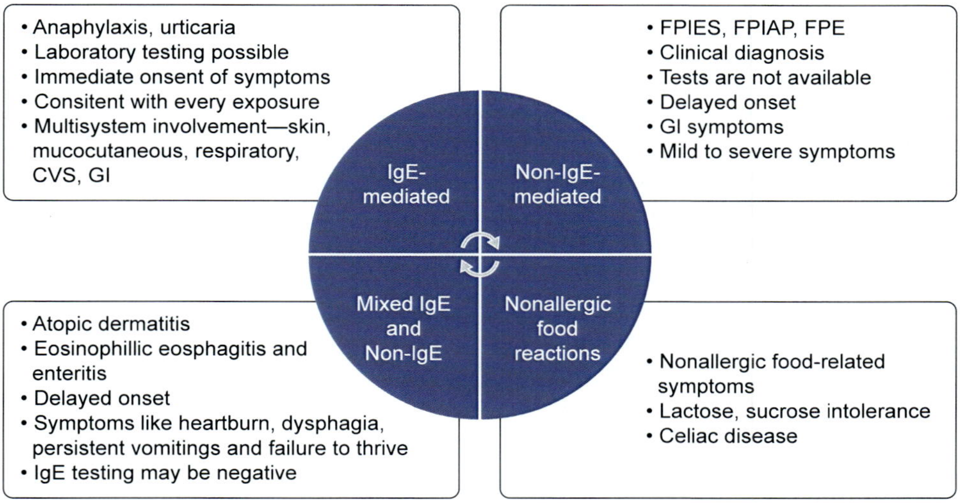

Fig. 3: Summary of drug allergy. (CVS: central nervous system; FPE: food protein-induced enteropathy; FPIAP: food protein-induced allergic proctocolitis; FPIES: food protein-induced enterocolitis syndrome; GI: gastrointestinal; IgE: immunoglobulin E)

a graded drug challenge, most patients with a history of allergies can be administered the offending drug. However, this approach is not typically practiced in cases of anaphylaxis **(Fig. 3)**. Certain human leukocyte antigen (HLA phenotypes are associated with cell-mediated allergy to particular drugs. Susceptibility can be assessed in certain cases, such as carbamazepine is associated with Stevens-Johnson syndrome and toxic epidermal necrolysis (SJS-TEN) in HLA B15-02* positive patients.

Historical elicitation includes the timing of symptoms, the route of administration, detailed descriptions of symptoms, whether anaphylaxis occurred, and the patient's history of drug allergies and allergies to other medications.

Intradermal testing is validated for assessing allergic reactions, particularly for penicillin allergy. A negative intradermal test followed by a negative oral challenge helps to rule out false-positives for penicillin allergy.

By employing a graded drug challenge, most patients with previous allergies can receive the offending drug. However, this practice is not recommended in cases of a history of anaphylaxis.

Venom Allergy

Insect bites can lead to severe systemic allergic reactions. Initial large local reactions to stings increase the probability of severe reactions on subsequent bites. Venom skin tests and specific IgE (sIGE) in serum are the gold standards for testing and diagnosis. Honeybees, wasps, and red ants are common insects known to cause allergies in humans. History regarding the time of the bite, details of symptoms, and a past history of large local reactions following stings should be elicited.

PHYSICAL EXAMINATION (GENERAL AND SYSTEMIC EXAMINATION)

General Examination

Signs of atopy: Upon examination, a child with allergies may present entirely normal general and systemic findings, particularly when assessed between episodes. However, after prolonged allergic manifestations, following signs may commence to appear.

- *Allergic shiners:* These are dark circles under the eyes caused by venous stasis due to nasal congestion.
- *Dennie–Morgan folds:* Also known as Dennie–Morgan lines, these are extra creases of skin running parallel to lower eyelids. They are caused by continuous spasms of the Muller eyelid muscles due to hypoxia.
- *Allergic salute:* This refers to habitual rubbing of the nose using hands in an upward movement in an attempt to wipe it or reduce the itch. The upward movement of the hand gives an impression of a salute.
- *Inflamed nonsuppurative conjunctiva:* This refers to allergic conjunctivitis, which causes redness of the eyes. Watering is often associated with AR.
- *Adenoid facies:* These are observed in cases of chronic airway obstruction associated with adenoid hypertrophy. Adenoid facies refer to the elongation of the lower face, an open mouth with two upper incisors visible, giving a hair-teeth appearance. This occurs due to changes in face structure that follow perpetual mouth breathing. It is sometimes associated with crowded and large teeth as well as dental caries.
- *Barrel-shaped chest (in chronic asthma):* Children with long-standing asthma have air trapping in their lungs, thereby expanding the anterior–posterior (AP) diameter of the chest, giving it a shape that resembles a barrel.
- Dry, scaly skin with thickening may be present in cases of associated dermatitis. Infants with AD have dry, scaly, red, and itchy skin, usually affecting the face and extensor aspects of the limbs. However, older children and adults present with similar and sometimes darker and thicker skin, and they are involved in the flexural aspect as in folds of the arms, neck, and legs. Genital areas are usually spared in AD.

Nasal examination: Nasal examination can be conducted by direct observation of the nose using a torch, with gentle lifting of the nasal tip. However, the use of a nasal endoscope provides a more comprehensive view of the turbinates and adenoids. An otoscope can also be employed in pediatric outpatient department (OPD) practice to visualize the turbinates and nasal mucosa. During examination, the following findings may be observed:

- Pale and boggy nasal mucosa
- Hypertrophied turbinates
- Nasal polyps

Chest examination: Wheezing can be heard in patients with asthma during an episode, typically expiratory and terminal. Wheezing observed during both phases of respiration indicates severe bronchoconstriction. Chest examinations may be completely normal between episodes.

Skin examination: Dry scaly, lichenification, hyperpigmented, itchy, or oozy skin can be seen in AD.

Other systems: Examination of CVS, CNS, and GI systems are normal.

INVESTIGATIONS

Laboratory Tests

- Hemogram
- Phadiatop
- sIgE test
- Molecular allergy test
- Cellular test—basophil activation test (BAT)

Hemograms: Hemogram results are typically normal. Occasionally, eosinophilia may be observed, but it is neither a specific nor a sensitive indicator.

Screening for allergies:

- *Total IgE:* IgE antibodies tend to rise during allergic reactions, but their sensitivity and specificity are limited. They can also increase

TABLE 1: Screening for allergies.

	Normal total IgE level	*High total IgE level*
Absent sIgE	Nonallergic patient	Parasitic infestation, active viral or post-viral infectious state, malignancy, due to effects of pollution and hyper IgE syndrome (HIES) etc.
Present sIgE	Patients with sensitization	Need to rule out false positivity of specific IgE due to high total IgE

(sIgE: specific immunoglobulin E)

in nonallergic conditions **(Table 1)** and a slight increase in sIgE may not be reflected in the total IgE report **(Table 1)**.

Phadiatop: Phadiatop is a conglomeration of sIgEs against common allergens. Consequently, it can detect false-negative reports of an increase in sIgEs against common allergens with greater accuracy. So, it can be employed as a screening test for atopic diathesis.

Diagnostic Tests for Allergies

Skin prick tests (SPTs): The skin prick test is employed to confirm allergic sensitization to suspected allergens and diagnose immediate IgE-mediated allergies. Sensitization with an allergen generates two types of IgE antibodies: Circulating and mast cell bound.

Circulating antibodies are detected through blood tests utilizing various methods. Mast cell-bound IgE antibodies are considered better markers of allergies, as they are directly involved in symptom production. In sensitized individuals, IgE is bound to mast cells. When these adjacent IgE antibodies on mast cells encounter an allergen, it bridges the two, leading to the release of mediators from mast cells. This results in symptoms such as itching, inflammation, swelling, and wheezing.

The SPT serves as a direct indicator of this process. The procedure involves placing a small amount of allergen on the volar aspect of the skin of arm or upper back, followed by pricking it with a lancet to deliver the allergen to the mast-cell-rich dermis. If the mast cell is already sensitized and carries adjoining IgE antibodies on its surface, the allergen will connect with both, forming a bridge and initiating an inflammatory cascade. This can be observed with the naked eye.

This when compared with positive and negative control of saline and histamine can give positive and negative results to inciting allergens. Knowledge of cross reactivity amongst allergens is important while interpreting results

Procedure: Place a drop of saline and histamine solution on the skin and gently prick with a 1 mm lancet. Saline should not cause a reaction. Histamine will form a small papule indicating an inflammatory reaction and vasodilatation. Place a drop of allergen extract on the skin, prick the epicutaneous gently, and read after 15 minutes. Measure the wheal size with a scale and compare it to the positive control. A wheal larger than the positive control is positive; smaller is negative, indicating no sensitization to the allergen.

Allergens to be tested: Testing multiple allergens is possible, but it is best to limit the number based on the patient's history—such as seasonality, indoor/outdoor symptoms, school/vacation periods, time of day for symptoms, and regional pollen calendar. Common allergen tested are given as follows:

House dust mites: Mite allergies can cause year-round symptoms, often worsening during the monsoon season and in early mornings. Common mites are *Dermatophagoides farinae*, *Dermatophagoides pteronyssinus*, and *Blomia tropicalis*.

Pollens: Pollen allergies cause symptoms in patients during certain plants' pollination seasons, leaving them symptom-free for the rest of the year. It is essential to obtain a detailed history regarding the seasonality of patients' symptoms and correlate this with the appropriate pollen calendar of that region before ordering tests. Various pollens that cause allergies include tree pollens, grass pollens, and weed pollens.

Molds: Aspergillus is a common indoor fungus that can cause primary allergies or worsen existing AR or asthma. Outdoor fungi, with seasonal variations based on the region, include *Cladosporium herbarium* and *Alternaria tenuis.*

Animal danders: Both pet and farm animals such dogs, cats, cows, horses, and camels can cause allergies and can be evaluated based on the history of exposure.

Insects: Cockroaches are the most common allergen in India found in most households. Among these two species of American and German are well identified. Testing is recommended if there is a history of perennial symptoms and exposure.

Food: Food allergies are tested only in cases with a history of anaphylaxis. Isolated respiratory symptoms are not associated with food allergies and therefore should not be tested routinely.

Prick-to-prick test: A prick-to-prick test using the actual food should be preferred instead of relying on commercial extracts, as their stability is often unreliable. Common food allergens in children include cow's milk, hen's egg, peanuts, tree nuts, fish, crustaceans, and mollusks.

Vegetables and fruits: Standardized automated skin prick test device may improve test output and reduce human errors in testing.

Indications of SPT ***(Table 2)****:*

- Asthma
- Rhinitis, rhinoconjunctivitis, conjunctivitis
- Eczema/AD (associated with other atopic manifestations)
- Suspected food allergy (oral allergy syndrome, anaphylaxis, acute onset urticaria, eczema correlated with food ingestion)
- Suspected drug allergy
- Hymenoptera venom allergy
- Suspected occupational disease or exposure to selected potential allergens
- Chronic urticaria in rare, selected cases
- Less common disorders—eosinophilic esophagitis (EoE), allergic bronchopulmonary aspergillosis (ABPA)

Skin prick test is not indicated in:

- Food intolerance
- Chronic urticaria in absence of allergic features
- Obesity and desire to lose weight
- Food associated symptoms to additives/preservatives/colorants
- Evaluation of allergen immunotherapy (AIT)
- Nonspecific respiratory symptoms to irritants (smoke, perfumes, detergents, chemicals and other strong odors)
- Nonspecific cutaneous rash
- Chronic fatigue syndrome

Advantages of SPT: It gives immediate results, IgE attaches to mast cells, and its degranulation is observed, which makes the detection more specific.

Disadvantages of SPT:

- Limited number of allergens can be tested.
- Drugs or recent anaphylaxis can modify results by reducing histamine release or consuming mast cells.
- Cannot be used in patients of dermographism
- Standard allergen solutions are not widely available for testing.
- Cannot be performed in younger children and certain medical conditions like chronic renal failure (CRF), cerebrovascular accident (CVA), diabetic neuropathy, and advanced age, which can reduce skin reactivity

TABLE 2: Stop these medicines before SPT.

Drugs	*Generic drug*	*Days suppressed*
Antihistamines	Chlorpheniramine	
	Cyproheptadine	
	Diphenhydramine	
	Hydroxyzine	
	Promethazine	
	Azelastine nasal	
	Ebastine	
	Cetirizine	
	Fexofenadine	
	Loratadine	
	Desloratadine	
	Levocetrizine	
	Bilastine	
Tricyclic antidepressants and tranquilizers	Imipramine	
	Doxepin, local and systemic	
H2 antagonist	Ranitidine	
Anti-IgE monoclonal antibodies	Omalizumab	6 weeks to 1 year
Cysteinyl leukotriene antagonist	Montelukast and zafirlukast	Do not suppress skin tests
Short-term OCS	30 mg of prednisolone daily for one week	Do not suppress skin tests
Long-term high dose	>20 mg/day	Possible suppression of immediate skin test reaction
Potent topical corticosteroids	>3 weeks	Suppress SPT at site of application
Local anesthetic	EMLA	1 hour before tests; only suppresses erythema

Source: Adapted from Ansotegui IJ, Melioli G, Canonica GW, Caraballo L, Villa E, Ebisawa M, et al. IgE allergy diagnostics and other relevant tests in allergy, a World Allergy Organization position paper. World Allergy Organ J. 2020;13(2):100080.
(IgE: immunoglobulin E; OCT: oral corticosteroids; SPT: skin prick test)

Examples of skin test concentrations advised by world allergy organization: Standard concentrations in skin prick test solutions will yield correct and reproducible results. Certain standardization based on dilutions and concentrations are advised by World Allergy Organization, which are described in **Table 3**.

Intradermal testing: It is used for both immediate IgE-mediated allergy and delayed-type hypersensitivity. Though it is more sensitive than SPT, it is less specific and has a higher risk of allergic reactions. Intradermal testing can be utilized for diagnosing allergies related to insect venom, beta-lactam drugs, and certain vaccines.

TABLE 3: Standardization of World Allergy Organization.

Allergen product	*Skin prick test concentration*	*Intradermal test concentration*
Standardized short ragweed	1:20 w/v	1:1,000 w/v
Standardized cat hair	10,000 BAU/mL	200 BAU/mL
Standardized grass pollens	10,000–100,000 BAU/mL	200 BAU/mL
Standardized hymenoptera venoms	100 µg protein/mL	0.1–1 µg protein/mL
Standardized mites	10,000 AU/mL	200 AU/mL
Nonstandardized allergens	1:40 to 1:20 w/v	1:1,000 w/v

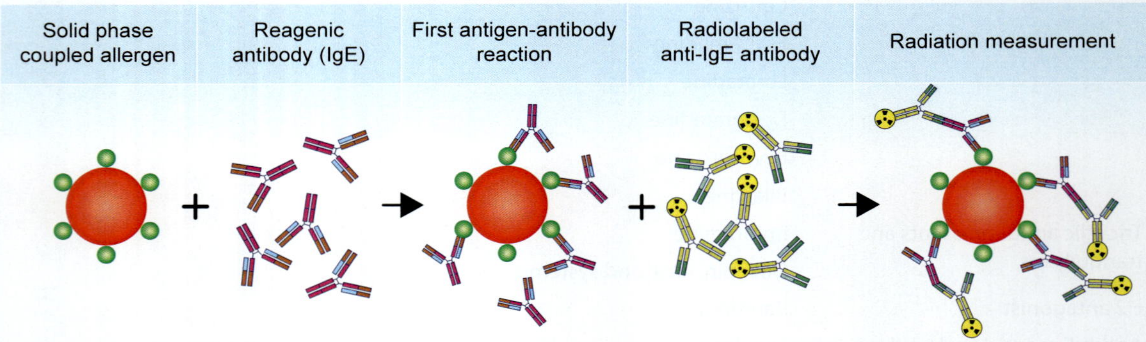

Fig. 4: Sequences of enzyme-linked immunosorbent assay (ELISA) test.

Patch testing: This test used to diagnose contact hypersensitivity and not useful test for immediate IgE response

In Vitro Testing

Specific IgE testing: Specific IgE testing quantifies circulating IgE antibodies to identify sensitization to allergens. It distinguishes sensitization from clinical allergies. Tests can be singleplex (targeting a single allergen) or multiplex (targeting multiple predefined allergens). Advancements in diagnostic techniques have led to improved results over time.

Radioallergosorbent test (RAST): RAST assays is a quantitative method for sIgE assessment; however, it is now replaced by more sensitive tests like ELISA (enzyme-linked immunosorbent assays).

Enzyme-linked immunosorbent assays: The assay for detection of sIgE uses the classic sandwich technique. The main components include the solid phase, the allergen conjugated with the solid phase, the patient's serum, the anti-IgE antibody, and labeling of anti-IgE with enzymes. It is a valid alternative to fluorescent enzyme immunoassay (FEIA) as it is relatively simple and inexpensive **(Fig. 4)**.

Fluorescent enzyme immunoassay: Fluorescent enzyme-labeled assays involve a fluorescent antibody binding to the patient's sIGE. The amount of sIGE is calculated based on the fluorescence observed. Its clinical value has been documented in scientific literature, and it is considered a reference standard for in vitro diagnosis. Commonly available Immunocap is based on FEIA technique and is considered as gold standard for in-vitro allergy diagnosis.

Component-Resolved Diagnostic

Component-resolved diagnosis identifies the allergenic epitopes of sensitizing allergen molecules. It enhances sensitivity by detecting concealed, small, degraded, or masked epitopes that ELISA may overlook, thereby preventing false negatives. Nonallergenic epitopes could result in false positives in skin prick tests and ELISA. Although it increases diagnostic accuracy, the test is costly and is incomplete due to limited identification of all allergen components. Accurate interpretation necessitates comprehensive knowledge of these components. This test measures IgE response but does not capture clinical manifestations of allergies.

Cellular Assays

Basophil activation test is in vitro test of documentation of actual allergic process **(Fig. 5)**. Here the sera are mixed with allergen, allergen not only binds the bridging antibodies basophils, which express high affinity FcεRI receptor on its surface and releases inflammatory mediators which can be detected and quantified by flow cytometry. BAT has gained significant interest in past few decades; however, it is not available for commercial use as of now.

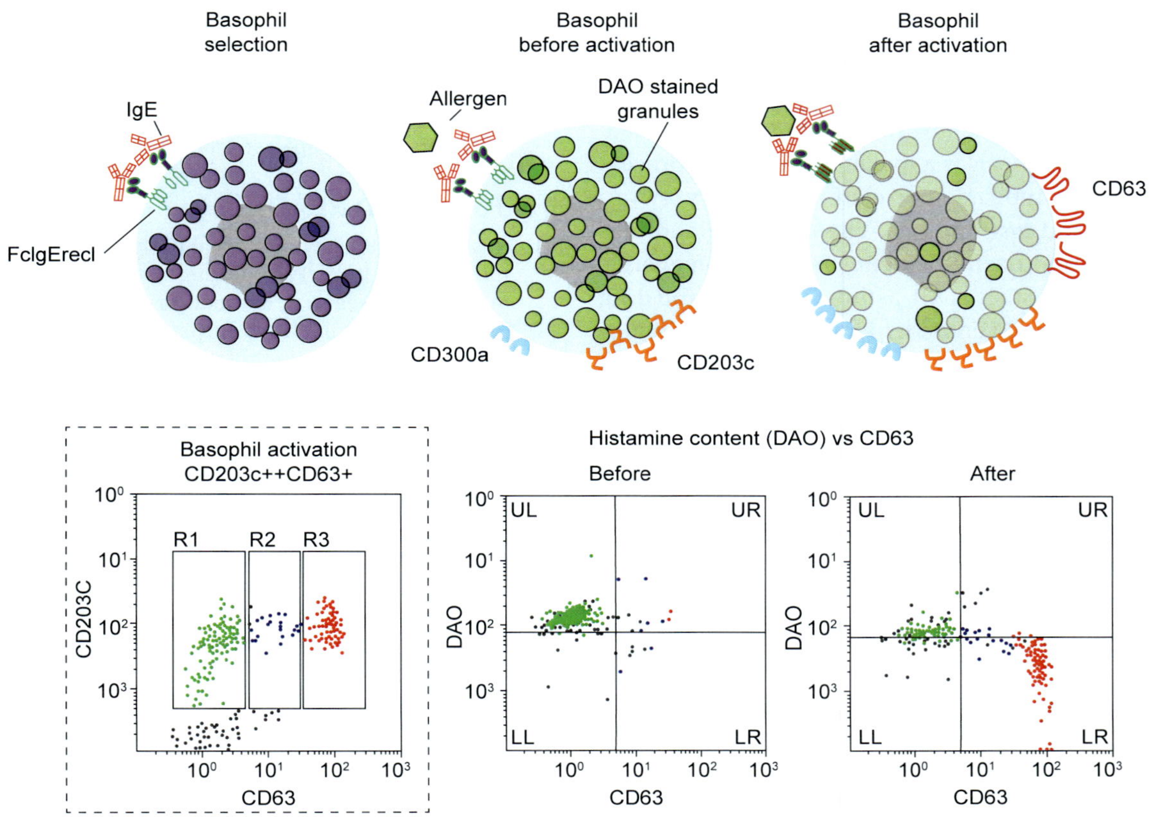

Fig. 5: Basophil activation test.

Source: Ansotegui IJ, Melioli G, Canonica GW, Caraballo L, Villa E, Ebisawa M, et al. IgE allergy diagnostics and other relevant tests in allergy, a World Allergy Organization position paper. World Allergy Organ J. 2020;13(2):100080.

Allergen Provocation Testing

Applying allergen extract to conjunctiva or nasal mucosa, or inhaling it in asthma cases, can cause symptoms of allergic conjunctivitis, rhinitis, or asthma, confirming the inciting allergen. It carries risk of inducing serious clinical reaction and standardized protocols for provocation tests are not yet available.

Allergen exposure chambers replicate real-life allergen exposure for sensitized individuals, but proper validation and limited availability restrict their use in clinical practice.

SUMMARY

This chapter provides a comprehensive framework for the diagnosis of allergic diseases, emphasizing the critical role of clinical history, targeted physical examination, and rational selection of diagnostic investigations. It highlights that allergy diagnosis is a dynamic, nonlinear process requiring repeated correlation of history, symptoms, and test findings. The chapter elaborates on the approach to diagnosing common allergic conditions such as AR, asthma, AD, food and drug allergies, and venom hypersensitivity. It outlines the indications, advantages, and limitations of various investigations—ranging from SPT, sIgE assays, and component-resolved diagnostics to cellular assays like the BAT. The chapter also stresses the contextual relevance of allergen exposure (e.g., dust mites, pollens, molds, foods, insect venom) and the importance of region-specific pollen calendars in test interpretation. Ultimately, it reaffirms that a meticulously taken clinical history remains the cornerstone of allergy diagnosis.

Key Learning Points

- *History is the foundation of diagnosis:*
  - Accurate diagnosis relies heavily on a detailed patient history, including symptom patterns, seasonality, environmental exposures, and personal/family history of atopy.
- *SPT as a gold standard:*
  - SPT is the most specific test for diagnosing IgE-mediated allergies. It offers immediate results and reflects mast cell-bound IgE reactivity, provided it is performed under proper protocols and interpretation.
- *Rational use of in vitro tests:*
  - sIgE testing, including ELISA and FEIA, is useful in selected scenarios, but total IgE lacks diagnostic specificity. Component-resolved diagnostics offer advanced insights but are costly and require expertise.
- *Integration of clinical features and physical signs:*
  - Allergic shiners, Dennie–Morgan folds, nasal mucosal changes, and wheeze support clinical suspicion of allergic diseases such as AR and asthma. Physical signs complement, but do not replace, history and investigations.
- *Emerging diagnostic tools and precautions:*
  - Newer tests like the BAT and allergen exposure chambers offer promise but require further standardization. Drug and food allergy evaluation should follow validated protocols with precautions against anaphylaxis.

SUGGESTED READING

1. Australasian Society of Clinical Immunology and Allergy. (2016). Skin Prick Testing for the Diagnosis of Allergic Disease: A Manual for Practitioners. [online] Available from https://www.allergy.org.au/images/stories/pospapers/ASCIA_SPT_Manual_March_2016.pdf [Last accessed August, 2025].
2. Ansotegui IJ, Melioli G, Canonica GW, Caraballo L, Villa E, Ebisawa M, et al. IgE allergy diagnostics and other relevant tests in allergy, a World Allergy Organization position paper. World Allergy Organ J. 2020;13(2):100080.
3. Bernstein IL, Li JT, Bernstein DI, et al. Allergy diagnostic testing: an updated practice parameter. Ann Allergy Asthma Immunol. 2008;100 (Suppl 3): S1-S148.227.
4. Robert E. Selection of allergen products for skin testing. In: Dolen WK (Ed). Immunology and Allergy Clinics of North America, volume 21, number 2. Philadelphia: Saunders; 2001.
5. Salazar A, Velazquez-Soto H, Ayala-Balboa J, Jiménez-Martínez MC. Allergen. [Internet]. InTech; 2017. Available from http://dx.doi.org/10.5772/65229 [Last accessed August, 2025].

CHAPTER 4

Advanced Diagnostic Methods

Mitesh Kakkad
Reviewer: *Neeraj Gupta*

INTRODUCTION

In recent years, the field of pediatric allergy and pulmonology has witnessed tremendous advances in diagnostic methodologies. The increasing prevalence of allergic diseases in children, driven by urbanization, pollution, dietary changes, and genetic susceptibility, has necessitated improved diagnostic approaches that are child-friendly, accurate, and non-invasive. Traditional tools such as spirometry and skin prick testing, though still central, are now complemented by more sophisticated technologies such as impulse oscillometry, fractional exhaled nitric oxide (FeNO), nasal cytology, and tympanometry. These diagnostic methods not only assist in identifying disease phenotypes but also help in tailoring therapies and monitoring disease progression more precisely. A robust understanding and application of these tools are critical for every clinician involved in the care of allergic and respiratory disorders in children.

LUNG FUNCTION ASSESSMENT

Spirometry

Principle and parameters: Spirometry remains the gold standard for assessing lung function. It measures the volume and flow of air that can be inhaled and exhaled, providing critical insight into obstructive and restrictive patterns of lung disease. Key spirometry parameters as shown in **Figure 1** include:

- *FVC (forced vital capacity):* Maximum volume of air exhaled after deep inhalation.
- *FEV1 (forced expiratory volume in 1 second):* Volume exhaled in the first second.
- *FEV1/FVC ratio:* Indicator of airflow obstruction
- *Peak expiratory flow (PEF) and forced expiratory flow (FEF) 25–75%:* Assess large and small airway function, respectively.

Indications:

- Chronic cough, wheezing, suspected or diagnosed asthma
- Monitoring progression in cystic fibrosis (CF) and primary ciliary dyskinesia (PCD)
- Diagnosis of restrictive lung diseases (ILDs, scoliosis, and neuromuscular conditions)

Contraindications:

- Acute exacerbations of asthma or respiratory infections
- Recent thoracic, abdominal, or ocular surgery
- Risk of pneumothorax

Pre-test requirements and procedure:

- Withhold bronchodilators for specified durations (e.g., *SABA:* 6 hours, *LABA:* 24 hours)
- Perform in seated position with nose clips
- *Ensure proper technique:* Deep inspiration followed by forced expiration and complete exhalation
- Minimum of three acceptable and reproducible attempts needed

Interpretation **(Flowchart 1 and Fig. 2)**

- *Obstructive pattern:* FEV1/FVC <85% predicted
- *Reversibility test:* Post-bronchodilator increase in FEV1 by ≥12% or ≥200 mL indicates asthma
- *Restrictive pattern:* Normal FEV1/FVC with reduced FVC

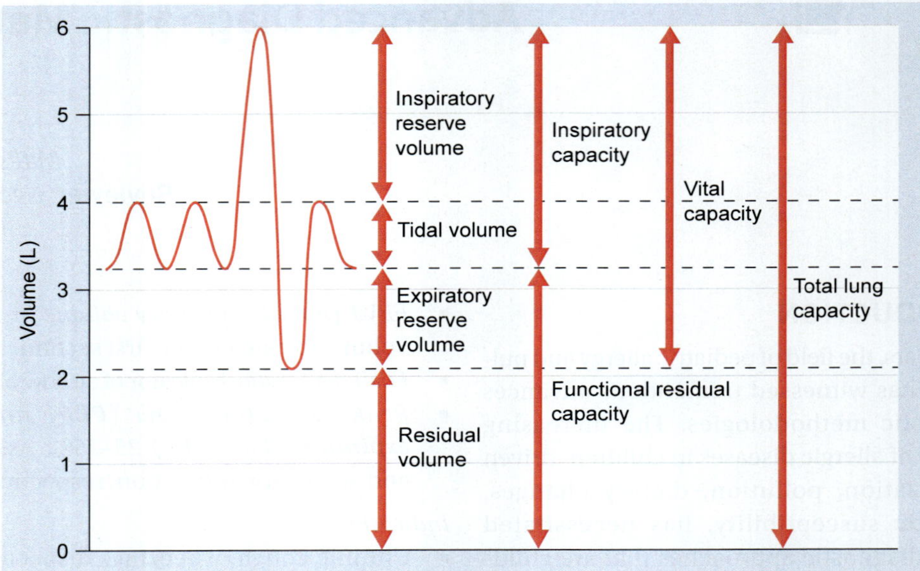

Fig. 1: Lung volumes and capacities—residual volume, functional residual capacity (FRC), and total lung capacity (TLC) cannot be measured by spirometry.

Flowchart 1: Spirometry interpretation (by numbers).

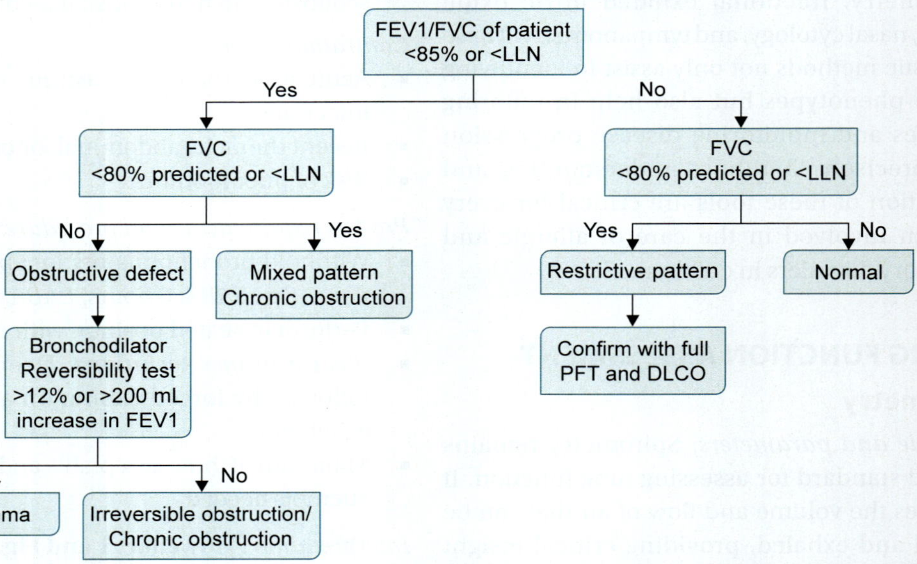

(DLCO: diffusing capacity of lungs for carbon monoxide; FEV1: forced expiratory volume in 1 second; FVC: forced vital capacity; LLN: lower limit of normal; PFT: pulmonary function test)

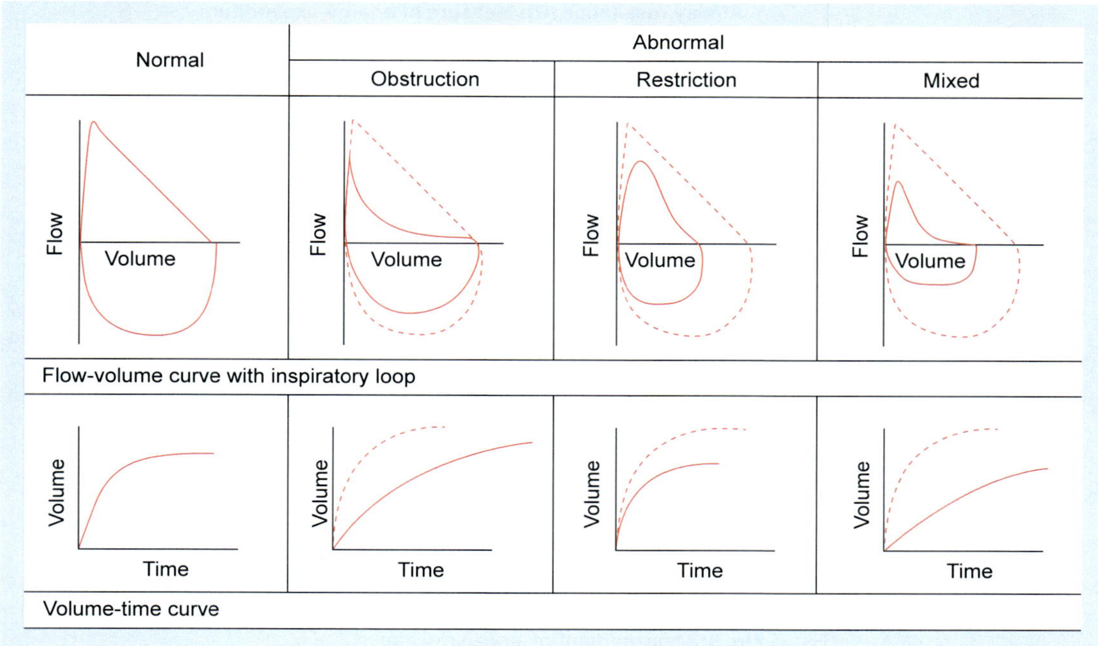

Fig. 2: Spirometry interpretation (by graphs).

Challenges in pediatrics:

- Requires active cooperation, making it difficult in children <6 years
- Interpretation must consider age, height, ethnicity, and sex-based normative values

Impulse Oscillometry

Principle: Impulse oscillometry (IOS) based on the forced oscillation technique (FOT), applies sound waves of varying frequencies to measure respiratory impedance during tidal breathing. It evaluates both resistance (R) **(Fig. 3)** and reactance (X) **(Fig. 4)**, making it particularly suited for young children who cannot perform spirometry **(Table 1)**.

Parameters:

- *R5:* Total airway resistance (central + peripheral)
- *R20:* Central airway resistance
- *R5–R20:* Peripheral airway resistance
- *X5:* Reactance at 5 Hz (reflects lung compliance and small airway function)
- *Fres:* Resonant frequency where elastic and inertial forces equalize.
- *AX:* Area under the reactance curve (marker of lung stiffness)

Advantages:

- It requires minimal cooperation.
- Non-invasive and easy to perform in children >3 years
- It detects early small airway involvement.
- Safe in children with low respiratory drive or neuromuscular weakness

Bronchodilator reversibility criteria **(Fig. 5)**:

- R5 ↓ ≥40%, X5 ↑ ≥50%, AX ↓ ≥80%

Clinical relevance:

- It helps in asthma diagnosis and monitoring.
- It complements spirometry in younger age groups.
- Limited normative data in Indian children; further research is needed.

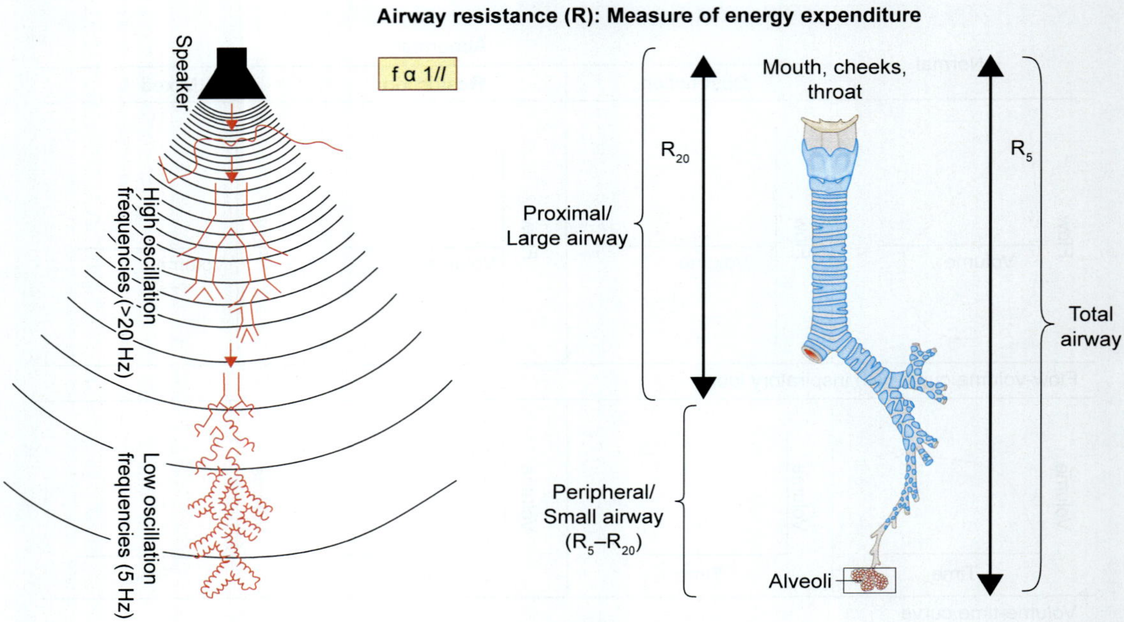

Fig. 3: Measurement of airway resistance.

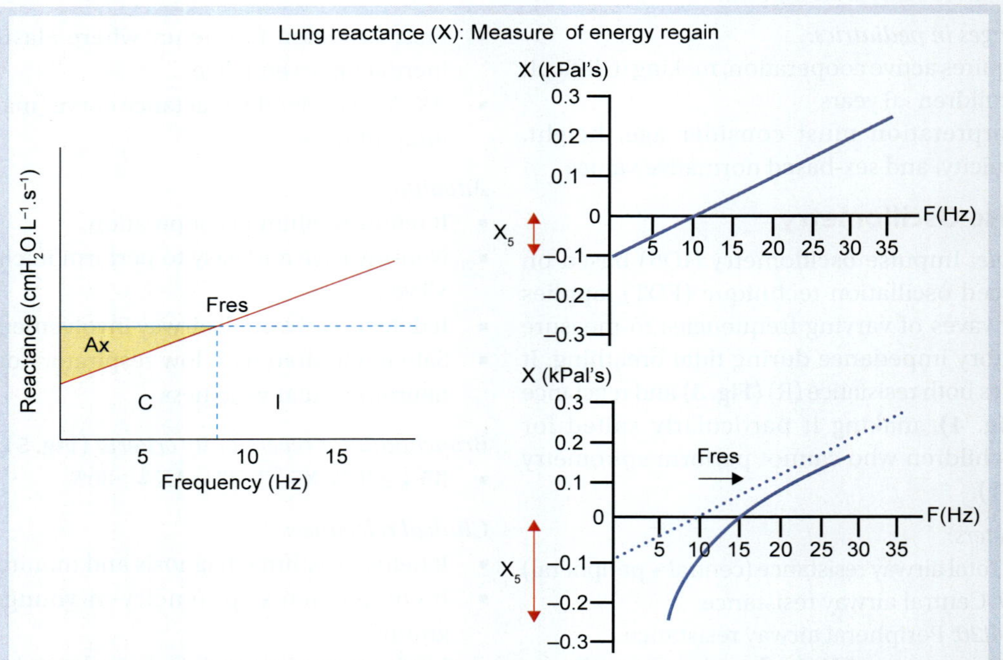

Fig. 4: Measurement of lung reactance.

Pathophysiology	Resistance	R_5	R_{20}	$R_5–R_{20}$	Reactance	X_5	Fres
Peripheral obstruction	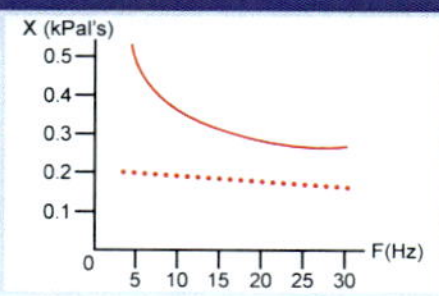	↑↑↑	N/↑	↑↑	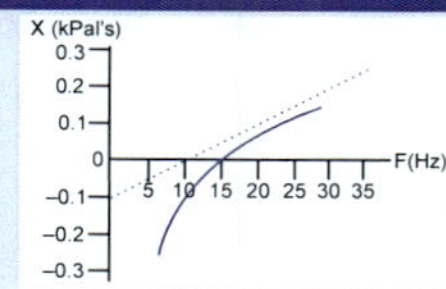	More negative	↑↑
Proximal obstruction	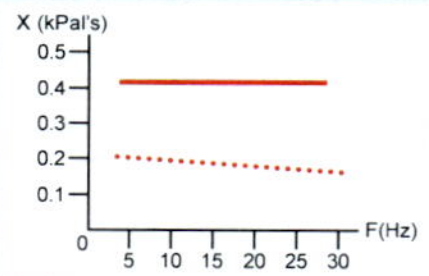	↑↑	↑↑	N	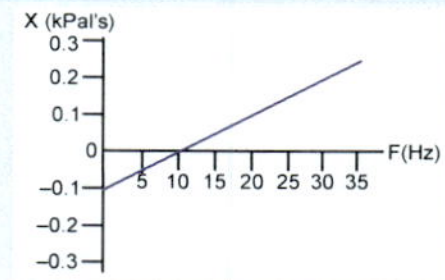	N	N
Restrictive lung disease	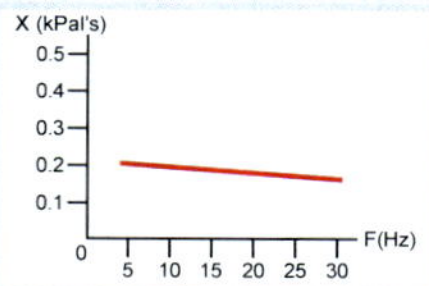	N	N	N	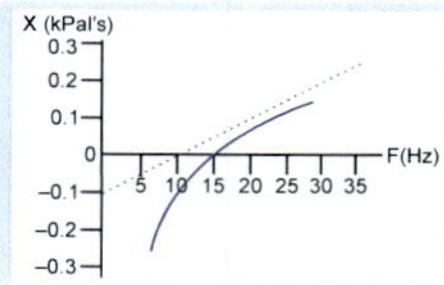	More negative	↑↑

Fig. 5: Interpretation of oscillometry.

TABLE 1: Comparison of spirometry with lung oscillometry.

Feature	*Spirometry*	*Impulse oscillometry (IOS)*
Maneuver	Forced expiration	Tidal breathing
Age suitability	>6 years	>2–3 years
Small airway detection	Moderate	High
Cooperation needed	High	Minimal
Cost	Low	Variable
Reference values	Available	Limited (especially in Indian population)

INFLAMMATORY BIOMARKERS

Fractional Exhaled Nitric Oxide

Role of Nitric oxide (NO): NO is a gaseous signaling molecule involved in bronchodilation, ciliary movement, and immune defense. In allergic airway inflammation, Th2-mediated processes upregulate inducible NO synthase (iNOS), leading to elevated NO levels in exhaled breath **(Flowchart 2)**.

Fractional exhaled NO testing:

- Non-invasive and simple
- Performed using chemiluminescence or electrochemical sensors **(Fig. 6)**
- Suitable for children >4 years

Flowchart 2: Synthesis of nitric oxide (NO).

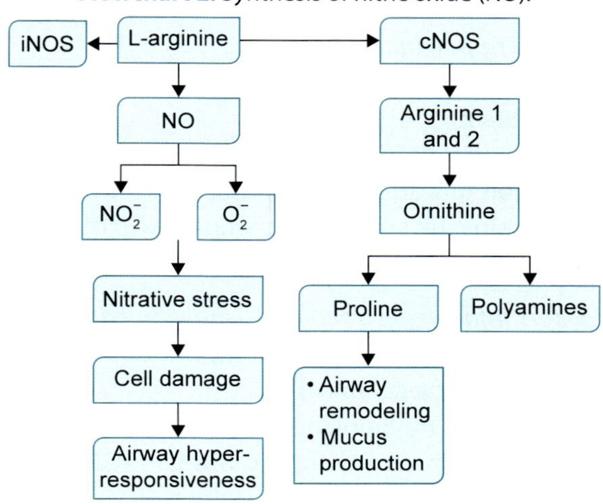

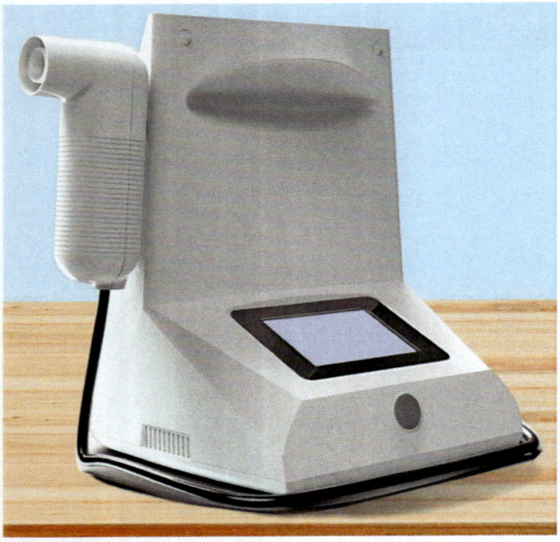

Fig. 6: Electrochemical sensors detect nitric oxide (NO) by measuring the electrical current generated when NO reacts with electrodes in the sensor.

TABLE 2: Interpretation of fractional exhaled nitric oxide (FeNO) (ATS guidelines).

*FeNO level**	*Children*	*Interpretation*
<20 ppb	Low	Unlikely eosinophilic inflammation
20–35 ppb	Intermediate	Possible
>35 ppb	High	Likely

*A change of 20% (in adults) and 10 ppb (in children) from baseline is considered as significant.

Clinical applications:

- Initial diagnosis of eosinophilic asthma **(Table 2)**
- It predicts corticosteroid responsiveness.
- It monitors adherence to ICS.
- It helps in step-up or step-down therapy decisions.

Factors influencing fractional exhaled nitric oxide:

- *Increased by:* Viral infections, nitrate-rich diet (e.g., leafy vegetables)
- *Decreased by:* Smoking, inhaled corticosteroids (ICS) use, obesity, cystic fibrosis (CF), and human immunodeficiency virus (HIV)

Strengths and limitations:

- High sensitivity for eosinophilic inflammation
- Not useful for neutrophilic or non-Th2 asthma
- It should be interpreted alongside clinical context.

UPPER AIRWAY ASSESSMENTS

Nasal Cytology and Nasal Eosinophils

Nasal cytology is a useful, non-invasive technique for evaluating the type and severity of inflammation in allergic rhinitis. The presence of nasal eosinophils is a hallmark of allergic inflammation and correlates with disease severity.

Technique:

- Collect sample from the medial surface of the inferior turbinate using a sterile swab
- Spread onto glass slides, fix with 95% alcohol
- Stain using May Grunwald-Giemsa
- Examine under high-power microscopy

Clinical use:

- It helps in differentiating allergic rhinitis from infectious or non-allergic forms.
- It identifies NARES (non-allergic rhinitis with eosinophilic syndrome).
- Useful for assessing treatment response in allergic rhinitis.

Nasopharyngoscopy

Nasopharyngoscopy allows direct visualization of the nasal cavity, adenoids, and nasopharynx using a flexible fiberoptic endoscope.

Indications:

- Recurrent nasal obstruction or discharge
- Suspected adenoid hypertrophy
- Nasal polyps or mass
- Evaluation of turbinate hypertrophy or deviated septum

Procedure:

- Performed under topical anesthesia (2% xylocaine spray)

- Child seated upright or slightly reclined
- Insert flexible endoscope through nostrils

Grading of adenoid hypertrophy:

- *Grade 1:* 25% obstruction
- *Grade 2:* 50%
- *Grade 3:* 75%
- *Grade 4:* >90%

Nasopharyngoscopy provides valuable structural information and can guide both medical and surgical management in children with chronic nasal symptoms.

MIDDLE EAR FUNCTION

Tympanometry

Tympanometry is a simple, objective test that measures the mobility of the tympanic membrane and status of the middle ear using sound waves and pressure changes.

Principle: A probe tone (typically 226 Hz) is introduced into the ear canal, and the compliance of the tympanic membrane is measured as air pressure in the ear canal is varied.

Clinical applications:

- Detecting middle ear effusions
- Diagnosing otitis media with effusion (OME)
- Evaluating eustachian tube function

Tympanogram types:

- *Type A:* Normal compliance and pressure
- *Type As:* Reduced compliance (e.g., tympanosclerosis)
- *Type Ad:* Hypermobile tympanic membrane (e.g., ossicular discontinuity)
- *Type B:* Flat trace (e.g., middle ear effusion)
- *Type C:* Negative pressure (e.g., eustachian tube dysfunction)

Age-specific norms:

- *Pediatric compliance range:* 0.2–1.6 mL/cm^3

Limitations:

- Requires intact tympanic membrane
- May be uncomfortable in small children

Acoustic Reflex Testing

The acoustic reflex is the involuntary contraction of the stapedius muscle in response to loud sounds. It provides information about the integrity of the auditory pathway.

Procedure:

- It uses the same equipment as tympanometry.
- A sound stimulus is delivered, and the presence or absence of reflex is recorded.

Clinical use:

- It determines type and degree of hearing loss.
- Reflex is usually absent in sensorineural or conductive hearing loss.
- Useful in detecting retrocochlear pathologies

Acoustic reflex thresholds generally range from 70 to 90 dB HL in normal ears. Absence of the reflex can help in identifying auditory neuropathy or facial nerve dysfunction.

CELLULAR AND MOLECULAR DIAGNOSTIC TOOLS

Sputum Eosinophilia

Induced sputum analysis provides direct insight into airway inflammation by quantifying eosinophils and other inflammatory cells. It helps in phenotyping asthma (eosinophilic vs. neutrophilic), guiding corticosteroid therapy, and predicting exacerbation risk.

Procedure:

- Patient inhales hypertonic saline to induce sputum production.
- Sample collected is processed with dithiothreitol (DTT) to break mucus.
- Centrifuged and stained for eosinophil counts.

Interpretation:

- *Eosinophilic asthma:* ≥3% eosinophils
- *Neutrophilic asthma:* ≥60% neutrophils
- *Paucigranulocytic asthma:* Normal cell counts

Clinical applications:

- Useful in identifying patients likely to benefit from corticosteroids or biologics (e.g., anti-IL-5)
- It monitors response to anti-inflammatory therapy.
- It predicts exacerbation risk, especially in uncontrolled asthma.

Limitations:

- Not feasible in young children (<8 years)
- Procedure may trigger bronchospasm.
- It requires laboratory infrastructure and trained personnel.

Emerging Biomarkers in Allergy Diagnosis

Recent advances in immunology and molecular diagnostics have introduced several novel biomarkers to identify allergic inflammation and endotypes:

- *Blood eosinophil count*:
  - Elevated levels (>300 cells/μL) indicate Th2 inflammation
  - Easily available and reproducible
- *Serum immunoglobulin E (IgE) (total and specific):*
  - Total IgE indicates overall atopic status.
  - Allergen-specific IgE helps in allergen identification and immunotherapy planning.
- *Periostin:*
  - Secreted by epithelial cells in response to IL-13
  - Marker of airway remodeling and eosinophilic inflammation
  - High levels predict response to anti-IL-13 therapy (e.g., lebrikizumab)
- *Eosinophil cationic protein:*
  - Released by activated eosinophils
  - It correlates with disease severity and steroid responsiveness.
- *Basophil activation test:*
  - It measures CD63/CD203c upregulation on basophils in response to allergens.
  - Useful in food allergy, drug allergy diagnosis when conventional tests are inconclusive.
- *Component-resolved diagnostics:*
  - It identifies specific allergenic protein components (e.g., Ara h2 in peanut allergy).
  - It helps in assessing cross-reactivity and severity risk.
  - It guides allergen immunotherapy more precisely.

SUMMARY

Advanced diagnostic methods in pediatric allergy and pulmonology provide a multidimensional understanding of airway diseases. These tools help in identifying disease endotypes, assessing inflammation, and tailoring therapy to the individual needs of the patient. From simple techniques such as FeNO and nasal eosinophil counts to sophisticated tools such as impulse oscillometry and component-resolved diagnostics, each modality adds value in optimizing care. Integration of these diagnostics into routine clinical practice ensures timely interventions, reduced exacerbation rates, and improved long-term outcomes in children with allergic diseases.

Key Learning Points

- *Impulse oscillometry* is an effective tool for assessing small airway function in children >3 years, requiring minimal patient effort.
- *Fractional exhaled nitric oxide testing* serves as a reliable, non-invasive marker of Th2 inflammation and assists in asthma management and adherence monitoring.
- *Tympanometry and acoustic reflex testing* provide objective assessment of middle ear function, crucial in recurrent upper respiratory symptoms.
- *Nasal cytology and nasopharyngoscopy* help evaluate the upper airway's structural and inflammatory status.
- *Molecular biomarkers* such as serum IgE, periostin, eosinophil cationic protein (ECP), and component-resolved diagnostics (CRD) offer precise endotyping and guide-targeted therapies and immunotherapy.

SUGGESTED READING

1. British Thoracic Society, Scottish Intercollegiate Guidelines Network. British Guideline on the Management of Asthma. Thorax. 2008;63:Suppl 4, iv1-iv121.
2. Cooper BG. An update on contraindications for lung function testing. Thorax. 2011;66:714-23.
3. Gendeh BS. Clinical Atlas of Nasal Endoscopy. Malaysia: Penerbit Universiti Kebangsaan; 2009.
4. Global Initiative for Asthma. Global Strategy for Asthma Management and Prevention, New York: GINA, 2008.
5. Guidelines for the measurement of respiratory function. Recommendations of the British Thoracic Society and the Association of Respiratory Technicians and Physiologist. Respir Med. 1994; 88:165-94.
6. Kaminsky DA, Simpson SJ, Berger KI, Calverley P, de Melo PL, Dandurand R, et al. Clinical significance and applications of oscillometry. Eur Respir Rev. 2022;31:210208.
7. Kedgule R, Salvi S. Exposure to biomass smoke as a cause for airway disease in women and children. Curr Opin Allergy Clin Immuno. 2012;12: 82-90.
8. Miller MR, Hankinson J, Brusasco V, Burgos F, Casaburi R, Coates A, et al, Standardisation of spirometry. Eur Respir J. 2005;26:319-38.
9. Ricciardolo FL, Sorbello V, Ciprandi G. A pathophysiological approach for FeNO: A biomarker for asthma. Allergol Immunopathol (Madr). 2015; 43(6):609-16.
10. Salman SD. An Atlas of Diagnostic Nasal Endoscopy (Encyclopaedia of Visual Medicine Series). CRC Press; 2003.
11. Salvi S, Barnes PJ. Is exposure to biomass smoke the biggest risk factor or COPD globally? Chest. 2010;138:3-6.
12. Shiota S, Katoh M, Aoki S, Mastsuoka R, Fukuchi Y. Predictive equations and the reliability of the impulse oscillometry system in Japanese adult subjects. Respirology. 2005;22:64-71.
13. Song TW, Kim KW, Kim ES, Park JW, Sohn MH, Kim KE, et al. Utility of impulse oscillometry in young children with asthma. Pediatr Allergy Immunol. 2008;19:763-8.
14. Stanojevic S, Kaminsky DA, Miller MR, Thompson B, Aliverti A, Barjaktarevic I, et al. ERS/ATS technical standard on interpretive strategies for routine lung function tests. Eur Respir J. 2022; 60:2101499.
15. Wang Z, Pianosi P, Keogh K, Zaiem F, Alsawas M, Alahdab F, et al. The Clinical Utility of Fractional Exhaled Nitric Oxide (FeNO) in Asthma Management. Rockville (MD): Agency for Healthcare Research and Quality (US); 2017. Report No.: 17(18)-EHC030-EF.

CHAPTER 5

Pharmacotherapy for Allergies: Current Status, Diagnosis, and Management in Pediatric Patients

Sanjukta De

Reviewer: *Sowmya Arudi Nagarajan*

INTRODUCTION

Allergy is an umbrella term encompassing a wide spectrum of immune-mediated disorders collectively called allergic diseases [e.g., allergic rhinitis (AR), asthma, seasonal allergies, and food allergy], usually resulting from heightened immune response that are influenced by the complex interplay of genetic, environmental, and socioeconomic factors. The allergy landscape in India reflects a significant burden with high level of exposure to particulate matter owing to pollution, urbanization, climatic conditions, and high rates of infection, diet, diverse socioeconomic status, ethnicity, and literacy.

There are no defined guidelines on pediatric allergy management; therefore, the allergy protocols and pharmacotherapy guidance are primarily adapted from international guidelines such as those from the Global Initiative for Asthma (GINA), World Allergy Organization (WAO), American Academy of Allergy, and in the Indian scenario from protocol of the Indian Academy of Pediatrics (IAP), the Allergy and Immunology Chapter of IAP.

Owing to confounding factors that result in complex nature of allergic reactions in the pediatric population in India, a parallel cannot be drawn on the allergy management between Western countries and India.

This chapter focuses on the common pharmacotherapies for allergic diseases in pediatric patients and the specific challenges faced such as misuse of over-the-counter (OTC) medications, steroid abuse, and lack of adherence by patients to follow up on the medications.

PHARMACOTHERAPIES FOR PREVALENT ALLERGIC DISEASES

The treatment and management of pediatric allergies have progressed significantly, with various options available to manage AR, asthma, atopic dermatitis (AD), and food allergies. Currently, the approach is to focus on symptom control, reducing inflammation, and improving the child's overall quality of life (QoL) while minimizing adverse effects (AEs). This section covers the common pharmacotherapies available for some of the prominent allergic diseases.

Antihistamines

Biochemistry

Histamine is an essential by-product of histidine metabolic pathway that is produced by histidine decarboxylase in a vitamin B-dependent decarboxylation reaction. The mature histamine is stored in the granules of mature mast cells along with heparin, cytokines, and other enzymes. Once released, this ubiquitous amine interacts with G-protein coupled receptors (GPCRs) and initiates a cascade of allergic response. In addition, histamines are implicated in other physiological and pathophysiological conditions.

Histamines interact with four different types of GPCRs, viz., H_1R, H_2R, H_3R, and H_4R; of which their allergic and inflammatory symptoms are activated via the H_1R GPCRs, which are widely distributed throughout the body. H_1R-medicated allergic response include bronchoconstriction, nociception, vasodilatation, and cellular migration. Antihistamines belong to a class of pharmaceutical drugs that are H_1R antagonists that competitively bind to the H_1R receptors. H_1R-mediated competitive antagonism not only prevents and neutralizes the effects of histamine but also further exerts the opposite effect by suppressing the receptor signaling cascade, thereby mediating the antiallergic effects observed with antihistamines. Since their first development in 1937, antihistamines have undergone many modifications and are therefore classified as first-generation and second-generation antihistamines.

Antihistamines are primarily administered orally and used in a lot of allergic conditions such as nasal allergies, seasonal AR (hay fever), urticaria, AD, pruritus, and insect bites and stings. Intravenous (IV) and intramuscular (IM) administrations are also possible but are mostly reserved for in-patient treatment. Topical and intranasal applications of antihistamines have also been tried in different settings. Another third generation of antihistamines for the treatment of AR and chronic urticaria have also been discussed here.

Indications

In AR, topical antihistamines are generally the first line of treatment based on its severity as per Allergic Rhinitis and its Impact on Asthma (ARIA) guidelines. In intermittent AR, oral antihistamines are as well as intranasal histamines are required to relieve the symptoms. In chronic or persistent AR, only short courses are prescribed to relief symptoms with intranasal corticosteroids (INS) as the preferred drug choice. In allergic conjunctivitis (AC), antihistamines are mostly used topically, and oral formulations are used when AC occurs in association with AR to relieve the symptoms of itchy eyes.

Histamines are useful in both chronic and acute urticaria with relieving of allergic wheals and reduction of skin lesions. As per European Academy of Allergy and Clinical Immunology (EACCI) guidelines, the second-generation histamines are the first line of treatment in chronic urticaria, and the doses can be increased up to 4× to control the symptoms.

In food allergy, antihistamines have been used in combination with other antihistamines particularly in early non-life-threatening reactions to food. Antihistamines are not recommended in anaphylaxis, AD (except to provide relief from short-term pruritus), asthma, and hereditary angioderma.

First-Generation Antihistamines

The first-generation antihistamines were primarily developed from the anticholinergic drugs more than eight decades back. Since the first-generation antihistamines bind to both central and peripheral histamine-1 receptors nonspecifically, they exhibit poor receptor selectivity and can cause severe side effects by interacting with receptors of other biologically active amines causing antimuscarinic, anti-adrenergic, and antiserotonin effects. The existing data on the use of antihistamines, particularly first-generation antihistamines, in pediatric population is scanty and is mostly derived from data on adult or adolescent population assuming it to be effective in children as well. However, an important consideration often overridden is that the immune system of a child below 2 years of age is not fully developed or is immature and therefore their effectiveness toward a particular drug will be distinct from the adult.

Adverse effects associated with first-generation antihistamines: Some of the common side-effects of first-generation antihistamines mostly include dry mouth, urinary retention, constipation visual disturbances (mydriasis, photophobia), tachycardia, drowsiness, and confusion and agitation upon high-dose administration. Use of hydroxyzine has been reported in pediatric population with AD and eczema. However, as per European Medicines Agency (EMA) data, it has been reported that hydroxyzine is associated with small-risk QT interval prolongation, cardiovascular disease, and family history of sudden cardiac death, severe electrolyte imbalance, and bradycardia. Again, children under 6 years should not be prescribed OTC cough and cold medications containing promethazine and chlorphenamine. First-generation antihistamines used in pediatric population are sometimes also classified as "sedating" antihistamines. Some of the common sedating antihistamines, their indications and dose, contraindications, and side effects are summarized in **Table 1**.

Second-Generation Antihistamines

Advantages: The second-generation antihistamines came to advent to circumvent the AEs of the first-generation antihistamines. Introduced around 1980, this group of antihistamines was expected to offer an improved safety profile and be relatively less sedative or nonsedative in nature owing to low permeability across the blood–brain barrier (BBB). Some of the widely used second-generation antihistamines in children include cetirizine, desloratadine, levocetirizine, fexofenadine, rupatadine, loratadine, and bilastine.

Drug metabolism: The efficacy of antihistamine is determined by its affinity toward H_1R. Between desloratadine, levocetirizine, and fexofenadine, desloratadine is the most potent in terms of its affinity toward H_1R. Most of the antihistamines are well absorbed; however, fexofenadine exhibits variable absorption owing to its ability to bind to plasma proteins (~60–70% are bound to plasma proteins). The volume of distribution of desloratadine on the other hand is larger than fexofenadine and levocetirizine. Four-hour plasma concentrations of fexofenadine and levocetirizine are 174 nM and 28 nM, respectively, while desloratadine is barely 1 nM. Levocetirizine and desloratadine exert longer duration of action, despite the latter being relatively less active in wheal and flare reaction.

Information on drug metabolism is important as it will provide insights on what drugs to prescribe to patients on the basis of clinical evaluation and previous medical history.

Drug metabolism processes are similar in adults and pediatric population; however, in case of certain antihistamines, they are relatively accelerated in children and therefore the dosing in pediatric population needs to be adjusted accordingly. Levocetirizine, for example, is prescribed twice a day in kindergarten children. It has been observed that in children, the plasma concentration of drugs reaches near maximum within 30 minutes, however, it takes >1.5 hours to exert its clinical effect.

Adverse effects associated with second-generation antihistamines: No cardiac toxicity has been reported with loratadine, fexofenadine, mizolastine, ebastine, azelastine, cetirizine, desloratadine, and levocetirizine. However, in the 1990s, two second-generation antihistamines, astemizole and terfenadine, were associated with cardiac AEs and therefore have been removed from majority of the countries. Owing to this AE, new antihistamines are required to pass stringent safety measures before being approved by regulatory authorities.

However, some second-generation antihistamines might penetrate to a small extent particularly at high doses and thereby cause somnolence. Levocetirizine, for example, may cause drowsiness in some susceptible patients and somnolence has been reported in children whom higher doses have been prescribed.

Indications and use: In the last two decades significant clinical studies employing second-generation antihistamines in treating AR in pediatric population have been reported, thereby

TABLE 1: First-generation/sedating antihistamines for pediatric patients.

	Indications and dose	*Unlicensed use*	*Contraindications*	*Cautions*	*Side effects*
Alimemazine tartrate	• *Urticaria/pruritus* *Oral route:* – 6 months to 1 year (specialist use only): 0.25 mg/kg 3–4 times a day (maximum per dose—2.5 mg) – 2–4 years: 2.5 mg 3–4 times a day – 5–11 years: 5 mg 3–4 times a day – 12–17 years: 10 mg 23 times a day (doses up to 100 mg have been administered) • *Premedication to anesthesia* *Oral route:* – 2–6 years: Up to 2 mg/kg 1 dose, 1–2 h before OT	Reported to be used in urticaria and pruritus in children between 6 months to 1 year but it is not licensed for this age-group	• Epilepsy • Hepatic dysfunction • History of narrow angle glaucoma • Hypothyroidism • Myasthenia gravis • Neonate (due to antimuscarinic activity) • Parkinson's disease • Pheochromocytoma • Renal dysfunction	• Cardiovascular diseases • Exposure to sunlight should be avoided during treatment with high doses • Pyloroduodenal obstruction • Susceptibility to QT interval prolongation • Urinary retention • Volume depleted patients who are susceptible to orthostatic hypotension	• Agitation • Agranulocytosis • Amenorrhea • Thrombus formation • Autonomic dysfunction • Drug fever • Dry mouth • Eosinophilia • Galactorrhea • Gynecomastia • Hepatic disorders • Hyperprolactinemia • Hyperthermia • Hypotension • Insomnia • Leukopenia (prolonged high dose) • Movement disorder, muscle rigidity • Nasal congestion • Skin reactions, pallor • Ventricular tachycardia • Ventricular fibrillation *N.B.:* • Drowsiness may disappear after a few days • Children are more susceptible to side effects • To be avoided if there is renal impairment

Contd...

Contd...

	Indications and dose	*Unlicensed use*	*Contraindications*	*Cautions*	*Side effects*
Chlorphenamine maleate	• *Symptomatic relief against hay fever, urticaria, food allergy, drug reactions* *Oral route:* – 6–23 months: 1 mg twice daily – 2–5 years: 1 mg every 4–6 hours – 6–11 years: 2 mg every 4–6 hours – 12–17 years: 4 mg every 4–6 hours *IM or IV:* – 1–5 months: 0.25 mg/kg – 6 months to 5 years: 2.5 mg – 6–11 years: 5 mg 12–17 years: 10 mg *N.B.:* The IM/IV injections are single doses; however, irrespective of age can be scaled up to 4 doses per day if needed	May be used for children under 1 year of age for treatment of allergies and itch associated with chicken pox, but it is not licensed for this age-group *N.B.:* Children under 6 years should not be given over-the-counter cough and cold medicines containing chlorphenamine	Neonate due to severe antimuscarinic activity	• Epilepsy • Pyloroduodenal obstruction • Susceptibility to angle-closure glaucoma • Urinary retention	*General side effects:* • Drowsiness (specific) • Concentration impaired • Abnormal coordination • Dizziness • Dry mouth • Fatigue • Headache • Nausea • Blurred vision Other side effects with no known frequency • Agitation • Poor appetite • Blood disorders, hemolytic anemia • Increased bronchial secretion viscosity • Hypotension • Irritability • Arrhythmias • Chest tightness • Confusion • GI discomfort • Hepatic disorders • CNS stimulation • Urinary retention • Photosensitivity reactions *N.B.:* Hepatic impairment—manufacturer advises caution

Contd...

Contd...

	Indications and dose	*Unlicensed use*	*Contraindications*	*Cautions*	*Side effects*
Hydroxyzine hydrochloride	• Hydroxyzine is a sedating antihistamine which exerts its actions by antagonizing the effects of histamine *Oral route:* – 6 months to 5 years: 5–15 mg (divided doses adjusted according to body weight; maximum limit of up to 2 mg/kg per day) – 6–17 years (up to 40 kg): 15–25 mg – (divided doses increased as required, adjusted according to weight; maximum limit of up to 2 mg/kg per day) – 6–17 years (above 40 kg): 6 to 17 years (up to 40 kg): 15–25 mg – (divided doses increased as required – 12–17 years: 4 mg every 4–6 hours	—	Risk factors for QT interval prolongation includes significant electrolyte imbalance, bradycardia, cardiovascular disease, and family history of sudden cardiac death	• Bladder outflow obstruction • Breathing problems • Cardiovascular disease • Decreased GI motility • Dementia • Epilepsy • Hypertension • Hyperthyroidism • Myasthenia gravis • Pyloroduodenal obstruction • Stenosing peptic ulcer • Susceptibility to angle-closure glaucoma • Urinary retention *N.B.:* Children have an increased susceptibility to CNS effects	*Side effects with no known frequency:* • Agranulocytosis • Alopecia • Anticholinergic syndrome • Anxiety • Arrhythmias • Asthenia • Blood disorders, hemolytic anemia • Increased bronchial secretion viscosity • Chest tightness • Chills • Dry throat and dry mouth • Dizziness • Drowsiness • Dyskinesia (on discontinuation) • Fever, flushing • GI disorders • Hallucination • Headache • Hepatic dysfunction • Sleep disorders • Slurred speech • Tremors • Urinary disorders • Vertigo • Vomiting *N.B.:* • Hepatic impairment—manufacturer advises caution in mild to moderate impairment, avoid in severe impairment • Renal impairment—to be used with caution (reduce daily dose by half in moderate to severe cases)

Contd...

Contd...

	Indications and dose	*Unlicensed use*	*Contraindications*	*Cautions*	*Side effects*
Ketotifen	• Allergic rhinitis *Oral route:* – 3–17 years: 1 mg twice daily	—	Avoid use in acute porphyrias	• Epilepsy • Pyloroduodenal obstruction • Susceptibility to angle-closure glaucoma • Urinary retention	*Common:* • Anxiety • Insomnia • Irritability *Uncommon:* • Cystitis • Dizziness • Dry mouth • Skin reactions *Rare/very rare:* • Hepatitis • Sedation seizure • Stevens–Johnson syndrome • Increased weight *N.B.:* • Avoiding use in pregnancy, during breast feeding
Promethazine hydrochloride	• *Symptomatic relief of allergy such as hay fever and urticaria as well as insomnia associated with urticaria and pruritus* *Oral route:* • *2–4 years:* 5 mg twice daily, alternatively 5–15 mg once daily, to be taken at night • *5–9 years:* 5–10 mg twice daily, alter-natively 10–25 mg once daily, to be taken at night	Not licensed for use for sedation in children under 2 years	• Neonate due to severe antimuscarinic activity • Children under 2 years for fatal respiratory depression (only specialist use recommended)	• Epilepsy • Pyloroduodenal obstruction • Susceptibility to angle-closure glaucoma • Severe coronary artery disease • Susceptibility to angle-closure glaucoma • Susceptibility to QT interval prolongation • Urinary retention	*General side effects:* • Arrhythmias • Blood disorder • Confusion • Dizziness • Drowsiness • Dry mouth • Headache • Hypotension • Jaundice • Movement disorders • Palpitations • Photosensitivity reactions • QT interval prolongation • Urinary retention

Contd...

Contd...

	Indications and dose	*Unlicensed use*	*Contraindications*	*Cautions*	*Side effects*
	• *10–17 years:* 10–20 mg 2–3 times daily, alternatively 25 mg once daily, to be taken at night. Dose can be increased to 25 mg twice daily if necessary				*Specific side effects:* • Agranulocytosis • Angle closure glaucoma • Anti cholinergic syndrome • Anxiety • Insomnia • Leucopenia • Nasal congestion • Nausea • Rash • Seizure • Thrombocytopenia • Tinnitus • Tremor • Vomiting *With parenteral use:* • Decreased appetite • Epigastric discomfort • Fatigue • Hemolytic anemia • Hypersensitivity • Muscle spasms • Nightmare • Restlessness • Skin reactions *N.B.:* • Renal impairment—to be used with caution • Hepatic impairment—manufacturer advises caution

(CNS: central nervous system; GI: gastrointestinal; OT: operation theater) allowing its consolidated use in this population. Antihistamines, however, have shown to be less effective against nasal congestion. There are no clinical studies in children with nasal congestion wherein efficacy of antihistamines with nasal corticosteroids (CS) have been made. However in adults such combinations have been clinically studied.

In a clinical study it has been demonstrated that loratadine, a second-generation antihistamine, improved academic performance in children with respect to sedating histamine diphenhydramine HCl in conditions where long-term antihistamines were unavoidable.

Although antihistamines are extensively prescribed, it has been suggested that use of these medications should be avoided against common cold, seromucosal otitis, and random use of OTC cough medication in pediatric patients. Some of the common second-generation nonsedating antihistamines, their indications and dose, contraindications, and side effects are summarized in **Table 2**.

Third-Generation Antihistamines

Another advanced new-generation antihistamines have been categorized as third-generation antihistamines; however, different publications have referred to them interchangeably as second-generation or third-generation, such as fexofenadine and desloratadine. There is no unanimous definition of the third-generation antihistamines used and therefore a Consensus Group on New Generation Antihistamines (COGNA) was established with the help of British Society of Allergy and Clinical Immunology. According to this group, the new recommendations to classify a drug under this category should demonstrate the following properties: Anti-inflammatory, should be highly potent and effective with high benefit-to-risk ratio, should lack of cardiac toxicity, exhibit minimal drug interactions, and lack CNS effects, and exert additional effect other than being an H_1 blocker.

A second-generation antihistamine, ebastine, has shown most of the abovementioned properties but its therapeutic profile does not differ greatly from the other second-generation antihistamines. It would be beneficial to observe the interaction of antihistamines with the other histamine receptors in combination with its effect on H_1R. Norastemizole or tecastemizole is metabolically derived from astemizole, which is a second-generation antihistamine. This drug initially showed potency to be classified as a third-generation antihistamine; however, Food and Drug Administration (FDA) rejected its application owing to AEs such as phospholipidosis and cardiomyopathies in animals exposed to the drug.

Allergen Immunotherapy

The World Health Organization (WHO) along with other allergy, asthma, and immunology societies throughout the world unanimously achieved a consensus wherein they introduced the concept "allergen vaccine" instead of "allergen extract" to emphasize on the fact that allergen vaccines can be used as immunotherapy.

Pharmacology

Allergen immunotherapy (AIT) for established immunoglobulin E (IgE)-mediated hypersensitivity employs exposing small amounts of allergens such as dust mites, grass pollen, cat or dog dander, wasp venom extract, bee venom extract, etc. over several years to child's immune system to act as immune modifiers like any other vaccine thereby building long-term tolerance and reducing allergic reactions.

TABLE 2: Second-generation/nonsedating antihistamines for pediatric patients.

	Indications and dose	*Unlicensed use*	*Contra-indications*	*Cautions*	*Side effects*
Acrivastine	• *Symptomatic relief of allergy (hay fever, chronic idiopathic urticaria)* *Oral route:* – 12–17 years: 8 mg 3 times a day	—	• Avoid use in acute porphyrias	—	*Common/very common:* • Drowsiness • Dry mouth *Frequency not known:* • Dizziness • Rash *Side effects, further information:* • Less sedation and psychomotor impairment is probable *N.B.:* • Avoid use in severe renal impairment
Bilastine	• *Symptomatic relief of allergic rhinoconjunctivitis and urticaria* *Oral route:* – 12–17 years: 20 mg once a day	—	• Avoid use in acute porphyrias	• Epilepsy • Pyloroduodenal obstruction • Susceptibility to angle-closure glaucoma • Urinary retention	*General side-effects:* • Drowsiness • Headache *Uncommon:* • Anxiety • Increased appetite • Asthenia • Bundle branch block • Diarrhea • Dry mouth • Dyspnea • Fever • GI discomfort • Insomnia • Nasal complaints • Nausea • Oral herpes • Pruritus • QT interval prolongation • Sinus arrhythmia • Tinnitus • Vertigo • Increased weight *Side effects, further information:* • Less sedation and psychomotor impairment is probable

Contd...

Contd...

	Indications and dose	*Unlicensed use*	*Contra-indications*	*Cautions*	*Side effects*
Cetirizine hydrochloride	• *Symptomatic relief of allergy (hay fever, chronic idiopathic urticaria, atopic dermatitis)* *Oral route:* – 1 year: 0.25 mg/kg twice daily – 2–5 years: 2.5 mg twice daily – 6–11 years: 5 mg twice daily – 12–17 years: 10 mg once a day	Not licensed for use in children under 2 years		Epilepsy	*Uncommon:* • Agitation • Asthenia • Diarrhea • Malaise • Paresthesia • Skin reaction *Rare/very rare:* • Aggression • Angioderma • Confusion • Depression • Hallucination • Abnormal hepatic function • Insomnia • Movement disorders • Edema • Seizure • Syncope • Tachycardia • Altered taste • Tic • Tremor • Urinary disorders • Vision disorder • Increased weight *Side effects with no known frequency:* • Abdominal pain • Increased appetite • Dry mouth • Dizziness • Drowsiness • Headache • Memory loss

Contd...

Contd...

	Indications and dose	*Unlicensed use*	*Contra-indications*	*Cautions*	*Side effects*
					• Nausea • Pharyngitis • Suicidal ideation • Vertigo *N.B.:* Renal impairment avoid if estimated GFR is <10 mL/min/1.73 m^2; *reduce to half normal* dose if estimated GFR is 30–50 mL/min/1.73 m^2; *reduce to half normal and reduce frequency to alternate days* if estimated GFR is 10–30 mL/min/1.73 m^2
Desloratadine*	• *Symptomatic relief of allergy (allergic rhinitis, urticaria, and chronic idiopathic urticaria)* *Oral route:* – 1–5 years: 1.25 mg/kg once daily – 6–11 years: 2.5 mg once daily – 12–17 years: 5 mg once daily	—	—	—	*Common/very common:* • Asthenia • Dry mouth • Headache *Rare/very rare:* • Akathisia • Arrhythmias • Diarrhea • Dizziness • Drowsiness • GI discomfort • Hepatic disorders • Insomnia • Myalgia • Nausea • Palpitations • Seizure • Vomiting *Side effects with no known frequency:* • Abnormal behavior • Photosensitivity reaction • QT interval prolongation *N.B.:* • Contraindicated if history of hypersensitivity to loratadine • Renal impairment—use with caution

Contd...

Contd...

	Indications and dose	*Unlicensed use*	*Contra-indications*	*Cautions*	*Side effects*
Fexofenadine hydrochloride	• *Symptomatic relief of seasonal allergic rhinitis* *Oral route:* – 6–11 years: 30 mg twice daily – 12–17 years: 120 mg once daily • *Symptomatic relief of chronic idiopathic urticaria* *Oral route:* – 12–17 years: 180 mg once daily	—	—		*Common/very common:* • Dizziness • Drowsiness • Headache • Nausea *Uncommon:* • Fatigue *Frequency not known:* • Diarrhea • Nervousness • Palpitations • Skin reactions • Sleep disorders • Tachycardia *N.B.:* Avoiding use in pregnancy, during breast feeding
Levocetirizine hydrochloride†	• *Symptomatic allergy (hay fever, urticaria)* *Oral route:* – 2–5 years: 1.25 mg/kg twice daily – 6–11 years: 5 mg once daily		• Avoid use in acute porphyrias		*Common/very common:* • Asthenia • Constipation • Diarrhea • Drowsiness • Dry mouth • Sleep disorders *Uncommon:* • Abdominal pain *Frequency not known:* • Aggression • Agitation • Angioderma • Increased appetite • Arthralgia

Contd...

Contd...

	Indications and dose	*Unlicensed use*	*Contra-indications*	*Cautions*	*Side effects*
					• Depression • Dizziness • Dyspnea • Hallucination • Hepatitis • Myalgia • Nausea • Oedema • Palpitations • Paresthesia • Seizure • Skin reactions • Suicidal ideation • Syncope • Tachycardia • Tremor • Urinary disorders • Vertigo • Vision disorders • Vomiting • Increased weight *N.B.:* Renal impairment—avoid if estimated GFR is <10 mL/min/1.73 m^2; *reduce dose frequency to alternate days* if estimated GFR is 30–50 mL/min/1.73 m^2; *reduce dose frequency to every 3 days* dose if estimated GFR is 10–30 mL/min/1.73 m^2

Contd...

Contd...

	Indications and dose	*Unlicensed use*	*Contra-indications*	*Cautions*	*Side effects*
Loratidine	• *Symptomatic relief of allergy (hay fever, chronic* idiopathic urticaria) *Oral route:* – 2–11 years (body weight up to 31 kg): 5 mg once daily – 2–11 years (body weight >31 kg): 10 mg once daily – 12–17 years: 10 mg once daily	—	—	—	*Common/very common:* • Drowsiness • Fatigue • Headache • Nervousness *Uncommon:* • Increased appetite *Rare/very rare:* • Alopecia • Angioderma • Seizures • Dizziness • Dry mouth • Gastritis • Altered LFT • Tachycardia *N.B.:* Hepatic impairment—use with caution
Mizolastine	• *Symptomatic relief of allergy (hay fever, chronic idiopathic urticaria)* *Oral route:* – 12–17 years: 10 mg once daily		• Cardiac disease • Susceptibility to QT interval prolongation		*Common/very common:* • Increased appetite • Weight gain or loss • Diarrhea • Nausea • Dizziness • Drowsiness *Uncommon:* • Arrhythmias • Anxiety, depression • Arthralgia, myalgia *Rare/very rare:* • Hypersensitivity *Frequency not known:* • Exacerbated asthma • Bronchospasm • QT interval prolongation *N.B.:* • Hepatic impairment—avoid use in significant impairment

Contd...

	Indications and dose	Unlicensed use	Contra-indications	Cautions	Side effects
Rupatidine	• *Symptomatic relief of allergic rhinitis and urticaria* *Oral route:* *Tablet:* – 12–17 years: 10 mg once daily *Oral solution:* • 2–11 years (10–24 kg): 2.5 mg once daily • 2–11 years (≥25 kg): 5 mg once daily			• History of QT interval prolongation	*Common/very common:* • Asthenia • Dizziness • Drowsiness • Dry mouth • Headache *Uncommon:* • Increased appetite and weight • Arthalgia, myalgia • Back pain • Impaired concentration • Constipation • Cough, dry throat and nose • Diarrhea • Eosinophilia, neutropenia • Epistaxis • Fever • GI discomfort, nausea • Increased risk of infection *Rare/very rare:* • Palpitations • Tachycardia *N.B.:* Hepatic and renal impairment—avoid use/use with caution

[*] Desloratadine is a metabolite of loratadine.
[†] Levocetirizine is an isomer of cetirizine.

(GFR: glomerular filtration rate; GI: gastrointestinal; LFT: liver function test)

Indications

Allergen immunotherapy are especially effective in patients who have shown an incompetent response to anti-allergy medications or have shown AEs-associated-related medications. Allergen vaccines have shown to relieve symptoms of asthma, allergic rhinoconjunctivitis, and insect sting allergy in pediatric population.

Types of Allergen Immunotherapy

There are two main forms of allergy immunotherapy for aeroallergens: Subcutaneous immunotherapy (SCIT), or allergy shots, and sublingual immunotherapy (SLIT), which involves placing allergen extracts under the tongue. Both methods work by gradually desensitizing the immune system to specific allergens, reducing symptoms over time.

An oral preparation of grass pollen extract is licensed for the treatment of grass pollen-induced rhinitis and conjunctivitis; house dust mite licensed for disease-modifying treatment of AR/conjunctivitis in children above 12 years of age. In children, allergy immunotherapy offers long-term benefits, potentially preventing the progression of allergic diseases, such as AR developing into asthma. However, treatment duration can be lengthy (typically 3–5 years), and there is a risk of adverse reactions, including anaphylaxis in rare cases.

Oral immunotherapy (OIT) for children with food allergy such as peanuts might undergo desensitization treatment in order the alleviate symptoms in case of accidental exposure to the allergenic food. An approved oral peanut powder, Palforzia, is now licensed for use in clinical practice.

Patients who are at risk of anaphylaxis from insect stings are commonly offered SCIT.

Leukotriene Receptor Antagonists

Pharmacology and Mechanism of Action

Arachidonic acid (AA) and its metabolites derived from ω-6 polyunsaturated fatty acid (PUFA) are implicated in a variety of physiological processes and have been of particular interest owing to its role in the inflammatory pathway. The AA in turn is metabolized by three distinct enzyme systems: Cyclooxygenases (COXs) or prostaglandin G/H synthases (PGHS), lipoxygenases (LOXs), and cytochrome P450 (CYP) enzymes (ω-hydroxylases and epoxygenases).

The LOX pathway was the second eicosanoid and inflammatory pathway to be of therapeutic interest. The AA in the LOX pathway is oxidized by 5-lipoxygenase (5-LO) into hydroperoxides and other lipid mediators, particularly leukotrienes (LTs). LTs can be classified into two groups:

1. LTB_4 that binds to BLT receptors, which are seven-transmembrane domain GPCRs.
2. Cysteinyl LT (Cys-LT) such as LTC_4, LTD_4, and LTE_4, bind to cys-LT receptors (Cys-LTR); which are further classified into $Cys\text{-}LT_1R$ and $Cys\text{-}LT_2R$ receptors. $Cys\text{-}LT_1R$ has high affinity for LTD_4 and is a therapeutic target for montelukast, zafirlukast, and pranlukast. Since these receptors are expressed in platelets, drugs targeting these receptors could result in excessive bleeding.

Antagonists targeting the 5-LO inhibitors and cys-LT receptor antagonists are useful for the treatment of asthma, AR, and AD. Cys-LT are associated with early- and late-phase reactions in asthma. They are potent bronchoconstrictors, mediate vascular permeability, induce mucus secretion, mast cell activation, eosinophil recruitment, and chronic inflammation. The arachidonate 5-LOX (ALOX5) and LT receptor antagonists are primarily of interest in therapeutic interventions such as asthma and allergy.

Environmental stimuli such as cold, or antigen–antibody receptor activation or any stimulation that increases intercellular calcium could result in the production of LTs. This in turn sets in an inflammatory cascade resulting in clinical symptoms such as bronchoconstriction, airway hyperresponsiveness, mucus secretion, and increased influx of eosinophils into airway tissue.

Indications

Leukotriene antagonists are implicated in the treatment of not only asthma but also other allergic conditions such as AR, AD, and chronic urticaria. The drugs used in allergy are either LT antagonists or act by inhibiting LT synthesis. Leukotriene receptor antagonists (LRTAs) are not meant to be used for immediate relief of asthma symptoms during an acute attack. The LT receptor antagonists are zafirlukast (Accolate) and montelukast (Singulair); inhibitor.

Whereas, the only known LT synthesis inhibitor is Zileuton (Zyflo).

All these drugs are orally administered. Montelukast is used for AR, prophylaxis and chronic treatment of asthma, and prevention of exercise-induced bronchospasm. It is prescribed once a day, particularly in the evening and needs to be taken 2 hours before exercise to avoid exercise-induced asthma. Zafirlukast has to be taken 2 hours prior to meals as food can reduce the bioavailability of the medicine unlike montelukast where there is no stringency of consuming it before or after meals. Zafirlukast can be used in children ≥5 years. It can be used off-label for AR and prophylaxis of exercise-induced bronchospasm.

Adverse Effects Associated with Leukotriene Receptor Antagonists

Since AEs have been reported in children and adolescents using LRTAs, an extensive systematic review "PROSPERO" was conducted to understand the side effects associated with the use of this class of drugs in this population. Out of 7,012 patients recorded, 6,853 patients received an LTRA. A wide spectrum of adverse drug reactions (ADRs) ranging from anxiety to mood and sleep disorders were reported. Some common ADRs reported were agitation, hyperactivity, irritability, nervousness, aggression, and headache. The frequencies of ADRs were reported in seven out of eight studies. It is therefore necessary to use these LRTAs under stringent clinical supervision, especially in pediatric population. Recently, US FDA has issued a warning against the use of montelukast on the basis of post-marketing surveillance (PMS) of neuropsychiatric events such as agitation, anxiety, nightmares, depression, insomnia, and suicidal thoughts.

Other AEs associated with LRTAs include:

- Zileuton is implicated in inducing liver toxicity and drug reactions. Common AEs include headache, viral infections, abdominal pain, cough, diarrhea, nausea, dyspepsia, myalgias, leucopenia, sleep disorders, and behavioral changes. It is not used in younger children but only adults and children
- Zafirlukast is well tolerated and associated with minimal side effects with respect to montelukast

Steroids

Pharmacology

Corticosteroids are synthetic analogs of cortisol which are natural steroid hormones produced in the adrenal glands and can be further subdivided into glucocorticoids (GC) and mineralocorticoids. GC are of prime importance in allergy and inflammation owing to their immunosuppressive, anti-inflammatory, and vasoconstrictive effects.

Since their isolation and synthesis over roughly eight decades, GC have revolutionized the treatment of inflammatory diseases and are currently the most widely prescribed drugs used in a wide variety of conditions particularly in allergy such as asthma, AR, AC, angioedema, eczema, certain types of food allergy, and anaphylaxis, and to prevent a delayed response.

Mechanism of Action

Corticosteroids exert their effect by both endocrine and nonendocrine mechanisms; the latter is involved in the anti-inflammatory property. The anti-inflammatory and immunosuppressive effects of CS are mediated through their ubiquitously distributed glucocorticoid receptors (GR), which are transcription factors that belong to the steroid receptor subfamily. In the target cell, when the GC binds to the human (h) GR, transcription of the target genes occurs that promote the production of growth factors and inflammatory cytokines thereby mediating anti-inflammatory and immunosuppressive effects.

In clinical practice, GC are classified by their duration of action, such as short-acting to medium-acting steroids such as hydrocortisone, prednisolone, and methylprednisolone; intermediate-acting steroids such as triamcinolone; and long-acting steroids such as betamethasone and dexamethasone.

As per GINA guidelines, inhaled corticosteroid (ICS) preparations have been given preference. In children between age-groups of 6 and 11 years old, ICS are used as maintenance therapy to prevent recurrent episodes of asthma attacks. Short-acting β_2 agonists are used as maintenance and reliever therapy (MART) in this age-group. In adolescents, a combination of both ICS and long-acting β_2 agonists are used as MART. The doses of ICS in different age-groups have been presented in **Table 3**.

Uses of CS are as follows:
- Orally in short courses for 3–5 days at 1–2 mg/kg/day in acute asthma exacerbation
- ICS in various stages of GINA guidelines
- INS in AR
- Topical in AD

Administration and Indication

Allergic rhinitis: As per the ARIA guidelines, the drugs preferably used are INS. Since AR develops early in childhood, use of INS early in life prevents development of AR into asthma in adolescents and adults. INS have been used in combination with antihistamines in AR. The doses of ICS in different age-groups have been presented in **Table 4**.

TABLE 3: Doses of inhaled corticosteroids.

Drug	*Low dose (µg/day)*	*Medium dose (µg/day)*	*High dose (µg/day)*
Budesonide (DPI) 6–11 year	100–200	200–400	>400
Budesonide (DPI) >11 year	200–400	400–800	>800
Budesonide (nebules)	250–500	500–1,000	>1,000
Fluticasone propionate (pMDI) 6–11 year	100–250	250–500	>500
Fluticasone propionate (pMDI) >11 year	50–100	100–200	>200
Beclomethasone dipropionate (pMDI) 6–11 year	100–200	200–400	>400
Beclomethasone dipropionate (pMDI) >11 year	200–500	500–1,000	>1,000
Mometasone furoate (pMDI) 6–11 year	100	100	200
Mometasone furoate (pMDI) >11 year	200–400	200–400	>400

(DPI: dry powder inhaler; pMDI: pressurized metered-dose inhaler)

TABLE 4: Doses of intranasal corticosteroids.

Drug	*Dosing*	
	2–11 years	*>11 years*
Mometasone (50 µg/spray)	1 spray in each nostril OD	2 sprays in each nostril OD
Fluticasone furoate (27.5 µg/spray)	1 spray in each nostril OD	2 sprays in each nostril OD
Fluticasone propionate (50 µg/spray)	>4 years only—1 spray each nostril	2 sprays in each nostril OD
Triamcinolone acetate (55 µg/spray)	1 spray in each nostril OD	2 sprays in each nostril OD

Atopic dermatis: Topical steroids are the mainstay to prevent inflammation and itch. Most of the steroids used vary from mild to moderately potency depending on the severity of the condition. In some severe cases, stronger doses are required to maintain remission. Mild and moderate CS are used in body sites where the skin is thin such as face, axillae, groin, and anogenital area. Steroid creams are usually applied depending on the amount of cream taken which is measured by "finger tip unit" or FTU. 1 FTU = 0.5 g of cream.

Urticaria: It is commonly known as hives, results in the occurrence of recurrent wheals over the skin with pruritus. It can be acute (lasting <6 weeks) or chronic (lasting longer than 6 weeks) depending on the duration of the disease. As per EACCI guidelines, topical steroids are not recommended except for pressure urticaria on soles as alternative therapy where evidence is low. In chronic urticaria, stronger doses of steroids such as prednisolone at 20 mg/day or 50 mg/day for a longer duration are required. This is, however, associated with AEs on long-term use. Therefore, CS is generally not a choice in chronic urticaria. In acute urticaria, and acute exacerbations of chronic urticaria, short courses of CS up to 10 days might be helpful

Allergic conjunctivitis: Steroids in AC have been reported when antihistamines do not respond. Despite their anti-inflammatory effects, AEs such as cataract and raised intraocular pressure limit their use for shorter durations. Commonly used steroid is loteprednol etabonate 0.2% four times a day for shorter durations in seasonal AC. Prednisolone acetate 1% has greater absorption and penetration properties and more favored owing to its superior anti-inflammatory properties than dexamethasone 0.1%. In AC combined with AR, INS used to treat AR can also help control the AC symptoms.

In case of anaphylaxis and owing to delayed onset action of steroid treatment, their use makes them inappropriate for immediate control of anaphylaxis.

Adverse Effects Associated with Steroids

Adverse effects associated with use of steroids may be musculoskeletal which include osteoporosis, myopathy, and avascular necrosis of head femur. They may also affect the cardiovascular system and cause symptoms such as edema, fluid retention, hypertension, and atherosclerosis (on prolonged dosing). Steroids can also cause metabolic AEs such as hyperglycemia and weight gain. Their effect on hypothalamic–pituitary axis and adrenal hormone suppressions can cause symptoms such as fatigue, malaise, nausea, vomiting, fever, abdominal pain, anorexia, hypoglycemia, seizures, etc. They can also various other AEs such as GI, dermatologic, ophthalmologic infections, behavioral and cognitive, local AEs (oral thrush, dysphonia, epistaxis, etc.).

Important Consideration When Using Steroids

It is recommended that children receiving high steroid doses (prednisolone >2 mg/kg/day or for those >10 kg, 20 mg/day or equivalent) for >2 weeks should not receive live vaccines. In addition, blood sugar, blood pressure, and weight check should be done on regular intervals.

Bronchodilators

Bronchodilators are employed to improve or optimize airflow through lungs, thereby reducing bronchospasm and improve breathing in patients with asthma or chronic obstructive pulmonary disease (COPD). Classical bronchodilators are subclassified into sympathomimetics or β2-adrenoreceptor agonists, theophylline or methylxanthine, and muscarinic receptor antagonists or anticholinergic agents.

The first report of inhaled selective β agonist to be used as aerosol therapy for asthma dates back to 1950s. Thereafter, salbutamol as rapid- and short-acting therapy (SABA) in asthma was introduced. Ipratropium was the first approved anticholinergic agent introduced in 1987, and long-acting β2 agonists (LABA) was introduced around mid-1990s.

Classification and Mechanism of Action of Bronchodilators

Beta 2-adrenergic agonists are the most effective bronchodilators with reported minimal side effects. Two types of β2-adrenoreceptor agonists have been reported; SABA such as salbutamol and terbutaline act immediately and peak within half an hour and their action lasts for 3–5 hours. They are prescribed as needed. Another is LABA such as salmeterol, formoterol, and indacaterol show prolonged action usually >12 hours and are used in adjunct with GC. Formoterol show both rapid onset of 2–3 minutes and also a long duration of action up to 12 hours and is therefore recommended as a reliever medication in combination with low-dose ICS. Indacaterol show efficacy beyond 24 hours and are more effective against bronchoconstriction than twice daily LABA and more-frequent SABAs and is used in COPD. In 2003, there was a study on safety and efficacy of OD dose of indacaterol acetate.

Beta-2 agonists act by targeting the β2-adrenoceptor, which is a GPCR present in the smooth muscles of lungs. This activates the adenylate cyclase and increase cyclic adenosine monophosphate (cAMP) in the bronchial smooth muscles which phosphorylates several regulatory proteins that mediate bronchodilation, thereby relaxing the smooth muscles of the airways. Additionally cAMP is increased in mast cells and inhibits release of chemical mediators that secondarily cause bronchoconstriction. Bronchodilators are administered in various formulations for oral use, injections and also metered-dose inhalers, dry powder inhalers (DPIs) and nebulizers for inhalation use. Inhaled formulations have reported better efficacy at low doses than oral doses. Subcutaneous and inhaled routes are reported to be better than oral therapy. IV route is prescribed in severely ill patients but are generally associated with AEs owing to high plasma influx.

Methylxanthines such as theophylline are widely used in the developing nations for being cost-effective despite being less effective than the β2 agonists. In some countries two classes of theophylline, enprofylline, and doxofylline are also available and despite being less effective than adenosine antagonist, they have demonstrated a favorable safety profile. The exact mechanism of action of theophylline is still vague, but its bronchodilator action is attributed mainly to nonselective inhibition of phosphodiesterase. Competitive antagonism of adenosine at adenosine receptor might contribute to bronchodilator effect to a certain extent; however, this may be associated with some serious (S) AEs. Theophylline exerts additional anti-inflammatory, immunomodulatory, and bronchoprotective effects that contribute to its efficacy in controlling chronic asthma and COPD.

Anticholinergic or *antimuscarinic agents* act as competitive inhibitors of muscarinic receptors. Muscarinic receptor M1 is expressed in lymphocytes and mast cells, M3 in eosinophils, macrophages, and neutrophils, M4 in eosinophils and neutrophils, whereas M5 is exclusively expressed in neutrophils. Activation of muscarinic receptors on inflammatory cells and production of acetylcholine (Ach) from non-neuronal sources increase inflammatory activity. ACh induce bronchoconstriction and tracheobronchial mucus secretion. Competitive muscarinic agents inhibit the constrictor effect on bronchial smooth muscle mediated via the M3-Gq-PLC-IP3-Ca^{2+} pathway, leading to bronchodilation and increased mucus secretion. Antimuscarinic agents exhibit poor absorption profile and thus are associated with minimal systemic AEs. Two types of muscarinic antagonists have been classified into short-acting muscarinic antagonist (SAMA) such as ipratopium acts within 15 minutes and its maximal potency is achieved at approximately 1.5 hours, with an overall duration of action lasting up to 6 hours. It is generally prescribed 3 to 4 times a day on a regular basis. The duration of SAMA is longer compared to SABA. The other is long-acting muscarinic antagonist (LAMA) such as tiotropium is longer-acting (up to 24 hours). Newer drugs exhibit faster onset of action compared to tiotropium.

Various formulations of bronchodilators are available; however, inhaled formulations are preferable over oral doses owing to their lower AEs. Improved drug delivery methods, longer-acting medications and effective aerosol delivery devices have led to their preferred use owing to a better safety profile. The available bronchodilators and their features have been compared below **(Table 5)**.

Biologics

Biologics belong to a class of advanced drugs which are derived from diverse biological sources, from microorganisms such as yeast cultures to human cells or tissues. Biologics can also be proteins or peptides or cellular products or can be produced using biotechnological processes. The biologics function by targeting specific elements of the inflammatory pathway in an allergic reaction. The early biologics focused on developing monoclonal antibodies (mAbs) to target free IgE that was released following an allergic inflammation. Omalizumab was the first approved drug for treating allergic asthma.

Classification and Mechanism of Action of Biologics

Since their introduction in the past two decades, several more biologics have been introduced to treat allergic diseases and they function by either of the following methods, such as,

Inhibition of IgE: These biologics which are mostly mAbs quench free IgE in the bloodstream thereby preventing IgE from binding to their high-affinity FcεRI receptors present on mast cells and basophils thereby preventing their activation.

Cytokine blocking: Most of the biologics in this group either block or prevent the formation of pro-inflammatory cytokines such as interleukin 4 (IL-4)/IL-13, IL-5, IL-17 thereby preventing the activation of eosinophils and T helper 2 (Th2) cells.

Inhibition of eosinophils: Anti-IL-5 biologics such as mepolizumab, reslizumab, and benralizumab specifically target eosinophil in allergic inflammation such as asthma and eosinophilic disorders.

TABLE 5: Available bronchodilators and their comparative features.

	Beta agonist	*Methylxanthines*	*Anticholinergics*
Agents and available medications	• *SABA:* Salbutamol terbutaline • *LABA:* Salmeterol, fenoterol, formoterol, pirbuterol, indacaterol	Theophylline, aminophylline, enprofylline, doxofylline	• *SAMA:* Ipratropium bromide • *LAMA:* Tiotropium, glycopyrronium bromide, umeclidinium bromide, aclidinium bromide, revefenacin
Mechanism of action	• β2-adrenergic agonist	• Inhibition of PDE-3,4 • Adenosine receptor antagonism • IL-10 release	• Muscarinic M3 receptor antagonist
Route of administration	• By inhalation • Oral • Parenteral	• Intravenous aminophylline • Oral immediate-release theophylline tablets	• By inhalation
Efficacy and response	• Most effective bronchodilators • Quick onset of action when administered by inhalation	• Less effective than β2 agonist nebulizers • Rapid onset with IV route	• More effective in COPD • Less effective in asthma • Response slower compared to β2 agonist
Safety	• Dose-related AE • Tremor, tachycardia	• Dose-related headache, nausea, vomiting, increased acid secretion, abdominal discomfort and restlessness • High dose related cardiac arrhythmia and seizures • Requires monitoring	• Safest with minimal AE • Dry mouth, glaucoma • Urinary retention rare, tachycardia

(AE: adverse effect; COPD: chronic obstructive pulmonary disease; LABA: long-acting β2 agonist; LAMA: long-acting muscarinic antagonist; PDE: phosphodiesterase; SABA: short-acting β2 agonist; SAMA: short-acting muscarinic antagonist)

Inhibition of inflammatory receptors: Biologics such as dupilumab binds to and blocks the IL-4 receptors α subunit thereby blocking both IL-4 and IL-13 production.

Modulation of itch and pruritus: Some biologics such as anti-IL31 antibodies can modulate symptoms of itch and pruritus associated with AD.

Vascular endothelial growth factor (VEGF) inhibition: Biologic such as aflibercept inhibits the actions of VEGF which is involved in blood vessel growth and inflammation thereby enabling their management in allergic eye disorders such as AC.

Some of the biologics are also approved for allergy in pediatric population; however, more studies are required to ensure their safety and efficacy in this population.

Asthma: Omalizumab is possibly the first biologic to be approved by FDA in 2003 for treating moderate-to-severe persistent asthma in patients aged ≥6 years. Dupilumab is another biologic approved to reduce bronchoconstriction and airway inflammation by targeting IL receptors such as IL-4 and IL-13 thereby improving the asthma symptoms. Mepolizumab and reslizumab are IL-5 inhibitors while benralizumab blocks the IL-5 receptors, thereby preventing the eosinophil production. This helps in the management of airway inflammation and asthma symptoms in eosinophilic asthma. Sometimes biologics are also used in combination with other medicines to treat asthma, such as omalizumab used as an additional therapy in patients who are already on high-dose inhaled CS and long-acting β-agonists.

Atopic dermatitis: Dupilumab was approved by FDA to treat moderate-to-severe AD in patients with little or no response to topical treatments. The European Commission approved its use in children ≥6 months for severe AD. Dupilumab prevents the binding of IL-4 and IL-13 to the α-subunit of IL-4 receptor thereby down-regulating the signaling cascade involving Th2 cells and thereby helps in reducing inflammation, pruritus, and skin lesions thereby improving eczema symptoms. Dupilumab and nemolizumab (IL-31 inhibitor) significantly improve the QoL in patients with AD by relieving the severe itch associated with AD. Dupilumab has also shown to improve skin barrier function by improved hydration and reduced inflammation. Combination therapy such as dupilumab with topical medications have also been reported.

Allergic rhinitis: Since omalizumab is a potent IgE blocker, it has been reported to act effectively in AR and allergic symptoms such as sneezing, running nose, and nasal congestion. Biologics in AR have reportedly improved the QoL of the patients by improving their sleep and performance in daily activities. Omalizumab has shown to be potent in managing both AR and asthma offering an all-inclusive therapy.

Chronic urticaria: Omalizumab has been approved by FDA to treat chronic spontaneous urticaria (CSU) in patients aged >12 years, which helps reduce IgE and therefore controls hives and angioderma. Omalizumab has shown to be effective in the long-term use thereby significantly improving the patients' QoL.

Food allergy: Approximately a year back, FDA approved omalizumab injection for IgE-mediated food allergy in certain adults and children ≥1 year and also in reducing the risk of anaphylaxis that might be associated with the exposure to one or more food. Since it is used to reduce the risk of allergy, it is not approved for immediate emergency treatment of allergic reactions such as anaphylaxis. Biologics are aimed to supplement OIT owing to their safe and effective profile. OIT in combination with omalizumab has shown to induce tolerance to food allergen more effectively.

Chronic rhinosinusitis: Dupilumab has shown to be promising in reducing inflammation and decreasing the nasal polyp size in chronic rhinosinusitis with nasal polyp (CRSWNP) and hence reduces nasal inflammation and improves nasal airflow. Biologics in combination with INC or surgery have also been successfully implemented.

EPINEPHRINE IN ANAPHYLAXIS: A SPECIAL NOTE

Anaphylaxis is a serious manifestation of an immediate allergy reaction or hypersensitivity reaction that exhibits rapid onset and is often potentially fatal. Clinical presentation and severity varies not only among patients but also in the same patient from one episode to another. Epinephrine is the first line of treatment in anaphylaxis **(Box 1)** and has been used by physicians for over a century, yet the patients and physicians are

BOX 1: Anaphylaxis management.

Early intramuscular (IM) adrenaline is the first drug of choice.

Doses:

- IM adrenaline: 10 µg/kg 90.01 mg/kg
- Maximum dose: 0.5 mg/dose
- IM into anterolateral aspect of thigh
- Striated muscle is very vascular—faster absorption compared to subcutaneous

inadequately informed or mostly unaware about its proper dosing and administration.

Dose Administration and Associated Adverse Effects

Delays in epinephrine administration can result in poor outcomes or even severe adverse effect (SAE) such as respiratory or cardiac arrest. Epinephrine is administered at 0.1 mg/kg via IM in children ≤30 kg and the dose can be increased up to 0.3 mg in prepubertal children. Adolescents are administered at 0.5 mg. The epinephrine is administered into the deltoid or the vastus lateralis muscle of the mid-outer thigh and can be repeated within 5–15 minutes. Autoinjectors are effective, single-use, prefilled syringes and are available in the following doses: 0.3 mg for adults and for children and adolescents weighing >30 kg, and 0.15 mg for children weighing between 15 and 30 kg.

EpiPens are not available in India owing to cost involved and therefore it is advisable to carry adrenaline injections for patients who are prone to develop anaphylaxis. Errors in administration, such as IV administration or wrong dosages, are often reported and can result in severe hypertension, angina, myocardial infarction (MI), cardiogenic shock, stroke, and potentially fatal tachyarrhythmias. In addition, it is often difficult to diagnose anaphylaxis during anesthesia and delayed injection or delayed diagnosis can be fatal and also lead to hypoxic-ischemic encephalopathy and death.

Intravenous infusions of epinephrine should be used only for refractory anaphylaxis, wherein patients exhibit symptoms despite two doses of IM epinephrine; reported in about 1% of patients with anaphylaxis. With the help of specialized clinical care, 1 μg/mL of crystalloid solution of epinephrine infused at 5–20 mL/min is administered.

SUMMARY

This chapter provides a detailed overview of the pharmacological management of allergic diseases in children, tailored to the Indian context. It addresses the common allergic conditions—such as AR, asthma, AD, food allergy, and anaphylaxis—and their therapeutic options, including antihistamines, CS, LRTAs, bronchodilators, biologics, and immunotherapy. The chapter emphasizes the differentiation between first-, second-, and emerging third-generation antihistamines, and their respective roles, side effect profiles, and dosage considerations in the pediatric population. It critically explores the safety and effectiveness of ICS in asthma, LT antagonists like montelukast, and the growing utility of biologics such as omalizumab and dupilumab in severe cases. Special focus is given to misuse of OTC medications and steroids in India, the high cost and limited access to biologics, and the importance of individualized treatment. Epinephrine use in anaphylaxis is highlighted as a life-saving intervention. The chapter underscores that optimal pharmacotherapy in pediatric allergy requires rational drug use, caregiver education, adherence support, and vigilant monitoring for AEs.

Key Learning Points

- *Early and accurate diagnosis* is essential to distinguish allergic conditions from other pediatric diseases and to guide targeted therapy.
- *Second-generation antihistamines* and *INS* remain first-line treatments for most allergic conditions in children due to their safety and efficacy.
- *ICS* are the cornerstone of asthma management, with stepwise escalation and de-escalation based on symptom control and risk factors.
- *Biologic therapies* (e.g., omalizumab, dupilumab) have transformed the treatment of severe allergic diseases and are increasingly being used in pediatric patients.
- *Montelukast use is declining* due to neuropsychiatric concerns, reinforcing the need for individualized treatment planning.

- *Immunotherapy* (SCIT and SLIT) offers long-term benefits for selected patients with AR and asthma.
- *Patient and caregiver education*, adherence to therapy, and environmental control are critical components of successful allergy management.
- *Ongoing research* and pharmacovigilance are needed to expand safe options for children and optimize long-term outcomes.

SUGGESTED READING

1. Bousquet J, et al. Next-generation Allergic Rhinitis and Its Impact on Asthma (ARIA) guidelines. Journal of Allergy and Clinical Immunology, 2025; 155(1):1-12.
2. Global Initiative for Asthma. (2025). Global Initiative for Asthma (GINA) 2025 Report. [online] Available from https://ginasthma.org [Last accessed August, 2025].
3. Pawankar R, Canonica GW, Holgate ST, Lockey RF, Blaiss MS. (2013). WAO White Book on Allergy. [online] Available from https://www.worldallergy.org [Last accessed August, 2025].
4. Tsabouri S, Arasi S, Beken B, et al. A European survey of management approaches in chronic urticaria in children: EAACI pediatric urticaria taskforce. Pediatr Allergy Immunol. 2022;33(1): e13674.
5. US Food & Drug Administration (FDA). (2020). FDA requires boxed warning for serious mental health side effects for asthma and allergy drug montelukast (Singulair); advises restricting use for allergic rhinitis. [online] Available from https://www.fda.gov [Last accessed August, 2025].
6. Zuberbier T, Abdul Latiff AH, Abuzakouk M, et al. The international EAACI/GA²LEN/EuroGuiDerm/APAAACI guideline for the definition, classification, diagnosis, and management of urticaria. Allergy. 2022;77(3):734-66.

CHAPTER

6

Allergen Immunotherapy

Gayatri S Pandit
Reviewer: *Vinay Mehta*

INTRODUCTION

Allergen immunotherapy (AIT) is a disease-modifying treatment available for several common allergic disorders. While globally established for more than a century, AIT is recently gaining structured momentum in India, particularly in the era of rising allergic disorders and growing awareness among clinicians and patients. Persistent allergen exposure to house dust mites, pollens, fungal spore, and animal dander can prevent symptom control despite environmental control measures and optimal pharmacological treatment.

In this setting, AIT offers transformative potential. By inducing long-term tolerance, it addresses the underlying pathophysiology more than merely suppressing symptoms. AIT has demonstrated efficacy in reducing symptom burden and medication burden and improving patient's quality of life. More importantly, in children, early intervention with AIT has shown the potential to alter the natural course of disease by preventing progression from allergic rhinitis to asthma.

Despite its potential, several challenges remain in India. These include variability in diagnostic procedures, access to standardized allergens, and a limited number of allergy training programs. Fortunately, recent advances in diagnostic tests, recent availability of standardized house dust mite tablet, and emerging SLIT options are paving way for wider and safer adoption. AIT stands at a pivotal juncture in Indian allergy practice. Hence, establishing India-specific practice parameters can ensure safety, efficacy, and foster integration of AIT in to mainstream pediatric and adult allergy care.

INDICATIONS FOR ALLERGEN IMMUNOTHERAPY

- Allergic rhinitis
- Allergic conjunctivitis
- Allergic asthma
- Atopic dermatitis

Allergen immunotherapy is not recommended for:

- Non-immunoglobulin E (IgE)-mediated allergic disease
- Patients on beta blockers
- AIT is not initiated during pregnancy, although it may be continued in women who were receiving therapy prior to becoming pregnant.

Ideal patient for AIT: The ideal patient for AIT is one with documented and clinically relevant IgE-mediated allergy, persistent symptoms despite optimal medical therapy, and the willingness and ability to adhere to a structured treatment plan. Careful patient selection ensures high efficacy, safety, and long-term disease control.

It is essential to note that asthma must be well-controlled before initiating AIT. Young patients are typically good responders to AIT, while elderly patients may not benefit as significantly due to the forementioned factors.

The decision to begin AIT might depend on several other factors, including but not limited to the patient's preference/acceptability, adherence, medication requirements, response to avoidance measures, and adverse effects of medications.

Allergen immunotherapy can be started from the age of 5 years onward.

IDEAL ALLERGENS FOR IMMUNOTHERAPY

One should consider obtaining a second history to ascertain the clinical relevance of positive allergy tests when selecting allergens for immunotherapy. One needs to consider the prevalence of the allergens in the patient's locality, potential cross-reactivity to other allergens, and clinical correlation with the patient's symptoms. In general, the fewer the number of allergens selected, the better the efficacy of immunotherapy.

Allergen immunotherapy is highly effective for house dust mites, tree pollen, grass pollen, weed pollen, cat dander, dog dander, *Alternaria*, and *Cladosporium*. Its efficacy with other molds, cockroach, and other animals (rodent, horse) has not been rigorously studied.

Mold and cockroach extracts contain proteases that can degrade other types of allergens. Therefore, they should not be mixed with each other or with other allergens in the same treatment vials.

EFFECTIVE DOSE OF IMMUNOTHERAPY

The effectiveness of AIT is dose-dependent. The optimal dose range is specific to each type of allergen and varies significantly among allergens. Optimal doses have been determined for many of the major inhalant allergens. Information about effective doses is presented separately for standardized and nonstandardized allergens in **Table 1**.

ROUTES OF IMMUNOTHERAPY

Allergen immunotherapy has traditionally been administered by subcutaneous injections. Subcutaneous immunotherapy (SCIT) has proven efficacy in allergic rhinoconjunctivitis and asthma, but it requires regular injections at a clinician's office and carries a potential risk of anaphylaxis. Sublingual immunotherapy (SLIT) is an alternate approach of administering allergens in which the allergen is given as either a dissolvable tablet (under the tongue) or as an aqueous or liquid extract. SLIT can be self-administered at home and carries a much lower risk of anaphylaxis.

Subcutaneous Immunotherapy

Subcutaneous immunotherapy is the most extensively studied and widely practiced form of AIT. It involves the administration of gradually increasing doses of specific allergen extract to modulate the immune response and induce long-term tolerance.

Subcutaneous immunotherapy schedules differ in the number of injections per visit, number of visits per week, and the rapidity with which the patient reaches the maintenance dose. Conventional immunotherapy schedules involve 1–3 injections per week during a buildup phase that lasts several weeks, followed by a maintenance phase, during which injections are given every 2–4 weeks for 3–5 years **(Fig. 1)**. Example of conventional schedule of Indian SCIT preparation has been given in **Figure 2**.

Accelerated schedules involve shortening the length of the buildup phase, while the maintenance phase remains the same. They are associated with higher rates of systemic allergic reactions compared with conventional schedules, and therefore premedication with H1 and H2 antihistamines and montelukast is recommended.

Cluster

Cluster schedules involve the administration of several injections (two to three) of increasing dose at 30-minute intervals in 1 day. The patient typically returns on one or more nonconsecutive

TABLE 1: Probable effective dose range for standardized and nonstandardized US licensed allergen extracts.

Allergenic extract	*Labeled potency or concentration*	*Probable effective dose range*	*Range of estimated major allergen content in US-licensed extracts*
Dust mites: *Dermatophagoides farinae* and *Dermatophagoides pteronyssinus*	3,000, 5,000, 10,000, and 30,000 AU/mL	500–2,000 AU	10,000 AU/mL 20–160 μg/mL Der p 1, Der f 1[*] 2–180 μg/mL Der p 2, Der f 2[*] 78–206 μg/mL Der p 1, Der f[†] 13–147 μg/mL Der p 2, Der f 2[†]
Cat hair	5,000 and 10,000 BAU/mL	1,000–4,000 BAU	10,000 BAU/mL 20–50 μg/mL Fel d 1[‡] 30–100 μg/mL cat albumin[§]
Cat pelt	5,000–10,000 BAU/mL	1,000–4,000 BAU	10,000 BAU/mL 20–50 μg/mL Fel d 1[*] 400–2,000 μg/mL cat albumin[§]
Grass, standardized	100,000 BAU/mL	1,000–4,000 BAU	100,000 BAU/mL 425–1,100 μg/mL Phl p 5[*] 506–2,346 μg/mL group[‖]
Bermuda	10,000 BAU/mL	300–1,500 BAU	10,000 BAU/mL 141–422 Cyn d 1 μg/mL[*]
Short ragweed	1:10, 1:20 w/v, 100,000 AU/mL	6–12 μg of Amb a 1 or 1,000–4,000 AU	1:10 w/v 300 μg/mL Amb a 1[‡] Concentration of Amb a 1 is on the label of w/v extracts
Nonstandardized AP dog	1:100 w/v	15 μg of Can f 1	80–400 μg/mL Can f 1[†] 10–20 μg/mL dog albumin
Nonstandardized extract, dog	1:10 and 1:20 w/v	15 μg of Can f 1	0.5 to 10 μg/mL Can f 1[†] <12–1,500 μg/mL dog albumin
Nonstandardized extracts: Pollen	1:10 to 1:40 w/v or 10,000–40,000 PNU/mL	0.5 mL of 1:100 or 1:200 w/v	NA
Nonstandardized extracts: Mold/fungi, cockroach	1:10 to 1:40 w/v or 10,000–40,000 PNU/mL	Highest tolerated dose	NA
Hymenoptera venom	100 μg/mL single venom 300 μg/mL in mixed vespid extract	50–200 μg of each venom	100–300 μg/mL of venom protein
Imported fire ant	1:10 to 1:20 w/v whole-body extract	0.5 mL of a 1:100 w/v to 0.5 mL of a 1:10 w/v extract	NA

[*]ALK-Abelló ELISA
[†]Indoor Biotechnology ELISA
[‡]FDA radial immunodiffusion assay
[§]Greer Radial Immunodiffusion assay
[‖]Greer ELISA
[¶]Hollister–Stier ELISA using Innovative Research, Inc., reagents
(NA: information not available)
Source: Adapted from Cox L, Nelson H, Lockey R, Calabria C, Chacko T, Finegold I, et al. et al. Allergen immunotherapy: a practice parameter third update. J Allergy Clin Immunol. 2011;127(1 Suppl):S1-55.

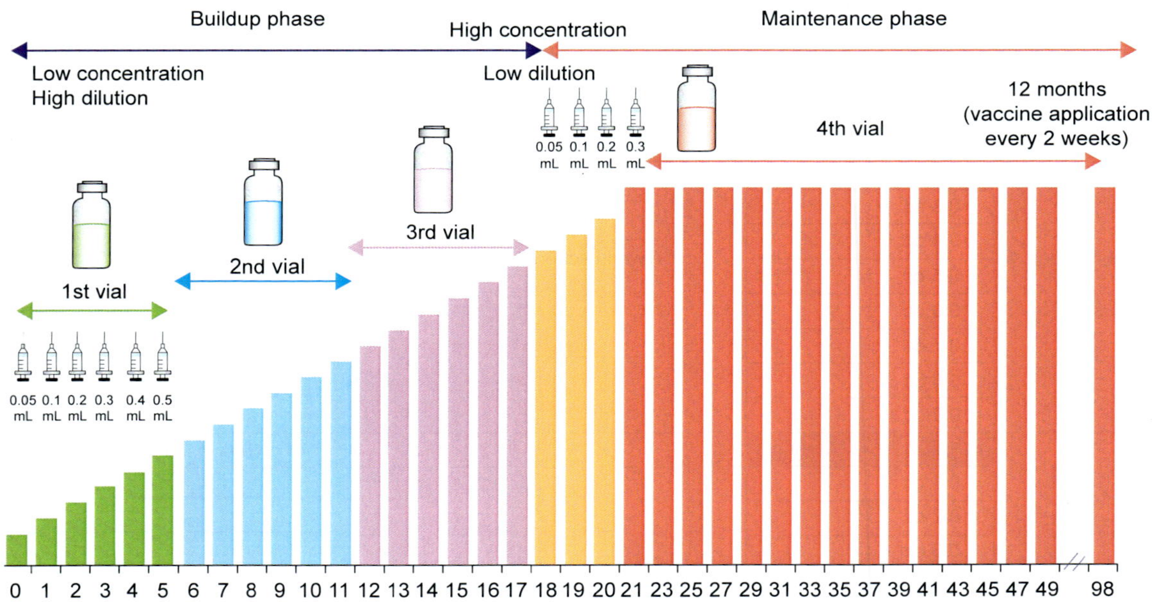

Fig. 1: Example of conventional immunotherapy schedule.
Source: Adapted from Pavón-Romero GF, Parra-Vargas MI, Ramírez-Jiménez F, Melgoza-Ruiz E, Serrano-Pérez NH, Teran LM. Allergen Immunotherapy: Current and Future Trends. Cells. 2022;11:212.

days, several days per week. Maintenance is achieved in 4–8 weeks, depending upon the spacing of the visits.

Rush

Rush schedules involve administering injections of increasing dose at 15- to 60-minute intervals over 1–3 consecutive days until a target dose is achieved. The remainder of the buildup phase proceeds using a traditional schedule until maintenance is achieved, usually in <8 weeks.

Comparison between all three schedules of SCIT has been mentioned in **Table 2**.

Allergoids

Allergoids are chemically modified allergens using formaldehyde or glutaraldehyde aimed to reduce IgE binding while preserving immunogenicity. They are designed to reduce the risk of systemic reactions, while still inducing the desired immune response.

Preparation of allergen extracts: In the Indian setup, the prescriber writes the prescription for AIT and the manufacturer dispenses the extract in fixed dilutions. SCIT preparations are aqueous-based and dispensed in the strength of 1:5,000 w/v, 1:500 w/v, and 1:50 w/v. SLIT preparations are glycerin-based and are dispensed in 1:500 w/v, 1:250 w/v, and 1:50 w/v

STANDARD OPERATING PROCEDURE FOR SUBCUTANEOUS IMMUNOTHERAPY

Prior to administration of injection:

- Verify that asthma is under good control
- Peak flow meter monitoring
- Check vitals
- Ask how well patient has tolerated the last dose.

Vial no:	Conc of antigen	S/C Injection	One line progress note regarding severity and frequency of asthma or rhinits	Mention quantities if using steroids and broncho dilators
Vial number: 1	1:5000	Date	Two injections in a week	Report if any reaction
	0.1 cc			
	0.2 cc			
	0.3 cc			
	0.4 cc			
	0.5 cc			
	0.6 cc			
	0.7 cc			
	0.8 cc			
	0.9 cc			
Vial number: 2	1:500	Date	Two injections in a week (after vial: 1)	Report if any reaction
	0.1 cc			
	0.2 cc			
	0.3 cc			
	0.4 cc			
	0.5 cc			
	0.6 cc			
	0.7 cc			
	0.8 cc			
	0.9 cc			
Vial number: 3	1:50	Date	One injections in a week (after vial: 2)	Report if any reaction
	0.1 cc			
	0.2 cc			
	0.3 cc			
	0.4 cc			
	0.5 cc			
	0.5 cc			
	0.5 cc			
	0.5 cc			
	0.5 cc			
	0.5 cc			
	0.5 cc			

Fig. 2: *Contd...*

	1:50	Date		Report if any reaction
Vial number: 4	0.6 cc		One injections in 2 weeks (after vial: 3)	
	0.6 cc			
	0.6 cc			
	0.6 cc			
	0.6 cc			
	0.6 cc			
	0.6 cc			
	0.6 cc			
	1:50	Date		Report if any reaction
Vial number: 5	0.7 cc		One injections in 3 weeks (after vial: 4)	
	0.7 cc			
	0.7 cc			
	0.7 cc			
	0.7 cc			
	0.7 cc			
	0.7 cc			
	1:50	Date		Report if any reaction
Vial number: 6	0.8 cc		One injections in 4 weeks (after vial: 5)	
	0.8 cc			
	0.8 cc			
	0.8 cc			
	0.8 cc			
	0.8 cc			
	1:50	Date		Report if any reaction
Vial number: 7	0.9 cc		One injections in 4 weeks (after vial: 6)	
	0.9 cc			
	0.9 cc			
	0.9 cc			
	0.9 cc			
	1:50	Date		Report if any reaction
Vial number: 8	0.1		One injections in 4 weeks (after vial: 7)	
	0.1			
	0.1			
	0.1			
	0.1			

Fig. 2: Conventional schedule Indian subcutaneous immunotherapy (SCIT).
Source: Adapted from Allvac Allergen Immunotherapy manufacturer schedule

TABLE 2: Comparison of immunotherapy schedules.

Feature	*Conventional SCIT*	*Cluster immunotherapy*	*Rush immunotherapy*
Buildup	12–24 weeks	4–8 weeks	1–3 days
Frequency in build up	1–2 injections/week	3–4 injections per sitting, multiple visits/week	
Setting required	Clinic with observation area and access to emergency	Specialized clinic with access to emergency	Hospital setup with emergency facility
Premedication	Not required	Required	Required
Advantage	Widely used, safe, well accepted	Faster buildup, fewer visits	Rapid desensitization
Disadvantage	Multiple clinic visits	Increased risk of systemic reactions	Increased risk of systemic reactions

Injection procedure:

- Confirm patient identity.
- Confirm the dosage schedule.
- Load injection in insulin syringe/tuberculin syringe and administer subcutaneously in mid-posterolateral upper arm.
- Apply compression on injection site.
- Patient sits in waiting area for 30 minutes; ask patient to report any new symptoms.

Post injection:

- Ask patient how he/she is feeling.
- Look for local reaction.
- Give cold compression for large local reaction.

REACTIONS TO SUBCUTANEOUS IMMUNOTHERAPY

Local reactions can be immediate or delayed. They consist of redness, pruritus, and swelling. Local reactions are fairly common, and are related to several factors, including allergen concentration, number of allergens per extract, and larger injection volumes. Large local reactions do not increase the risk of subsequent systemic reactions. They can be treated with oral antihistamines and application of cold packs. Local reactions can be reduced by premedication with oral antihistamines and rinsing the immunotherapy syringe with a solution of epinephrine (1 mg/mL).

Systemic reactions involve organ systems distant from the injection site. Most serious systemic reactions occur within 30 minutes after the injection. Factors that may increase the risk of systemic reaction include poor asthma control, prior systemic allergic reactions, dosing errors, dosing from new vials, dosing during active pollination season, and concurrent use of beta blockers. To minimize the risk, we recommend checking peak flow values in known asthmatics, verifying the patient's identity and dosage, and reducing the dose with new vials and during peak pollination season.

Dose Adjustments

There is no single, universally agreed-upon protocol for dose adjustments in AIT, and practitioners may vary their approach based on individual patient needs and experience. However, after a systemic reaction, one commonly reduces the next injection to the previously tolerated dose. In cases of very severe reactions, the clinician should determine with the patient whether the risk/benefit of AIT justifies continuation of therapy.

BOX 1: Subcutaneous immunotherapy (SCIT) buildup dose adjustment for skip dose.

- 1–14 day—Increase according to schedule
- 15–28 day—Repeat last dose
- 29–35 day—Decrease by 1 dose
- 36–42 day—Decrease by 2 doses
- 43–49 day—Decrease by 3 doses
- 50–56 day—Decrease by 4 doses
- 57–84 day—Decrease by 1 vial, same volume
- 85–112 day—Decrease by 2 vials, same volume
- >112 day—Start all over (e.g., 0.05 mL 1:1,000 v/v, green vial)

BOX 2: Subcutaneous immunotherapy (SCIT) maintenance adjustment for skip dose.

- 1–42 day—Repeat maintenance dose
- 43–49 day—Decrease by 1 dose
- 50–56 day—Decrease by 2 doses
- 57–63 day—Decrease by 3 doses
- 64–70 day—Decrease by 4 doses
- 71–84 day—Decrease by 1 vial, same volume
- 85–112 day—Decrease by 2 vials, same volume
- >112 day—Start all over (e.g., 0.05 mL 1:1,000 v/v, green vial)

Source: Adapted from Ebstein TE and Tankersly MS. Are Allergen Immunotherapy Dose Adjustments Needed for Local Reactions, Peaks of Season, or Gaps in Treatment? J Allergy Clin Immunol Pract. 2017;5(5):1227-33.

How to Manage Missed Doses?

It is customary to dose adjust for missed doses to reduce the risk of systemic reactions. An empiric schedule for missed doses outlined in the **Boxes 1 and 2**.

SUBLINGUAL IMMUNOTHERAPY

Sublingual immunotherapy offers several advantages compared with SCIT. It is safer, more convenient (as it is self-administered at home), and more comfortable (no needles involved). However, it must be administered daily, and therefore patient compliance is crucial. In addition to the contraindications associated with SCIT, SLIT is also contraindicated in patients with a history of eosinophilic esophagitis. Patients should discontinue SLIT temporarily if they develop gum or mouth ulcers or immediately following dental surgery or tooth extraction. In addition, patients with asthma should hold SLIT therapy during asthma exacerbations.

Sublingual immunotherapy typically contains one or two antigens, making it suitable for patients who are monosensitized rather than polysensitized.

Adverse Events

The most common adverse effects of SLIT include oral pruritus, ear pruritus, throat irritation, and swelling of the lips, tongue, and pharynx. These self-limited local reactions typically occur with the first dose of treatment and last up to 60 minutes. Symptoms tend to lessen in duration with continued therapy and resolve in the majority of patients within 1–2 weeks. Rarely, a patient may experience edema of the tongue, uvula, lip, or throat that requires epinephrine. Anaphylaxis is quite rare, occurring in 1.4/100,000 SLIT doses. The first dose of SLIT is recommended to be administered in the office under supervision.

Maintenance dose of different standardized allergens for sublingual preparation has been has been mentioned in **Table 3**.

Sublingual immunotherapy tablets are rapidly dissolving tablets that are held under the tongue until completely dissolved. SLIT tablet therapy is initiated with a full dose in most cases. SLIT drops are held under the tongue for 1–2 minutes, then swallowed. They usually involve a buildup phase before achieving maintenance dose.

Standardized house dust mite tablets are now available in India under the commercial name Sensimune. These tablets are approved for patients 12 years and older for allergic rhinitis. The tablets are to be stored in cool dry place below 30°C and administered daily. Different schedules of SLIT that are followed are mentioned in **Figure 3**.

TABLE 3: Optimal maintenance doses in the main dose finding studies.

Author, year	*Dose*	*Allergen source*	*Manufacturer*
Durham, 2006	15 µg Phl p 5/day	Grass	ALK-Abellò
Didier, 2007	25 µg Group 5/day	Grass	Stallergenes
Creticos, 2013	12 µg Amb a 1/day	Ragweed	MSD
Bergmann, 2014	(500 IR) 300 IR—approved: 16/68 Der p 1/Der f 1/day	Dust mite	Stallergenes
Mosbech, 2014	6 SQ7d (15 µg/day)	Dust Mite	ALK-Abellò
Nolte, 2015	12 DU/day (=6 SQ/day)	Ragweed	MSD
Virchow, 2016	6 or 12 HDM-SQ/day	Dust mite	ALK-Abellò
Demoly, 2017	6 or 12 HDM-SQ/day	Dust mite	ALK-Abellò

Source: Adapted from Passalacqua G, Bagnasco D, Canonica GW. 30 years of Sublingual Immunotherapy. Allergy. 2020;75:1107-20.

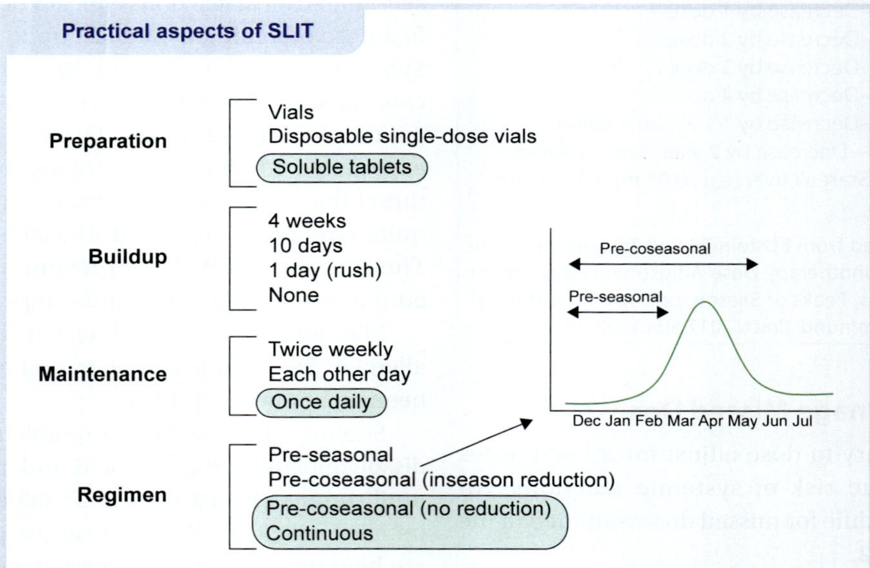

Fig. 3: Three different schedules of sublingual immunotherapy (SLIT).
Source: Adapted from Passalacqua G, Bagnasco D, Canonica GW. 30 years of Sublingual Immunotherapy. Allergy. 2020;75:1107-20.

COMPLIANCE

Patient compliance can be challenging, as therapy is self-administered at home. To improve adherence, it is important to clearly communicate the expected benefit and time course of improvement before starting therapy. Potential adverse effects should be thoroughly reviewed, and patients should be advised to consult their allergist regarding any questions or concerns that may arise. Regular follow-up visits should be encouraged to assess progress.

CHALLENGES IN INDIA

Allergen immunotherapy in India faces several unique challenges that hinder its integration into routine allergy care. First, there is a lack of standardized high-quality allergens, potentially leading to inconsistent treatment outcomes. Specifically, Indian-manufactured allergen extracts have been found to be less potent than those manufactured in the United States and Europe, which can impact the efficacy of immunotherapy. Second, the lack of comprehensive aerobiological data makes it difficult to accurately identify relevant regional allergens. Third, there is a shortage of trained allergists and limited awareness of AIT as a treatment modality among patients and healthcare professionals. Finally, challenges related to access and costs continue to be significant.

To fully leverage AIT, a comprehensive strategy is needed focusing on improving affordability through policy and insurance coverage, enhancing the quality of allergen extracts, training more allergy specialists, and establishing standardized practice parameters. This approach is necessary to address the rising incidence of allergic disorders in India.

SUMMARY

This chapter provides a detailed insight into AIT, a disease-modifying treatment for IgE-mediated allergic conditions such as allergic rhinitis, allergic asthma, and conjunctivitis. AIT works by inducing immune tolerance to specific allergens, thereby reducing symptom severity, medication need, and risk of disease progression—especially in children. It highlights the growing relevance of AIT in India amid increasing allergy prevalence and evolving diagnostic capabilities. The chapter explains the principles of patient selection, ideal allergens, administration routes (SCIT and SLIT), schedules (conventional, cluster, rush), and monitoring protocols. It emphasizes the importance of standard operating procedures, safety measures, and managing reactions. The practical challenges in India—such as inconsistent allergen extract quality, lack of trained personnel, and poor awareness—are discussed, with suggestions for overcoming these barriers. AIT, when practiced appropriately, promises long-term benefits and could become a cornerstone in allergy management in India.

Key Learning Points

- *AIT is the only disease-modifying therapy* for allergic diseases like allergic rhinitis and asthma, offering long-term tolerance and symptom reduction by targeting the underlying immune response.
- *Two main administration routes exist:* SCIT and SLIT, each with unique advantages, risk profiles, and suitability based on patient preference and clinical context.
- *Ideal candidates for AIT* are children over 5 years with well-controlled asthma and confirmed IgE-mediated allergy with poor symptom control despite pharmacotherapy and allergen avoidance.
- *Immunotherapy schedules vary* (conventional, cluster, rush), with accelerated schedules offering faster desensitization but higher risks of systemic reactions—requiring premedication and close monitoring.
- *India-specific challenges* like poor standardization of allergen extracts, limited allergy training, and affordability issues need urgent redressal to improve AIT adoption and outcomes nationwide.

SUGGESTED READING

1. Calderon MA, Waserman S, Bernstein DI, Demoly P, Douglass J, Gagnon R, et al. Clinical Practice of Allergen Immunotherapy for Allergic Rhinoconjunctivitis and Asthma: An Expert Panel Report. J Allergy Clin Immunol Pract. 2020;8(9):2920-36.e1.
2. Cox L, Nelson H, Lockey R, Calabria C, Chacko T, Finegold I, et al. Allergen immunotherapy: A practice parameter third update. J Allergy Clin Immunol. 2011;127(1 Suppl):S1-55.

3. Epstein TE, Tankersley MS. Are allergen immunotherapy dose adjustments needed for local reactions, peaks of seasons, or gaps in treatment? J Allergy Clin Immunol Pract. 2017;5(5):1227-33.
4. Gaur SN, Kumar R, Singh AB, Agarwal MK, Arora N. Guidelines for Practice of Allergen Immunotherapy in India: 2017—an Update. Indian J Allergy Asthma Immunol. 2017;31(1):3-33.
5. Pandit GS. Immunotherapy Practice in India. J Pediatr Pulmonol. 2023;2(Supplement 2).
6. Passalacqua G, Bagnasco D, Canonica GW. 30 years of sublingual immunotherapy. Allergy. 2020;75:1107-20.
7. Sub-lingual Immunotherapy: World Allergy Organization Position Paper 2009. Allergy. 2009;64 Suppl 91:1-59.

CHAPTER

7

Management of Asthma in Children and Adults

Krishna Mohan R
Reviewer: *Mohit Poddar*

INTRODUCTION

Asthma is one of the most common chronic respiratory conditions affecting children worldwide and represents a significant cause of morbidity, school absenteeism, and healthcare visits. Its presentation and management can vary widely due to underlying genetic, environmental, and social factors. Recognizing this, several international and national bodies have developed structured guidelines to aid in the diagnosis and management of asthma in pediatric populations. Notable among these are the Global Initiative for Asthma (GINA), the National Asthma Education and Prevention Program (NAEPP) in the United States, the British Thoracic Society/Scottish Intercollegiate Guidelines Network (BTS/SIGN), the Canadian Thoracic Society guidelines, and the Australian Asthma Handbook. While these documents share core principles—such as symptom-based assessment, stepwise pharmacotherapy, and the emphasis on long-term control—there are differences in their approach, particularly in age-specific recommendations, medication choices, and diagnostic tools.

Among these, the GINA guidelines are widely recognized and adopted across different regions for their evidence-based, regularly updated, and globally applicable recommendations. In India, GINA serves as the principal reference for pediatric asthma care, with endorsement from several national pediatric respiratory and allergy societies such as the IAP National Respiratory Chapter and the Pediatric Allergy Association of India. However, implementing these guidelines in the Indian context presents unique challenges which include clinical, socio-cultural, and systemic factors. Hence, while the GINA guidelines offer a valuable framework, their application in India requires thoughtful adaptation to address local healthcare realities. This chapter reviews the stepwise approach to managing pediatric asthma as outlined in the GINA 2025 update and explores how these strategies can be effectively tailored to the Indian setting.

Driven primarily by a chronic Th2-mediated inflammatory response, the management of asthma focuses on three key aspects:

1. *Acute management* of wheezing episodes
2. *Long-term control* of underlying airway inflammation
3. *Addressing comorbid conditions.*

GOALS OF LONG-TERM ASTHMA MANAGEMENT

The primary objectives of long-term asthma care include:

- Achieving and maintaining good symptom control
- Optimizing pharmacotherapy to balance effective control with minimal side effects
- Supporting normal levels of activity and ensuring restful sleep

GLOBAL INITIATIVE FOR ASTHMA-BASED STRATEGY FOR LONG-TERM MANAGEMENT

According to the GINA guidelines, a structured, three-step approach is recommended:

- *Assess:* This involves confirming the diagnosis of asthma, evaluating current symptom control, monitoring treatment response, and reviewing inhaler use and technique.
- *Adjust treatment:* Based on the level of control, treatment is either stepped up (when symptoms are not well-controlled) or stepped down (when good control is maintained).
- *Review response:* Ongoing reassessment is essential to evaluate treatment efficacy, detect side effects and modify therapy as needed.

INITIATION OF TREATMENT

In children who present with recurrent wheezing triggered by identifiable factors, diagnostic evaluation—including peak expiratory flow rate (PEFR), spirometry, and challenge testing—is essential to confirm asthma. Once diagnosed, symptom categorization is performed based on:

- *Daytime symptoms*
- *Nighttime (nocturnal) symptoms*
- *Frequency of short-acting beta-agonist (SABA) use*
- *Limitations in physical activity*

This classification helps determine the level of asthma control, which is categorized as:

- *Well-controlled asthma*
- *Partly controlled asthma*
- *Uncontrolled asthma*

MANAGEMENT GUIDELINES

Personalized Asthma Management—Global Initiative for Asthma 2025 Approach

The cornerstone of asthma care, as emphasized in *GINA 2025*, is *personalized asthma management*. The primary goal is to achieve and maintain optimal *symptom control*, prevent exacerbations, and minimize future risk, including airway remodeling.

This process involves two key phases:

1. *Initiation of appropriate therapy* based on the individual's level of symptom control and risk profile.
2. *Ongoing treatment adjustment* through a stepwise approach—stepping up treatment when control is poor and stepping down when good control is achieved and sustained.

COMPONENTS OF ASTHMA PHARMACOTHERAPY

Asthma treatment includes two major therapeutic components.

Maintenance Therapy

Focused on long-term control of airway inflammation, promoting healing, and preventing structural changes (airway remodeling). The primary agent remains *inhaled corticosteroids (ICS)*, which are the foundation of controller therapy.

Reliever Therapy

Aimed at providing quick relief during episodes of bronchospasm or acute symptoms. Options include:

- *Short-acting beta-2 agonists*—traditionally used as quick-relief medications.
- *Low-dose ICS-formoterol*—increasingly recommended in older children and adolescents as both *reliever* and *controller*, offering anti-inflammatory benefit with rapid onset.

THERAPEUTIC STRATEGIES COMBINING MAINTENANCE AND RELIEVER THERAPY

Global Initiative for Asthma 2025 outlines several flexible treatment models based on patient characteristics:

- *Maintenance and reliever therapy (MART):* The same combination of *low-dose ICS and formoterol* is used for both daily maintenance and as-needed symptom relief. This approach is recommended for individuals ≥12 years and children aged 6–11 years where appropriate, especially in those with moderate-to-severe asthma or frequent exacerbations.
- *Anti-inflammatory reliever (AIR):* In patients with *mild asthma,* daily maintenance therapy may not be needed. Instead, *as-needed low-dose ICS-formoterol* is used to relieve symptoms and provide anti-inflammatory action during exacerbations. This strategy reduces the risk of over-reliance on SABA.
- *Separate maintenance and reliever therapy:* In younger children (especially <6 years), where ICS–LABA combinations are not approved as relievers, treatment typically consists of:
    - A *daily controller* (usually ICS or ICS + leukotriene receptor antagonist)
    - A *separate reliever,* usually *SABA* as needed

This approach remains standard in preschool children due to age-specific medication approvals and developmental considerations.

STEPWISE LONG-TERM MANAGEMENT OF ASTHMA—GLOBAL INITIATIVE FOR ASTHMA 2025

Asthma management is tailored according to *age groups,* with specific stepwise algorithms:

- *Adolescents and adults (≥12 years):* Emphasis on ICS-formoterol as both MART or as-needed ICS-formoterol (AIR) in mild asthma. Traditional SABA-only strategies are no longer preferred due to increased risk of exacerbations.
- *Children aged 6–11 years:* Stepwise management includes ICS monotherapy, ICS + LABA, or MART where appropriate. Use of ICS-formoterol as a reliever is now supported in selected children.
- *Children <5 years (preschool wheezers):* Diagnosis is often clinical. Management depends on phenotype (e.g., episodic viral wheeze vs. multi-trigger wheeze), frequency of symptoms, and exacerbation history. Treatment involves low-dose ICS or montelukast for controller therapy, with SABA as the primary reliever.

Adolescents (>12 years)

Asthma management in adolescents follows principles similar to adult care, with an emphasis on *anti-inflammatory treatment even in mild disease,* abandoning the previous SABA-only approach. Adolescents are at increased risk of poor adherence, underreporting symptoms, and psychosocial factors affecting disease control. In the GINA 2025 guidelines for individuals aged 12 years and above, asthma management is structured into two tracks based on the choice of reliever medication. *Track 1,* which is the *preferred approach,* uses a combination of low-dose *inhaled corticosteroid (ICS)-formoterol* as both the controller and reliever. This approach provides better protection against severe exacerbations by addressing airway inflammation even during symptom relief. *Track 2,* the alternative option, uses a *SABA* as the reliever, alongside a regular maintenance controller such as ICS or ICS-LABA. Track 1 is prioritized due to its superior efficacy in reducing the risk of severe attacks and its simplified, flexible regimen that aligns better with real-world use patterns.

Stepwise Treatment (Steps 1–5)

- *Step 1:* As-needed low-dose ICS-formoterol is preferred for patients with infrequent symptoms. This "anti-inflammatory reliever" (AIR) strategy ensures that even mild asthma receives anti-inflammatory therapy during exacerbations, reducing reliance on SABA and preventing severe attacks.

- *Step 2:* Daily low-dose ICS with as-needed SABA, or as-needed low-dose ICS–formoterol (AIR), is recommended. The AIR strategy remains preferable due to better safety and fewer exacerbations.
- *Step 3:* Low-dose ICS–LABA as maintenance therapy with SABA as reliever, or low-dose ICS–formoterol used for both maintenance and relief (MART). MART simplifies treatment and improves adherence.
- *Step 4:* Medium-dose ICS–LABA (maintenance) with either SABA or low-dose ICS–formoterol as reliever. MART continues to be an option for eligible patients.
- *Step 5:* Referral for specialist evaluation. Consider add-on therapies such as tiotropium, biologics [e.g., anti-immunoglobulin E (anti-IgE) or anti-IL-5 agents], and phenotyping for severe asthma.

Monitoring and Step Adjustment

Treatment should be adjusted based on symptom control and risk reduction. Step-up is warranted for poor control, whereas a step-down should be considered after 3 months of good control. Regular review of inhaler technique and adherence is essential.

Children Aged 6–11 Years

Asthma in this age group requires a developmentally sensitive approach, considering the child's ability to use inhaler devices and adhere to therapy. GINA 2025 reflects an evolving paradigm that introduces anti-inflammatory reliever strategies in selected children.

Stepwise Treatment (Steps 1–5)

- *Step 1:* As-needed low-dose ICS taken with SABA at symptom onset is preferred. Alternatively, daily low-dose ICS may be started if symptoms occur more than twice a month.
- *Step 2:* Daily low-dose ICS with SABA as needed. A leukotriene receptor antagonist (LTRA) may be used in patients with poor ICS tolerance or allergic rhinitis, though efficacy is lower.
- *Step 3:* Low-dose ICS–LABA maintenance therapy with SABA as reliever. Alternatively, very low-dose ICS–formoterol as MART may be used in selected children who can manage the inhaler and demonstrate consistent symptom patterns. Another option is to use medium dose ICS maintenance therapy.
- *Step 4:* Medium-dose ICS–LABA or continue MART with a higher ICS dose if needed. Specialist referral should be considered for poor responders or frequent exacerbations.
- *Step 5:* Evaluation for severe asthma. Add-on biologics may be considered after confirming diagnosis, addressing modifiable factors, and assessing phenotypes.

Monitoring and Follow-up

Regular follow-up visits should assess symptom control, adherence, side effects, growth parameters, and psychosocial factors. Step-down therapy should be considered when control is sustained for at least 3 months.

Children Under 5 Years

Asthma diagnosis and management in preschool children are particularly challenging due to developmental limitations, overlapping viral wheeze syndromes, and the absence of reliable pulmonary function testing. GINA 2025 recommends a pragmatic, phenotype-driven, and response-based approach in this age group.

Stepwise Treatment (Steps 1–3)

- *Step 1:* Infrequent wheezing episodes (less than every 6–8 weeks and mild) may be managed with SABA alone. If the child is at risk of exacerbations, intermittent high-dose ICS for

7–10 days during episodes may be considered, though this should be used cautiously.

- *Step 2:* Daily low-dose ICS is the preferred controller therapy for persistent symptoms or frequent episodes. LTRA may be considered if there is poor ICS tolerance or coexisting allergic rhinitis.
- *Step 3:* Consider doubling the ICS dose or adding LTRA. Children who fail to respond should be referred to a specialist for reevaluation and to exclude alternative diagnoses.

Monitoring and Review

Monitor growth closely due to the systemic effects of ICS. Educate caregivers about proper inhaler technique and medication adherence. Reassessment every 3–6 months is recommended to decide on treatment adjustment or potential discontinuation in cases of sustained remission.

BIOLOGICALS IN PEDIATRIC ASTHMA

When conventional therapies fail despite rigorous adherence checks and comprehensive multidisciplinary evaluation, biologic agents become an option. These therapies are typically reserved for children with either truly severe, treatment-resistant asthma or those with refractory disease, where standard management flaws have been addressed to no avail.

Five biologics are currently licensed for pediatric use, although data from children, especially those <12 years, remains sparse compared to adults. These include omalizumab, mepolizumab, dupilumab, benralizumab, and tezepelumab. Of these, omalizumab is the most extensively studied in pediatric populations. The efficacy of these drugs is largely determined using biomarkers such as peripheral blood eosinophil count and fractional exhaled nitric oxide (FeNO), although these values vary naturally in children and are affected by infections and corticosteroid use.

Omalizumab: Anti-immunoglobulin E Therapy

Omalizumab, the first biologic approved for pediatric asthma, targets circulating IgE, thereby preventing its interaction with receptors on mast cells and basophils. This reduces mediator release and allergic inflammation.

As per GINA 2025, omalizumab should be considered in children aged ≥6 years with moderate-to-severe allergic asthma that is uncontrolled despite optimized inhaled therapy, and who have evidence of sensitization to perennial aeroallergens along with elevated serum IgE levels within the dosing range for omalizumab. The child should have a history of frequent exacerbations or persistent symptoms, and treatment should follow a confirmed diagnosis with assessment of adherence and inhaler technique.

Dosing is weight and IgE-dependent, and response is typically assessed after 16 weeks. Though considered safe, rare side effects include serum sickness-like reactions, thrombocytopenia, and unmasking of eosinophilic granulomatosis with polyangiitis following oral corticosteroids (OCS) tapering.

Mepolizumab: Anti-Interleukin-5 Therapy

Mepolizumab was the second biologic to gain approval for children. It works by binding to interleukin-5 (IL-5), a key driver of eosinophilic inflammation, thereby reducing eosinophil activation and survival. It is licensed for children 6 years and older with elevated eosinophil counts (usually >300–400 cells/μL) and a history of multiple exacerbations or prolonged OCS use. Dosing is 40 mg for children aged 6–11 years and 100 mg for those 12 years or older, administered every 4 weeks. Treatment continuation is typically based on reduction in exacerbation frequency or tapering of OCS.

Despite its established role, various studies have suggested that mepolizumab is less effective in children than in adults. Potential reasons include different inflammatory pathways, environmental factors such as air pollution, and the possibility that IL-5 plays a less prominent role in pediatric asthma. These findings emphasize that adult data should not be directly extrapolated to younger populations.

Dupilumab

Dupilumab is a monoclonal antibody approved for use in children aged 6 years and older with moderate-to-severe asthma characterized by type 2 inflammation, as defined by elevated eosinophils or FeNO. According to GINA 2025, it is considered an add-on therapy for patients who remain uncontrolled despite optimized standard treatment, including high-dose ICS-LABA. Dupilumab targets the IL-4 receptor alpha, thereby inhibiting both IL-4 and IL-13 signaling, which are key drivers of type 2 inflammation. Clinical trials have shown improvements in asthma control, lung function, and reduction in exacerbations in pediatric patients with appropriate biomarkers. It is particularly beneficial for children with co-existing severe eczema. Dupilumab increases nitric oxide synthesis in airways, making FeNO a useful biomarker for predicting response. Dosing varies by age and weight, with biweekly or monthly subcutaneous injections depending on these parameters. Response is evaluated after 16 weeks.

Tezepelumab

Tezepelumab represents a significant advance as it is effective even in non-TH2 asthma phenotypes. It blocks thymic stromal lymphopoietin (TSLP), an epithelial-derived cytokine involved in initiating and amplifying airway inflammation. TSLP acts upstream in the inflammatory cascade, affecting both TH2 and non-TH2 pathways. Tezepelumab is licensed for children aged 12 years and older with uncontrolled asthma despite high-dose ICS and additional therapy. Unlike other biologics, it does not require elevated eosinophils or FeNO for initiation.

Adverse Effects of Biologicals

Biological therapies have emerged as a significant advancement in the management of severe asthma, particularly in patients with type 2 inflammation who remain uncontrolled despite high-dose inhaled corticosteroids and additional controllers. While they have demonstrated substantial clinical benefits, it is important to be aware of their potential adverse effects, which may vary depending on the specific agent used. **Table 1** provides an overview of the commonly used biologicals in asthma and their associated adverse effects.

TABLE 1: Adverse effects of biologicals.

Biologicals	*Adverse effects*
Omalizumab	*Injection:* Site reactions Serum sickness-like reaction, thrombocytopenia anaphylaxis—rare
Mepolizumab	Headache, abdomen and back pain, fever, increased infection risk, and nasal congestion *Injection:* Site reactions
Dupilumab	*Injection:* Site reactions, arthralgia, increased upper respiratory tract infection (URTI) risk Transient blood eosinophilia (4–13% patients)
Tezepelumab	*Injection:* Site reactions, arthralgia, headache, and increased URTI risk Anaphylaxis—rare

OTHER KEY ASPECTS OF LONG-TERM ASTHMA MANAGEMENT

Optimal long-term asthma control extends beyond pharmacotherapy. It includes addressing modifiable risk factors and managing comorbid conditions that contribute to poor symptom control, increased exacerbation risk, and reduced quality of life.

Management of Comorbidities

- *Obesity:* Obesity is a systemic pro-inflammatory state that can worsen asthma symptoms and reduce treatment responsiveness. Individualized strategies involving nutritional counseling, increased physical activity, and behavioral support should be implemented to achieve and maintain healthy weight in children and adolescents with asthma.
- *Food allergy:* In children with coexisting food allergies, identifying and avoiding trigger foods are essential to prevent systemic allergic reactions and to improve overall asthma control. Coordination with allergy specialists and dieticians is often beneficial.
- *Allergic rhinitis:* Effective treatment of allergic rhinitis is critical, as upper and lower airways form a unified respiratory tract. Inflammation in the nasal mucosa can exacerbate asthma symptoms. Intranasal corticosteroids, antihistamines, and allergen avoidance are recommended to achieve good control, which in turn contributes to better asthma outcomes.

ADDRESSING MODIFIABLE RISK FACTORS

- *Tobacco smoke exposure:* Active smoking significantly impairs asthma control and increases the risk of severe exacerbations. Adolescents and adults should be supported through smoking cessation programs. Children must be protected from second-hand and third-hand smoke exposure, both of which are strongly linked to increased asthma symptoms and medication use.
- *Air pollution:* Exposure to both outdoor and indoor air pollutants can exacerbate asthma and reduce the effectiveness of treatment.
  - *Outdoor air pollution:* During periods of high air pollution (e.g., elevated Air Quality Index), children with asthma should be advised to remain indoors. Use of well-fitted masks while commuting or in polluted environments may help reduce inhalation of particulate matter. Families should avoid travel through highly polluted areas, especially during respiratory infections.
  - *Indoor air pollution:* Indoor pollutants such as incense sticks, mosquito coils, biomass fuels, scented candles, and air fresheners can worsen asthma symptoms. Families should be counseled to minimize or eliminate exposure to these irritants. The use of clean cooking alternatives and improving household ventilation is strongly recommended.
- *Allergen exposure:* For children with confirmed sensitization to indoor allergens (e.g., dust mites, pet dander, molds), targeted environmental control measures can help improve symptom control. While complete allergen avoidance is often impractical, specific interventions—such as controlling household dampness to prevent mold growth—can be beneficial.
- *Medication-related exacerbations:* Certain medications, notably non-selective beta-blockers and nonsteroidal anti-inflammatory drugs (NSAIDs) (especially aspirin), can trigger asthma exacerbations in susceptible individuals. In children with a history of medication-induced asthma worsening (e.g., aspirin-exacerbated respiratory disease),

these drugs should be avoided, and alternative therapies should be used under medical supervision.

CHALLENGES IN THE DIAGNOSIS AND MANAGEMENT OF PEDIATRIC ASTHMA IN INDIA

The management of pediatric asthma in India presents unique challenges that stem from a combination of clinical, socio-cultural, and systemic factors. One of the most pressing issues is the under-recognition and underreporting of asthma in children, which significantly impairs timely diagnosis and intervention. This is often due to low public awareness, both among caregivers and healthcare workers, about the varied clinical presentations of asthma, especially in younger children. Symptoms such as recurrent cough or wheeze are frequently attributed to common viral illnesses or allergic bronchitis, delaying appropriate management. Stigma and misconceptions surrounding the diagnosis of asthma further exacerbate this problem. Families may resist accepting the label of "asthma" due to fear of social judgment, long-term medication dependence, or concerns about the impact on the child's lifestyle and future prospects. This leads to underreporting, inadequate treatment adherence, and reluctance to use inhaled corticosteroids, which are the cornerstone of asthma control. Environmental factors significantly contribute to poor asthma control. High levels of ambient air pollution, particularly in urban areas, and indoor exposure to biomass fuel smoke, especially in rural and peri-urban households, are well-established triggers for airway inflammation and exacerbations. In many low-income settings, households rely on wood, cow dung, or charcoal for cooking, often in poorly ventilated spaces. Children, especially those <5 years of age, are particularly vulnerable to these exposures. Furthermore, frequent respiratory infections, common in crowded living conditions with poor sanitation, often mimic or exacerbate asthma symptoms, complicating both diagnosis and management.

The healthcare infrastructure poses additional barriers to optimal asthma care. Limited access to trained personnel, lack of diagnostic tools such as spirometry and peak flow meters at the primary care level, and inconsistent availability of essential medications hinder standardized care delivery. Many primary care physicians rely on symptomatic diagnosis without objective assessment, leading to both under- and overdiagnosis.

Moreover, cultural beliefs and traditional practices often conflict with evidence-based asthma management. Parents may prioritize herbal remedies or homeopathic treatments, delay seeking allopathic care, or discontinue inhaled therapies prematurely, believing them to be habit-forming or harmful. Economic disparities also affect access to care—while inhalers are the most effective mode of drug delivery, the perceived and actual cost of inhaled medications may deter families from initiating or maintaining long-term controller therapy. Another complicating factor is the symptomatic overlap between asthma and other common respiratory conditions such as pulmonary tuberculosis, recurrent bronchitis, and lower respiratory tract infections, especially in younger children. In regions with a high burden of tuberculosis, chronic cough or wheeze may prompt anti-TB treatment without adequate evaluation for asthma, leading to misdiagnosis, unnecessary therapy, and prolonged morbidity.

The management of pediatric asthma is undergoing a significant transformation, guided by a deeper understanding of disease mechanisms, age-specific needs, and the availability of newer therapies. Global frameworks such as the GINA guidelines offer valuable, adaptable strategies for clinicians across diverse healthcare settings. Despite these advances, real-world challenges—such as delayed diagnosis, suboptimal adherence, and disparities in access to specialized care—continue to affect outcomes in children. The advent of biologic therapies marks a pivotal step in treating severe, uncontrolled asthma, emphasizing the importance of identifying eligible patients through clinical and biomarker-based assessment. Ultimately, tailoring guideline recommendations to individual needs and local contexts remains essential for delivering effective, long-term asthma control in pediatric populations.

SUMMARY

This comprehensive chapter reviews the evidence-based approach to asthma management in children, guided primarily by the Global Initiative for Asthma (GINA) 2025 guidelines. It outlines a structured framework that includes accurate diagnosis, severity classification, stepwise pharmacotherapy, and ongoing monitoring. Key treatment strategies include anti-inflammatory reliever (AIR) therapy, maintenance and reliever therapy (MART), and biologic therapies for severe asthma. The chapter discusses age-specific protocols—from preschoolers to adolescents—and emphasizes the importance of controller medications (e.g., inhaled corticosteroids) over traditional reliever-only strategies. It highlights the challenges of asthma diagnosis and management in India, including environmental triggers, poor access to diagnostics, treatment hesitancy, stigma, and the growing relevance of biologics such as omalizumab, mepolizumab, dupilumab, and tezepelumab. Emphasis is also placed on addressing comorbidities, environmental control, and adherence counseling for holistic asthma care in Indian children.

Key Learning Points

- *Global Initiative for Asthma 2025 provides age-specific, flexible treatment tracks*—with ICS-formoterol preferred even for mild asthma in older children and adolescents to reduce exacerbation risk and improve outcomes.
- *Stepwise pharmacotherapy* remains central to asthma management, with treatment intensification or de-escalation based on regular assessment of symptom control, adherence, and inhaler technique.
- *Biologic agents* (e.g., omalizumab, mepolizumab, dupilumab, tezepelumab) are now viable options for children with severe, refractory asthma, guided by phenotype and biomarker evaluation.
- *Inhaled corticosteroids* are the cornerstone of long-term control across all age groups, with newer strategies (MART and AIR) optimizing their use to reduce SABA over-reliance and airway remodeling.
- *Indian-specific barriers* such as poor awareness, diagnostic delays, pollution exposure, and treatment stigma must be addressed through caregiver education, system strengthening, and policy support.

SUGGESTED READING

1. Aggarwal AN, Gupta D, Jindal SK. Prevalence of bronchial asthma in Indian children: Indian Study on Epidemiology of Asthma, Respiratory Symptoms and Chronic Bronchitis in Adults (INSEARCH). Indian J Pediatr. 2009;76(3): 241-6.
2. Asher MI, Montefort S, Björkstén B, Lai CK, Strachan DP, Weiland SK, et al. Worldwide time trends in the prevalence of symptoms of asthma, allergic rhinoconjunctivitis, and eczema in childhood: ISAAC Phases One and Three repeat multicountry cross-sectional surveys. Lancet. 2006;368(9537):733-43.
3. Bush A, Saglani S, Fleming L. Severe asthma: looking beyond the amount of medication. Lancet Respir Med. 2017;5:844-6.
4. Cook J, Beresford F, Fainardi V, Hall P, Housley G, Jamalzadeh A, et al. Managing the paediatric patient with refractory asthma: a multidisciplinary approach. J Asthma Allergy. 2017;10:123-30.

5. Global Initiative for Asthma (GINA) (2025). Global Strategy for Asthma Management and Prevention– 2025 Update. [Internet]. Fontana, WI: GINA. [online] Available from https://ginasthma.org [Last accessed August 2025].
6. Kabra SK, Lodha R. Pediatric asthma in India: prevalence, management and gaps in implementation. J Postgrad Med Educ Res. 2020; 54(1):9-15.
7. Lodha R, Kabra SK. Management of asthma in children in India: current perspectives. Indian J Pediatr. 2018;85(12):1040-7.
8. Martinez FD. Genes, environments, development and asthma: a reappraisal. Eur Respir J. 2007;29(1): 179-84.
9. Worldwide variations in the prevalence of asthma symptoms: the International Study of Asthma and Allergies in Childhood (ISAAC). Eur Respir J. 1998;12(2):315-35.

CHAPTER

8 Management of Allergic Rhinitis

Sinchana Bhat
Reviewer: *Saibal Moitra*

INTRODUCTION

Rhinitis is defined as inflammation of the nasal mucosa. It can be classified as allergic and non-allergic **(Flowchart 1)**.

Allergic rhinitis (AR) is a very common chronic inflammatory condition of the nasal mucosa triggered by allergen exposure, seen in school children and adolescents. It is immunoglobulin E (IgE)-mediated disorder seen in sensitized individuals to an allergen.

Allergic rhinitis is not just a disorder affecting the nasal passages, but it represents a component of the systemic airway disease (united airway disease). It can cause a significant impact that affects the quality of life (QoL) of an individual. 45% of children experience sleep disruption because of nasal allergy symptoms. It affects the work and school performance and creates an enormous economic burden on the family. AR can, by itself, introduce significant inattention, impairment of cognition, and decreased daytime school performance. These problems can be mitigated if AR is diagnosed in the early phase and managed appropriately.

Flowchart 1: Classification of rhinitis.

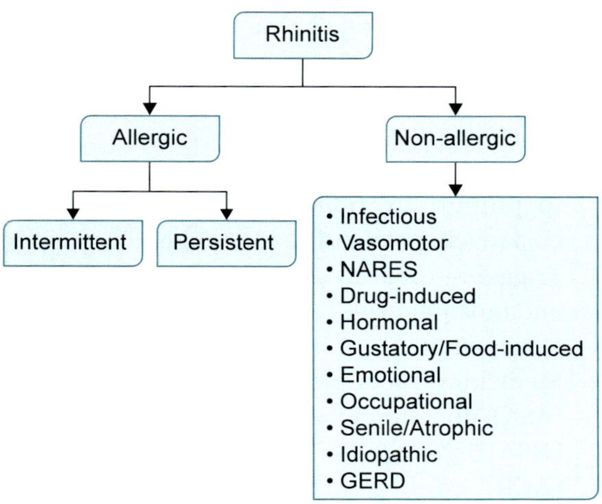

(GERD: gastroesophageal reflux disease; NARES: nonallergic rhinitis with eosinophilia syndrome)

PREVALENCE

The global prevalence ranges between 0.1 and 45%. The Global Asthma Network (GAN) reported the prevalence of AR among 6–7-year-olds was 7.7% and 23.5 % among 13–14-year-olds, with significantly higher prevalence among boys, and 9.8% in adults, with no gender-wise difference. Approximately, 20% of children experience AR symptoms by age 2–3 years, about 40% by age 6 years, and roughly 30% during adolescence.

This chapter describes the approach to a patient with rhinitis with special focus on allergic rhinitis. The treatment pathways for both adults and children remain the same.

The allergic rhinitis and its impact on asthma (ARIA) classifies AR based on the symptom duration and severity as follows **(Fig. 1)**:

SYMPTOMS

The cardinal symptoms of AR are:
- Sneezing
- Itching
- Rhinorrhea (runny nose)
- Nasal congestion

Secondary symptoms: Fatigue, headache, cognitive impairment, and sleep disturbance

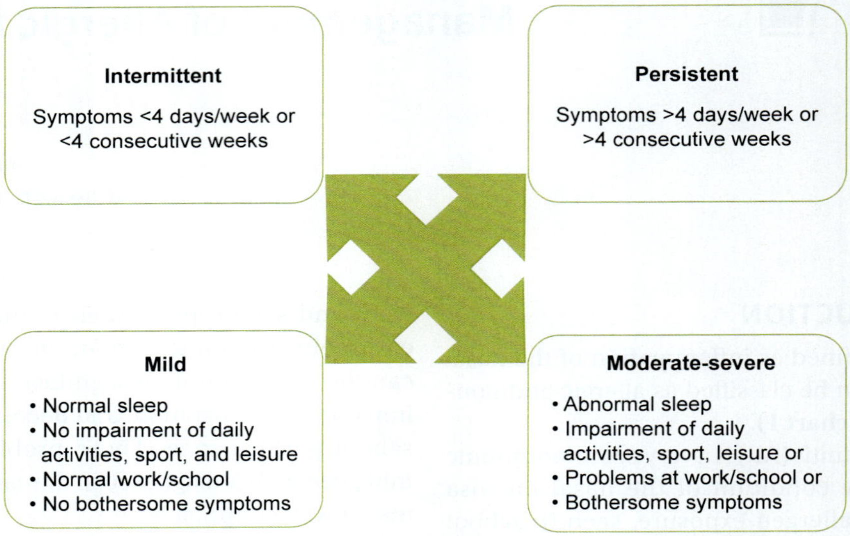

Fig. 1: Classification—the allergic rhinitis and its impact on asthma (ARIA).
Source: ARIA Guidelines, 2019.

Atypical presentation: Recurrent ear infections, reduced hearing due to eustachian tube dysfunction, poor control of asthma, sleep disturbances, prolonged, and frequent respiratory tract infections

The ARIA classification of allergic rhinitis which is based on symptom frequency and impact on QoL is shown in **Figure 1**.

The symptoms of AR can occur at any age however, most individuals develop symptoms at an early age, usually before 6 years of age. Studies have demonstrated that it requires at least two seasons of pollen exposure for a child to develop AR. Hence, the prevalence of AR is very low, below 2 years.

Alternative diagnosis should be considered in the presence of the following symptoms:

- Anosmia—nasal polyps
- *Persistent unilateral obstruction:* Anatomical defects such as deviated nasal septum, concha bullosa, and tumors
- Mucoid/mucopurulent discharge
- Recurrent epistaxis

DIAGNOSIS

Diagnosis of AR is usually clinical and should be arrived at with a good history and clinical examination. A thorough history and physical examination **(Table 1)** are the cornerstones of establishing the diagnosis of AR.

History

- Type and duration of symptoms
- Severity of the symptoms
- Seasonality
- Indoor/outdoor symptoms
- *Environment:* Focused history on exposure to potentially relevant allergens such as cockroach, pet dander, and molds
  Triggers—tobacco smoke, *agarbattis*, *dhoop*, and mosquito coil
- Occupation
- Medicines—beta-blockers, acetylsalicylic acid (ASA), non-steroidal anti-inflammatory drugs (NSAIDs), angiotensin-converting enzyme (ACE) inhibitors, hormone therapy, and recreational cocaine use can cause rhinitis.

TABLE 1: Examination.

Organ	*Salient findings*
Eyes	• *Dennie–Morgan folds* (Dennie lines)—prominent infraorbital skin folds that extend in an arc from the inner canthus beneath and parallel to the lower lid margin—a feature in AD • *Allergic shiners*—blue-gray to purple discolorations beneath lower eyelids, due to venous stasis—just a sign which suggests an allergic disease, not diagnostic • *Stringy or ropy eye discharge/conjunctival congestion and edema*—in AC • *Chemosis*—conjunctival edema seen in severe cases of AC • *Cobblestoning of the tarsal conjunctivae*—in VKD
Nose	• *Deviated nasal septum* • *Transverse nasal crease*—dark and horizontal line due to repeated rubbing of the nose and pushing it upward • *Mucosa*—pale to purple • *Inferior turbinate hypertrophy* • *Polyps*—have to rule out cystic fibrosis • *Allergic nasal secretions*—thin and clear • *Sinus tenderness*—in sinusitis
Ear	• Eczematous changes in postauricular area and base of the earlobe in AD • Otoscopy—otitis media with effusion is common in AR
Facies	• Adenoid facies—dull face, pinched nostrils, open mouth, protruding teeth, and high-arched palate • *Facial grimacing due to nasal congestion and adjusting the blocked airways*
Posterior pharynx	• Post-nasal drip • Cobblestoning—chronic postnasal drip and exposure to allergic mediators causing posterior pharyngeal lymphoid hyperplasia • Tonsillar and adenoid hypertrophy
Chest	Tachypnea, use of accessory muscles, wheeze/rhonchi—during flare-up of asthma
Skin	• Dry skin, hyperlinear palms, and soles • Keratosis pilaris seen on cheeks and extensor aspects of limbs in AD • Urticaria, angioedema, and dermatographism

- Presence of comorbidities (conjunctivitis, asthma, nasal polyps, sinusitis, otitis media, adenoid hypertrophy, impairment of smell/taste, sinus involvement, and nasal polyps atopic dermatitis)
- Family history of atopy
- Impact on QoL
- Response to previous medications

DIFFERENTIAL DIAGNOSIS

- Nonallergic rhinitis
- Local allergic rhinitis

Nonallergic Rhinitis

It is a heterogeneous group of disorders with symptoms similar to AR, such as sneezing, rhinorrhea, nasal congestion, and postnasal drip without a specific allergen trigger. Nasal congestion and rhinorrhea are the predominant symptoms. It is independent of an IgE-mediated mechanism. Patients with nonallergic rhinitis (NAR) are more likely to be older, and asthma is less prevalent in them. NAR can be classified into the following types **(Flowchart 1)**. The differentiating clinical features of AR and NAR are elicited in **Table 2**.

TABLE 2: Difference between allergic rhinitis (AR) and nonallergic rhinitis (NAR).

	AR	*NAR*
Triggers	Aeroallergens	Irritants
Symptoms	Rhinorrhea, sneezing, itching of the nose, and congestion	Nasal congestion and post-nasal drip
Nasal mucosa	Edematous, pale, and boggy with allergic shiners	Normal/erythematous/atrophic

"Nonallergic non-infectious rhinitis" is a term sometimes used to describe this group of patients. Usually, AR is present in conjunction with NAR, and this condition is known as mixed rhinitis.

Vasomotor Rhinitis/Non-allergic Rhinopathy/Idiopathic Rhinitis

This is the most prevalent type of NAR. It occurs due to an imbalance between the parasympathetic and sympathetic nerve stimulation, resulting in symptoms of congestion, rhinorrhea, and less sneezing and nasal pruritus.

Temperature and humidity changes, especially cold, dry air, airborne irritants, strong odors, including tobacco smoke, and/or exercise are the usual triggers for patients with the predominant symptom of nasal congestion. This occurs due to highly sensitive nociceptive neurons. Patients with predominant rhinorrhea (cholinergic rhinitis) appear to have enhanced cholinergic glandular secretory activity that can be effectively reduced with the use of atropine and ipratropium bromide.

Vasomotor rhinitis (VMR), often a diagnosis of exclusion, is frequently referred to as idiopathic rhinitis. History is the key determinant of diagnosis. Laboratory tests may vary, and nasal hyperresponsiveness is used only for research purposes and rarely in clinical practice. More recently, optical rhinometry with intranasal capsaicin challenge has been demonstrated to assist in the diagnosis of a subset of patients with VMR and nonallergic irritant rhinitis.

Infectious Rhinitis

Infectious rhinitis may range from self-limited rhinitis secondary to common viral upper respiratory infections to more severe disease caused by other pathogens, such as fungal infections in an immunocompromised patient. Viral infections account for as many as 98% of acute infectious rhinitis in young children. Secondary infections may occur, resulting in bacterial rhinosinusitis, which causes mucopurulent nasal discharge, nasal congestion, facial pain and pressure headache, postnasal drainage, and cough.

Children with anatomic abnormalities of the nares and sinuses, ciliary dysfunction cystic fibrosis, chronic rhinosinusitis with nasal polyps, and inborn errors of immunity are susceptible to persistent and refractory rhinosinusitis.

The presence of nasal and ocular pruritus and an obvious allergic trigger helps to differentiate AR from infectious (viral and bacterial) rhinosinusitis. A good history can help distinguish these conditions, thus preventing unnecessary prescription of antibiotics.

Gustatory Rhinitis

Rhinorrhea occurring after ingestion of hot and spicy food is induced due to the gustatory reflex. The mechanism is possibly due to a neurogenic reflex of the non-cholinergic non-adrenergic system.

Drug-induced Rhinitis

Drugs such as aspirin, non-steroidal anti-inflammatory drugs (NSAIDs), β-blockers and ACE inhibitors, central sympatholytic (clonidine, methyldopa) phosphodiesterase type 5-inhibitors (sildenafil), calcium-channel blockers, psychotropics (e.g., risperidone and chlorpromazine), gabapentin, oral contraceptives are known to cause symptoms of rhinitis. Overuse of topical decongestants can result in rhinitis medicamentosa, a form of drug-induced rhinitis.

Hormonal Rhinitis

Puberty, pregnancy, menopause, and hypothyroidism can cause rhinitis due to estradiol-mediated expression of H_1 receptor on nasal epithelium. This could be the reason for the increased prevalence and severity of rhinitis in females following puberty.

Local Allergic Rhinitis

Local allergic rhinitis (LAR), also referred to as *entopy*, is due to local production of IgE. The symptoms are similar to AR. It may start in childhood in 36% of patients, with a mean age of onset at 21 years, with a higher prevalence in women.

While most patients with LAR are monosensitized, most commonly to dust mite, up to 37% are polysensitized to seasonal and/or perennial allergens.

The *in vivo/in vitro* tests for the allergens are negative; however, nasal allergen provocation tests (NAPT) are positive. Increase in tryptase, eosinophilic cationic protein, and presence of nasal specific IgE in secretions are seen in 20–40% of patients.

The implications for the treatment of LAR are not well understood at this time, although some evidence suggests that allergen immunotherapy may be effective in this type of rhinitis.

INVESTIGATIONS

Although AR is a clinical diagnosis, further investigations are necessary to confirm the causative allergen. This helps in better management of the patient by focusing on allergen avoidance measures and also in selecting candidates for immunotherapy.

Skin prick test and allergen-specific IgE are the two tests that can be utilized for this purpose. Skin prick test is generally more cost-effective, sensitive, and gives quicker results than specific IgE. Sinonasal imaging is not advised in patients with symptoms suggestive of AR.

Treatment: The goals of therapy in AR are:

- To achieve symptom control and improve QoL
- To prevent recurrence
- To prevent the progression of atopic march

Symptom control can be achieved with pharmacotherapy and allergen avoidance measures.

Allergen avoidance measures are discussed in Chapter 12 of hand book.

The various medications which can be used for AR are:

- *Oral:* Antihistamines, decongestants, and leukotriene receptor antagonists
- Intranasal sprays—corticosteroid, corticosteroid + antihistamine, cromolyn sodium, anticholinergics

Oral antihistamines (OAH): Oral antihistamines block the H_1 receptors, thereby alleviating the symptoms of AR.

They are classified into 1st generation (chlorpheniramine, diphenhydramine, hydroxyzine, and promethazine) and 2nd generation (cetirizine, levocetirizine, loratadine, desloratadine, fexofenadine, and bilastine). The details of these drugs are mentioned in **Table 3**.

Though the 1st generation OAHs are effective in relieving the symptoms, they have been shown to negatively impact cognition and functioning. The advantages of 2nd generation over the 1st are that they are non-sedative due to their inability to cross the blood-brain barrier, and their duration of action is longer.

TABLE 3: Oral medications are commonly used to treat allergic rhinitis (AR).

Drug	*Dose*	*Monitor for*
First-generation H_1 antihistamines		
Hydroxyzine	2 mg/kg/day every 6–8 hours	Renal and liver dysfunction
Diphenhydramine	5 mg/kg/day every 6–8 hours	
Chlorpheniramine	*2–5 years:* 1 mg every 4–6 hours *6–11 years:* 2 mg every 4–6 hours *≥12 years:* 4 mg every 4–6 hours	Caution in asthma
Promethazine	0.1 mg/kg every 6 hours orally (maximum 12.5 mg/dose)	Dry mouth, dizziness, and constipation
Second-generation H_1 antihistamines		
Cetirizine	*6 months–5 years:* 2.5–5 mg OD *6–11 years:* 5–10 mg OD *≥12 years:* 10 mg OD	Dry mouth, drowsiness, tinnitus, and constipation
Levocetirizine	*≥6 years:* 5 mg OD	Same as cetirizine
Loratadine	*2–5 years:* 5 mg OD *6–10 years:* 10 mg OD	Sleepiness, diarrhea, headache, and liver dysfunction
Desloratadine	*6–11 months:* 1 mg OD *12 months–5 years:* 1.25 mg OD *6–11 years:* 2.5 mg OD *>11 years:* 5 mg OD	Sore throat, dry mouth, muscle pain, or drowsiness
Fexofenadine	*6 months–2 years:* 15 mg BD *2–11 years:* 30 mg BD *≥11 years:* 60 mg BD or 120–180 mg OD	Headache, drowsiness, and menstrual cramps
Bilastine	*4–11 years:* 10 mg OD *>11 years:* 20 mg OD	Headache, dizziness, dry mouth, and sore throat
Montelukast	*1–5 years:* 4 mg OD *6–14 years:* 5 mg OD *≥12 years:* 10 mg OD	Headache, mood changes, tremors, skin rash, and tiredness

Newer-generation formulations can be safely used for an extended period, including >1 year of continuous use in preschool-aged children.

Oral antihistamines effectively reduce histamine-mediated symptoms (sneezing, pruritus, and eye symptoms) when taken regularly at the time of maximal symptoms, but they are less effective in relieving nasal congestion. They are less efficacious than intranasal corticosteroids, however, they can be the preferred option for patients based on preference.

Oral decongestants: They are commonly prescribed medications for AR. Pseudoephedrine, phenylephrine, and phenylpropanolamine are the most commonly used. They relieve nasal congestion but are ineffective for other symptoms of AR.

Side effects: Insomnia, irritability, tachycardia, dizziness, and hypertension are some of the side effects that may be experienced. Hence, they should be used with caution in patients with heart disease and hypertension.

TABLE 4: Different intranasal corticosteroids available in India.

Drugs	*Age*	*Dose*
Mometasone furoate 50 ug/spray	2–12 years >12 years	One spray OD Two sprays OD
Fluticasone furoate 27.5 ug/spray	2–12 years >12 years	One spray OD Two sprays OD
Fluticasone propionate 50 ug/spray	4–12 years >12 years	One spray OD Two sprays OD

Leukotriene receptor antagonists (LTRA): Montelukast is the only LTRA approved to be used for the treatment of AR. However, it is inferior and less efficacious than intranasal corticosteroids (InCS).

Leukotriene receptor antagonists have been shown to improve nighttime control of rhinitis symptoms. If a patient has comorbid asthma, then an LTRA may be of benefit for both conditions.

Combination of LTRA with antihistamines is widely available however, there is no benefit when compared to using these agents alone.

Leukotriene receptor antagonists should be considered when alternatives are not well tolerated or are insufficient/ineffective in controlling the symptoms of AR.

Montelukast is also known to cause neuropsychiatric changes in children, such as anxiety, depression, mood changes, and suicidal tendencies.

INTRANASAL CORTICOSTEROIDS

Intranasal corticosteroids are the mainstay of treatment of persistent AR or AR with moderate-to-severe symptoms. They inhibit both the early and late phase reactions. They penetrate the cell membrane, bind to the cytoplasmic receptors, reach the nuclear DNA, and affect protein synthesis. This suppresses the activation of inflammatory cells such as eosinophils, mast cells, and T lymphocytes and downregulates the production of inflammatory mediators and interleukins IL-4, IL-5, and IL-13.

The therapeutic effect of InCS starts by 6–7 hours of administration and peaks by 2 weeks. It is shown to alleviate all the symptoms of AR and is superior to OAH and LTRA in controlling the symptoms. They have also been shown to improve ocular symptoms and reduce lower airway symptoms in patients with concurrent asthma and AR. However, choosing the appropriate type of corticosteroid is vital due to significant differences in absorption from the nasal mucosa and systemic bioavailability.

Common InCS available are fluticasone propionate, fluticasone furoate, mometasone furoate. The strength, dose, and other features are outlined in **Table 4**.

A common cause of treatment failure is poor technique when administering intranasal corticosteroids. Hence, it is important for physicians to spend time explaining the appropriate use of these devices.

These InCS possess a good local bioavailability with less systemic absorption. Fluticasone furoate has the highest local bioavailability.

Side effects: Nasal burning, stinging, dryness of the nose, throat irritation, and epistaxis.

Epistaxis may be related to drying and thinning of the nasal mucosa (4–8% in 2–12 weeks)

These side effects can usually be prevented by aiming the spray slightly away from the nasal septum.

INTRANASAL ANTIHISTAMINES

Azelastine and olopatadine are the two intranasal antihistamines available out of which azelastine is frequently available in combination with InCS. This combination can be tried when InCS alone is not effective.

Combination InCS and intranasal antihistamines (InAH) sprays are also superior to oral antihistamines used along with intranasal nasal steroids.

The combination has a greater efficacy than using either of the drugs alone. They have a very rapid onset of action, within 15–20 minutes of administration and can be used whenever the symptoms are severe or on demand.

It is recommended to use intranasal azelastine only in children >6 years in children. Olopatadine nasal spray is not available in our country.

Side effects: Azelastine has a bitter taste and can cause dryness of the nasal mucosa. Hence, it should not be used for a long time.

Anticholinergics: This group of drugs is useful when rhinorrhea is the predominant symptom. However, it is not effective in controlling the other symptoms of AR. Gustatory rhinorrhea and rhinorrhea due to cold exposure are the other indications for using anticholinergics.

Cromolyn sodium: It is a mast cell stabilizer which can be used before the onset of symptoms. The efficacy is inferior to both oral and InCS. It helps to relieve sneezing but is ineffective for nasal congestion. The recommended dose is four to six times a day, which may result in poor compliance. However, the safety profile of this drug is good in children and pregnant women.

Decongestants: They relieve nasal congestion very rapidly but do not alleviate the other symptoms of AR. This group should be used only if there is a severe nose block for a short duration.

Side effects include a burning sensation, stinging, or dryness in the nasal passages. There is a possible risk of rhinitis medicamentosa on prolonged use for >7 days.

The various drugs available to treat AR and their effect on the symptoms is summarized in **Table 5**.

SUPPORTIVE

Saline nasal irrigation: Research has shown that saline nasal irrigation improves symptoms,

TABLE 5: Effects of various pharmacological agents on symptoms of rhinitis.

Drug	*Sneezing*	*Itching*	*Congestion*	*Rhinorrhea*	*Eye*
OAH	++	+++	+/–	++	++
InAH	++	++	+	++	–
InCS	+++	+++	+++	+++	++
LTRA	+	+	++	+	+
Nasal decongestant	–	–	++++	–	–
Oral decongestant	–	–	+	–	–
Intranasal anticholinergics	–	–	–	++	–
Mast cell stabilizer nasal	+	+	+	+	–

(InAH: intranasal antihistamines; InCS: intranasal corticosteroids; LTRA: leukotriene receptor antagonists; OAH: oral antihistaminics)

reduces the requirement of medications in patients with AR. It aids in maintaining the nasal moisture and clearing the nasal mucus. It is an easy, low-cost option without any potential adverse effects. It can enhance the effectiveness of InCS. Commercially available preparations or boiled and cooled tap water can be used. It is safe for use in children >2 years. Devices such as neti pots or squeeze bottles should be used and regularly cleaned to maintain hygiene. Appropriate technique should be followed to minimize discomfort and ensure effectiveness.

DISEASE-MODIFYING THERAPY

Allergen immunotherapy is the only disease-modifying therapy in AR. It prevents the progression of the illness and sensitization to newer allergens. The duration of the therapy is 3–5 years. The benefits of the therapy persist even after discontinuation.

Indications:

- Severe disease
- Non-responsive to medications
- Inability to follow avoidance measures. Patients who do not wish to take long-term controller medicines.
- Patients with other allergies

Environmental control measures: Refer to Chapter 12 of hand book.

Approach to a patient with AR: ARIA guidelines 2019 recommend a systematic approach to a patient with AR based on visual analog score (VAS) **(Fig. 2 and Flowchart 2)**.

Monitoring the response to treatment: The response to therapy can be monitored using the VAS and algorithms in **(Flowcharts 3 and 4)** can be used to step up and step down the treatment. ARIA recommends the use of health applications on smartphones to develop and validate information

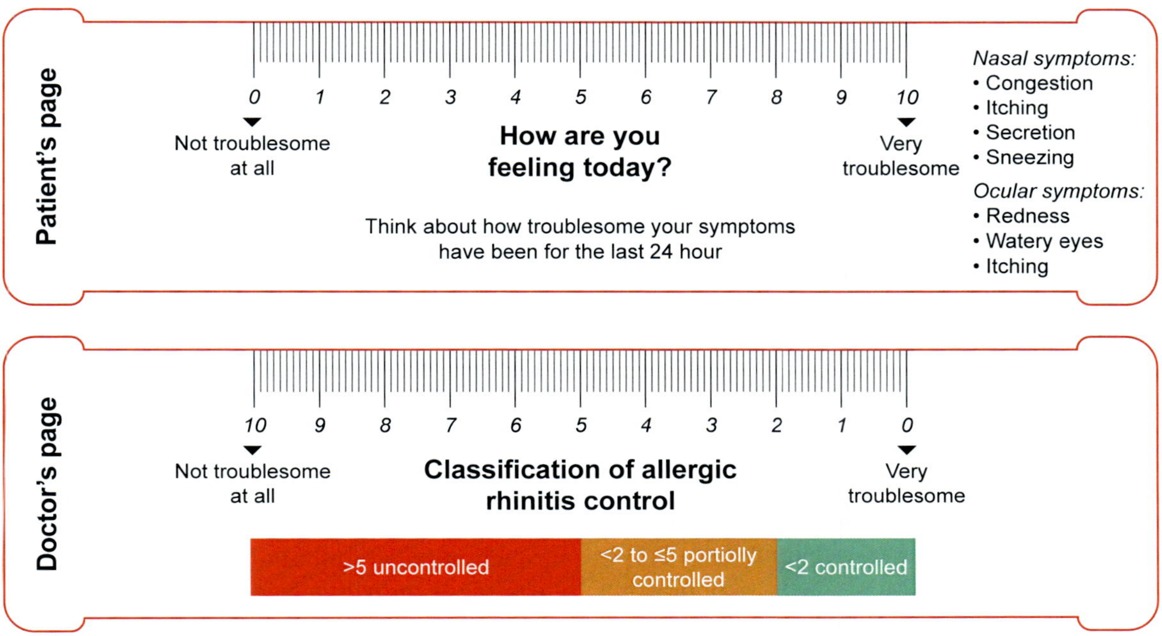

Fig. 2: Visual analog score.

Flowchart 2: Approach to a patient with allergic rhinitis (AR).

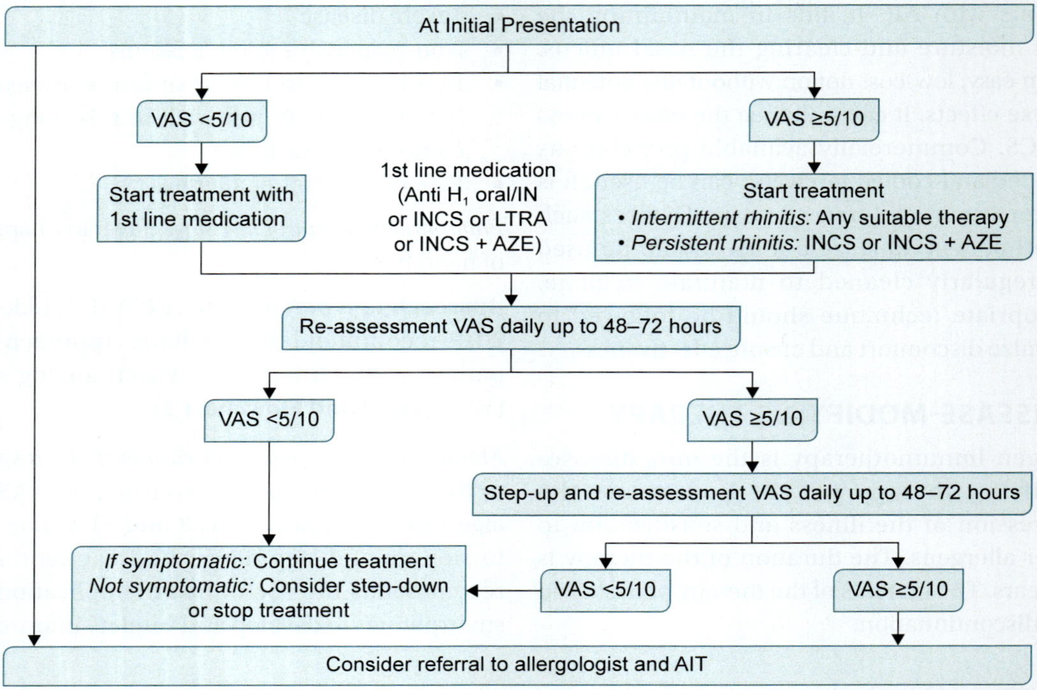

(AIT: allergen immunotherapy; AZE: azelastine; INCS: intranasal corticosteroids; LTRA: leukotriene receptor antagonists; VAS: visual analog score)
Source: ARIA guidelines 2019.

technology tools that strengthen self-medication management for AR patients and facilitate shared decision-making with healthcare professionals.

Mobile Airways Sentinel Network (MASK) stands as the most influential AR mHealth tool. The Control of Allergic Rhinitis/Asthma Test (CARAT) is also a powerful questionnaire-based tool for screening AR diagnosis and assessing disease control.

SUMMARY

This chapter provides an in-depth overview of the clinical approach to diagnosing and managing *AR*, a common IgE-mediated inflammatory disease affecting children and adolescents. Emphasizing AR's systemic impact as part of "united airway disease", the chapter explores the burden of symptoms such as sneezing, nasal congestion, itching, rhinorrhea, and their detrimental effect on sleep, cognition, and QoL. It outlines the ARIA classification system and discusses key differentials such as non-allergic rhinitis and local allergic rhinitis. A comprehensive section covers both diagnostic evaluation—including history-taking and allergy testing—and the stepwise pharmacologic management with oral antihistamines, leukotriene receptor antagonists, intranasal corticosteroids, decongestants, and other topical therapies. Emphasis is also placed on patient education, environmental control, nasal irrigation, and disease-modifying treatment through allergen immunotherapy. The chapter encourages individualized care and highlights when referral to an allergist is warranted for optimal control and improved outcomes.

Flowchart 3: Approach to a patient with allergic rhinitis using the visual analog score (VAS).

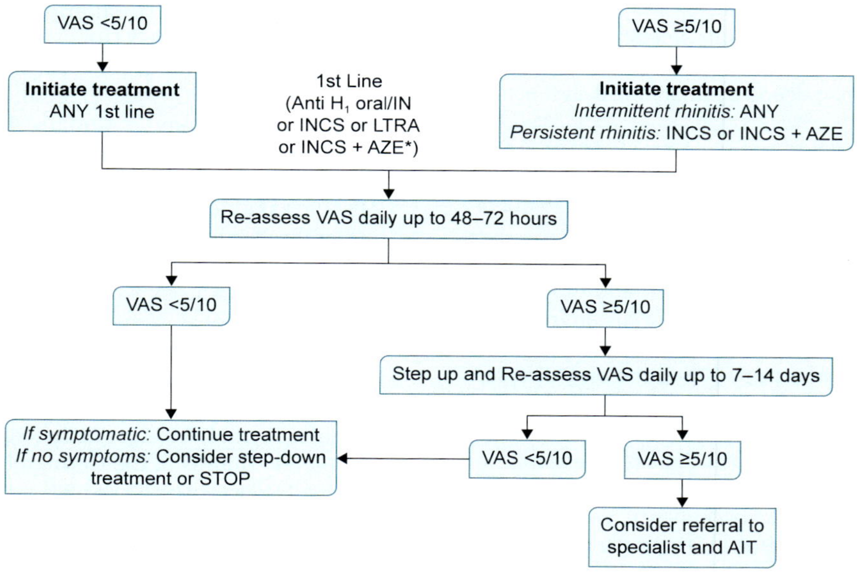

(AIT: allergen immunotherapy; AZE: azelastine; VAS: visual analog score)
Source: Abdul Latiff AH, Husain S, Abdullah B, Suppiah P, Tan V, Ing Ping T, et al. ARIA Care Pathways 2019: Next-Generation Allergic Rhinitis Care and Allergen Immunotherapy in Malaysia. J Pers Med. 2023;13(5):835.

Flowchart 4: Assessment of control in treated symptomatic patient.

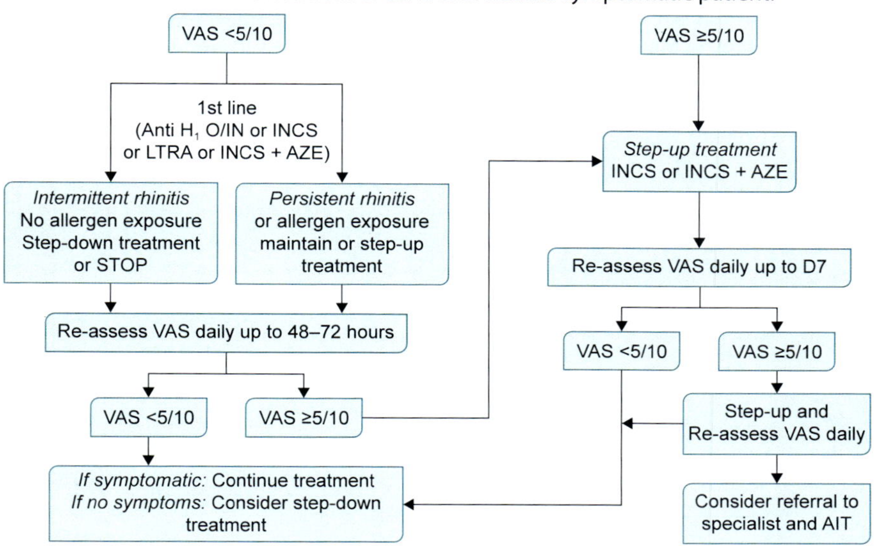

(AIT: allergen immunotherapy; AZE: azelastine; INCS: intranasal corticosteroids; LTRA: leukotriene receptor antagonists; VAS: visual analog score)
Source: Abdul Latiff AH, Husain S, Abdullah B, Suppiah P, Tan V, Ing Ping T, et al. ARIA Care Pathways 2019: Next-Generation Allergic Rhinitis Care and Allergen Immunotherapy in Malaysia. J Pers Med. 2023;13(5):835.

Key Learning Points

- *Allergic rhinitis is a systemic airway disorder*, often coexisting with asthma and conjunctivitis, significantly impairing sleep, cognition, and daily function in children.
- *Diagnosis is clinical*, based on detailed history and examination; skin prick testing and specific IgE assays help identify causative allergens to guide targeted management.
- *Intranasal corticosteroids are the cornerstone of therapy*, especially in persistent and moderate-to-severe cases, superior to antihistamines and leukotriene antagonists in symptom control.
- *Allergen immunotherapy (AIT)* is the only disease-modifying treatment option for AR, especially beneficial for severe, medication-unresponsive cases and those at risk of asthma progression.
- *Nasal irrigation, allergen avoidance, and correct technique with nasal sprays* enhance symptom relief and treatment adherence, especially in pediatric populations.

SUGGESTED READING

1. Abdul Latiff AH, Husain S, Abdullah B, Suppiah P, Tan V, Ing Ping T, et al. ARIA Care Pathways 2019: Next-Generation Allergic Rhinitis Care and Allergen Immunotherapy in Malaysia. J Pers Med. 2023;13(5):835.
2. Cheng M, Dai Q, Liu Z, Wang Y, Zhou C. New progress in pediatric allergic rhinitis. Front Immunol. 2024;15:1452410.
3. Dykewicz MS, Wallace DV, Amrol DJ, Baroody FM, Bernstein JA, Craig TJ, et al. Rhinitis 2020: A practice parameter update. J Allergy Clin Immunol. 2020;146(4):721-67.
4. Goniotakis I, Perikleous E, Fouzas S, Steiropoulos P, Paraskakis E. A Clinical Approach to Allergic Rhinitis in Children. Children (Basel). 2023;10(9):1571.
5. Hellings PW, Klimek L, Cingi C, Agache I, Akdis C, Bachert C, et al. Non-allergic rhinitis: Position paper of the European Academy of Allergy and Clinical Immunology. Allergy. 2017;72:1657-65.
6. Klimek L, Bachert C, Pfaar O, Becker S, Bieber T, Brehler R, et al. ARIA guideline 2019: treatment of allergic rhinitis in the German health system. Allergol Select. 2019;3(1):22-50.
7. Papadopoulos NG, Aggelides X, Stamataki S, Prokopakis E, Katotomichelakis M, Xepapadaki P. New concepts in pediatric rhinitis. Pediatr Allergy Immunol. 2021;32(4):635-46.
8. Rosenfield L, Keith PK, Quirt J, Small P, Ellis AK. Allergic rhinitis. Allergy Asthma Clin Immunol. 2024;20(Suppl 3):74.
9. Wise SK, Damask C, Roland LT, Ebert C, Levy JM, Lin S, et al. International Consensus Statement on Allergy and Rhinology: Allergic rhinitis–2023. Int Forum Allergy Rhinol. 2023;13:293-859.

CHAPTER

9

Food Allergies and Anaphylaxis

Sowmya Arudi Nagarajan, Rachna Mehta Shroff
Reviewer: *Mahesh PA*

INTRODUCTION

An immunological response to proteins in food that the immune system interprets as posing a risk to oneself, but which are generally safe for most people is known as a food allergy. It can be immunoglobulin (Ig)E-mediated or non-IgE-mediated. Food allergy affects populations around the world, which affects the quality of life and contributes to significant healthcare costs both to the patient and the healthcare system. Allergic food reactions contribute to a constellation of symptoms involving multi organ systems not limited to skin, gastrointestinal tract, and respiratory tract.

Food allergies represent a serious public health concern worldwide, including India, where unique cultural dietary habits and potential cross-reactivity of allergens present distinct challenges. Particularly pressing is the diagnosis and management of food allergies and associated anaphylaxis, alongside ensuring effective emergency protocols. Regulatory measures, such as food labeling laws, are pivotal in safeguarding consumers against hidden allergens in processed foods.

PREVALENCE OF FOOD ALLERGIES IN INDIA

With a population of around 1.4 billion, India accounts for 20% of the world's population.

Food sensitization is found in approximately 30% adults and about 20% children in India. Sensitization is most commonly found for shrimp, eggplant, banana, rice, and chickpea in India. Clinical food allergy appears to be not common in India, but many states lack prevalence studies.

A cross-sectional questionnaire study was conducted in New Delhi from 2022–2023 in 6–14 years school children found prevalence of parent-reported food allergy was 0.8% with overall prevalence of food allergy being low.

Chickpea, cabbage, eggplant, walnut, cumin, and betel leaf were the most commonly reported trigger foods in a prevalence survey done in Hyderabad, India.

CHALLENGES OF FOOD ALLERGIES IN INDIA

India's rich tapestry of culinary traditions encompasses a wide array of foods, including nuts, legumes, and diverse grains, some of which can trigger allergic reactions. Diagnosing food allergies is complicated by limited access to advanced diagnostic allergen testing facilities and affordability for most of the population. Moreover, cultural dietary habits often intertwine with food preparation, leading to cross-contamination risks. The phenomenon of cross-reactivity, where proteins in different foods or pollen can trigger similar allergic responses, adds further complexity to accurate diagnosis.

In India, some prevalent food allergens include dairy products, peanuts, tree nuts (such as cashew nuts and almonds), legumes (like chickpeas and lentils), sesame seeds, wheat, and soy. Seafood allergies, particularly to shellfish such as prawns and crabs, are also common.

Spices, fundamental to Indian cuisine, can also trigger allergic reactions, although spice allergies are relatively less common.

A significant barrier is the lack of awareness among both healthcare providers and the general population, leading to under-diagnosis and misdiagnosis. The actual prevalence of food allergies is less than the perceived food allergies in the Indian population. Cultural practices and dietary habits mean that allergens are often pervasive in everyday meals, making avoidance difficult. Additionally, labeling of packaged foods is not always comprehensive, with potential cross-contamination in processing facilities posing a hidden risk.

Furthermore, the social stigma associated with allergies can lead to a lack of understanding and empathy, especially in communal eating settings prevalent in Indian culture. There is also a scarcity of allergen-free foods in local markets, limiting options for individuals with food allergies.

Egg, milk, fish, shellfish, peanut, wheat, soyabean, and tree nut are the most common foods causing allergenic reactions reported globally. Self-reported adverse reaction to foods in adults in India was higher compared to other low- and middle-income countries mainly to wheat (11.9%) and peanut (2.2%). There was observed higher self-reported adverse reactions to fish (11%), milk (3.5%), egg (2.2%), tree nut (1.6%), and soybean (0.9%) in Vietnam. The highest self-reported adverse reaction to shellfish (24.4%) was observed in China.

In children, the highest prevalence of food sensitization (SPT) was in South Africa for the most common foods of global relevance except for shellfish which was most common in China. In India, wheat and soyabean had higher sensitization rates than other foods on SPT. In Indian children, higher IgE-mediated food sensitization to peanuts (6.3%), wheat (6.7%), soybean (5.4%), and tree nut (4.2%) was observed, while in Hong Kong, China, a higher prevalence of IgE-mediated food sensitization to eggs (5.4%) and milk (6.7%) was observed. The highest prevalence of sensitization to shellfish was seen in Shaoguan, China (13.1%) followed by India (10.3%).

DIAGNOSIS OF FOOD ALLERGIES IN INDIA

Diagnosing food allergies involves a combination of detailed medical history, physical examination, and specific tests such as the skin prick test and serum-specific IgE tests. However, these tests may not always be accessible in all parts of the country due to limited availability of allergy specialists and facilities. Some healthcare providers may resort to elimination diets to identify specific allergens, but this can be time-consuming and requires careful monitoring.

Food allergens can vary by region due to diverse dietary patterns and cultural practices across India:

- *North India:*
  - Lentils and pulses
- *South India:*
  - Coconut, found in curries, chutneys, and sweets
- *East India:*
  - Fish, especially in West Bengal and Odisha, and sesame
- *West India:*
  - Besan (chickpea flour)

Each region has its unique dietary features and allergens, making it important for individuals with food sensitivities to be aware of regional ingredients.

Genetic factors are also connected to the development of food allergies. An in-depth analysis of the most recent findings in the genetics of food allergy by Kanchan et al. revealed several genetic loci, genes, and variations that continue to support the significance of barrier and immune function genes in the development of food allergy. MALT1, FLG, and HLA have been shown to have the most significant influence on food allergy.

The lack of vitamin D has been identified as one of the potential risk factors for the development of food allergy because of its immunoregulatory properties.

According to Gideon Lack's "dual allergen exposure theory", the skin's compromised epithelial barrier facilitates the ability of allergens to sensitize the immune system and the development of IgE antibodies against it. In infants, a low dose of cutaneous exposure to a food allergen sensitizes the immune system, whereas oral exposure could potentially induce immunologic tolerance. Food allergy prevention recommendations now include adding specific foods such as peanuts to an infant's diet during their first year of life. Studies in India have shown a high prevalence of complementary feeding for infants starting between the ages of 6 and 8 months.

This, together with the high prevalence of fermented foods in traditional Indian diets, may protect against the development of food allergies. Applying oils to neonates' skin, such as mustard oil, sunflower oil, and coconut oil, is another common custom in India and whether this has the potential to explain the very low prevalence of atopic dermatitis seen in India is not clear. Further studies are needed on the effect of the daily application of these oils to the infant's skin on improving the skin barrier and the potential of reducing low-dose cutaneous exposure to food allergens needs to be explored.

The presence of early onset atopic dermatitis is an important risk factor for the development of primary food allergies. It is a component of the atopic march, in which the symptoms or illnesses develop in a certain order, beginning with the onset of atopic dermatitis, food allergies, then asthma and allergic rhinitis.

TESTING OF FOOD ALLERGIES

The diagnosis of food allergies is a multifaceted process involving a detailed clinical assessment, including history and physical examination—followed by allergy test to demonstrate IgE sensitization followed by second history and challenges if required.

Skin prick tests, which involve exposing the skin to small amounts of allergens and observing for reactions, are commonly used due to their simplicity and speed. Additionally, serum-specific IgE tests may be conducted to measure the levels of food-specific IgE antibodies in the blood, when SPT is not feasible.

Food allergens can generally be divided into heat-stable and heat-labile allergens. Heat-stable food allergens have molecular properties that confer conformational stability, such as disulfide bonds, protein glycation, and the ability to bind lipids. These properties can protect food allergens from degradation by heat, acid, and proteases, thereby enhancing uptake of intact protein in the gastrointestinal tract. In contrast, heat-labile allergens are highly sensitive to heat and acid. Sensitization to heat-labile allergens in plant-based foods is thought to result from exposure to homologous proteins in pollens, which leads to the development of pollen-food allergy syndrome.

When dealing with labile allergens, the prick-to-prick method is often preferred for SPTs. This involves using fresh, native food material (e.g., raw fruit or vegetable) instead of standardized extracts as standardized extracts may not always be available.

In certain cases, an oral food challenge may be deemed necessary, wherein the patient consumes increasing amounts of the suspected allergen under strict medical supervision to monitor any reactions. This gold-standard method provides precise confirmation of a food allergy, ensuring that both false positives and negatives from other tests are appropriately evaluated.

APPROACH TO A PATIENT WITH FOOD ALLERGY

To Identify the Symptoms of Food Allergy

Symptoms of Food Allergies

The symptoms of food allergies depicted in **Flowchart 1**.

To Recognize Whether it is Immunoglobulin E-mediated or Non-immunoglobulin-mediated Food Allergy

The immunoglobulin E vs. non-IgE-mediated food allergy depicted in **Table 1**.

Algorithm for Immunoglobulin E-mediated Food Allergy

The algorithm for immunoglobulin E-mediated food allergy depicted in **Flowchart 2**.

Algorithm for Nonimmunoglobulin E-mediated Food Allergy

The algorithm for non-immunoglobulin E-mediated food allergy depicted in **Flowchart 3**.

How do we Decide Between Choosing Skin Prick Test Versus Serum Specific Immunoglobulin E

The skin prick test vs. serum specific immunoglobulin E depicted in **Table 2**.

Spectrum of Food Allergy

The spectrum of food allergy depicted in **Figure 1**.

Food Allergies and Anaphylaxis

Anaphylaxis is a systemic life-threatening reaction that requires immediate medical attention. Symptoms are mentioned in the given chart. It is critical for individuals with known food allergies to carry emergency medication such as epinephrine, and to seek medical assistance immediately

Flowchart 1: Symptoms of food allergy.

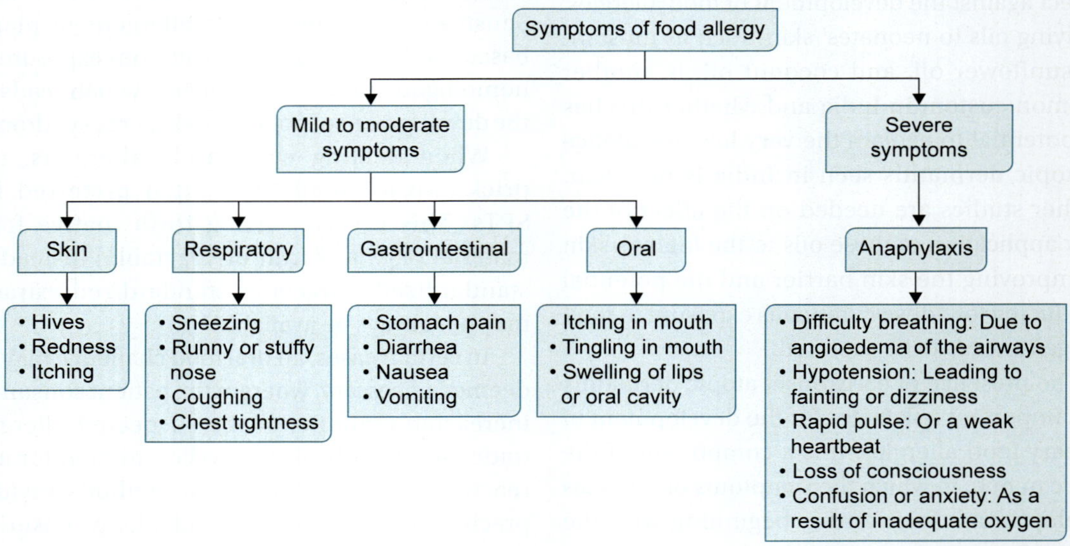

TABLE 1: Immunoglobulin E (IgE) vs. non-IgE-mediated food allergy.

	IgE mediated	*Non-IgE-mediated*
Onset of symptoms	Within seconds to minutes	Within hours to days
Severity	Can proceed to anaphylaxis rapidly	Variable, usually not life threatening
Pathogenesis	Type 1 hypersensitivity	Type 3 or 4 hypersensitivity
Most commonly systems involved	Skin, respiratory	Gastrointestinal
Symptoms	Skin—rash, pruritus, flushing Respiratory—runny nose, sneezing, chest tightness, and wheeze *Oral:* Tingling or itching in mouth, swelling on lips, oral cavity or face, *GI:* Nausea, vomiting, diarrhea, and abdominal cramps	Nausea, vomiting, diarrhea, and abdominal cramps
Examples:	Peanut, milk, and eggs	Food protein-induced enteropathy

Flowchart 2: Algorithm for immunoglobulin E (IgE)-mediated food allergy.

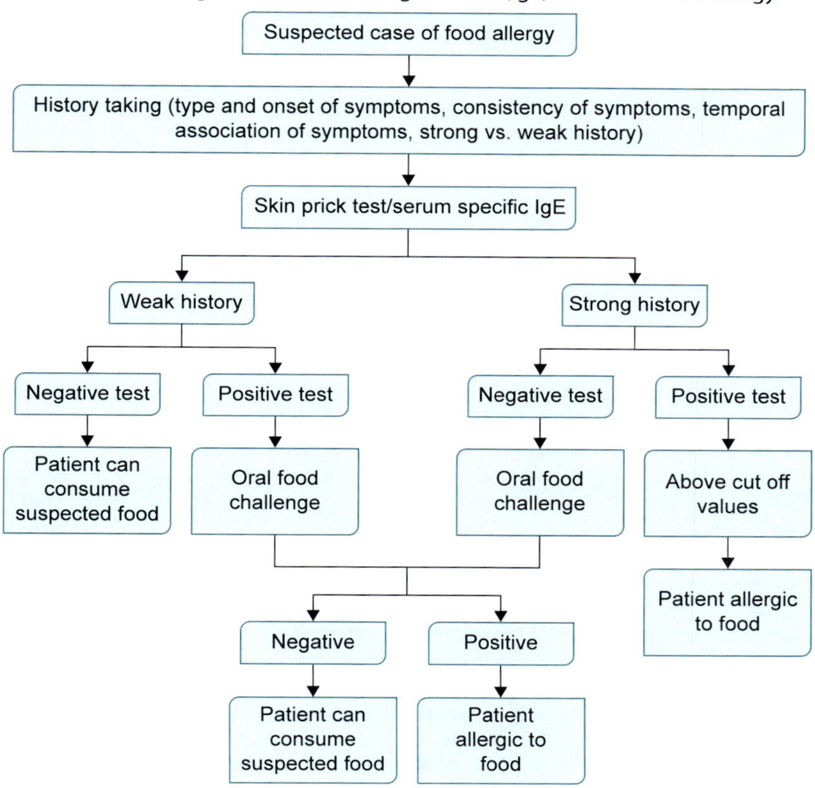

if they or someone else experiences symptoms of anaphylaxis.

In India, many remain unaware of anaphylaxis symptoms and the critical need for rapid intervention. Misdiagnosis or delayed diagnosis is all too common due to a lack of standardized protocols.

Flowchart 3: Algorithm for non-immunoglobulin E (IgE)-mediated food allergy.

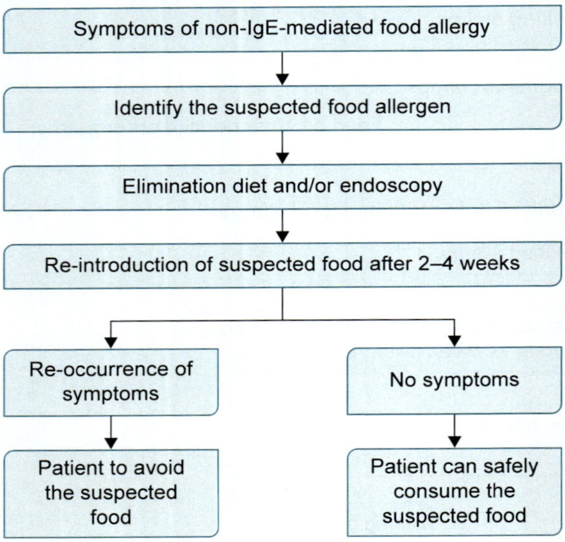

The WAO (World Allergy Organization) criteria for likelihood of anaphylaxis are followed when any one out of the following is fulfilled:

TABLE 2: Skin prick test vs. serum specific immunoglobulin E (IgE).

Skin prick test	*Serum-specific IgE*
Bound IgE	Circulatory IgE
First line of investigation	Can be considered when skin prick test is not a feasible option
Requires expertise	Does not require expertise
Needs to be off antihistamines for 5–7 days prior to testing	Not influenced by medication
Cost effective	Price varies
Concern of allergen quantity	Quality control is possible
Cannot be performed in eczema and other skin conditions	Can be performed in all skin conditions
Results within 30 minutes	Varies
Higher sensitivity	Higher specificity
Difficult to do in kids	Less difficult in kids
Severe allergic reaction chances in few cases	No severe allergic reactions

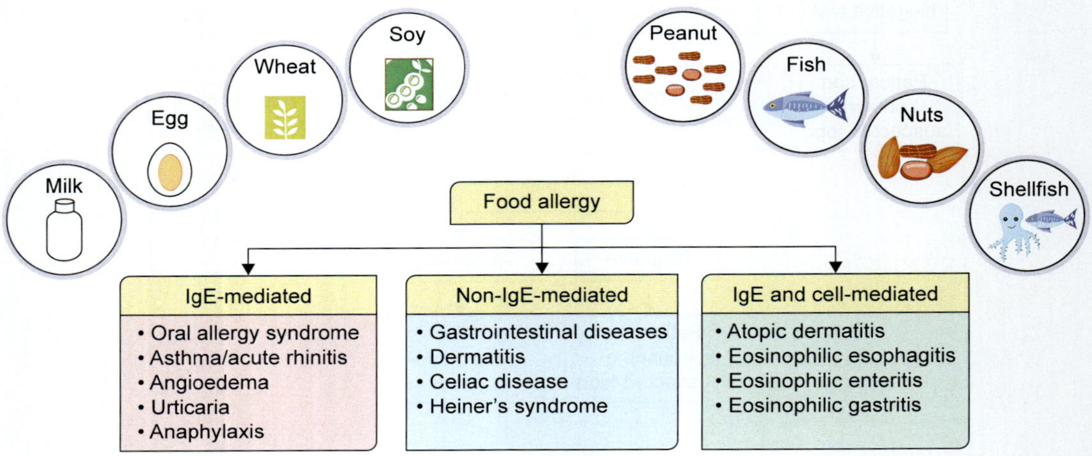

Fig. 1: Spectrum of food allergy.

Criteria 1:
Acute onset of an illness (minutes to several hours) with simultaneous involvement of the skin, mucosal tissue, or both (e.g., generalized hives, pruritus or flushing, swollen lips-tongue-uvula)

And at least one of the following:
- Respiratory compromise (e.g., dyspnea, wheeze-bronchospasm, stridor, reduced PEF, hypoxemia)
- Reduced BP or associated symptoms of end-organ dysfunction [e.g., hypotonia (collapse), syncope, and incontinence]
- Severe gastrointestinal symptoms (e.g., severe crampy abdominal pain, repetitive vomiting), especially after exposure to non-food allergens

Criteria 2:
Acute onset of hypotension or bronchospasm or laryngeal involvement after exposure to a known or highly probable allergy end for that patient (minutes to several hours), even in the absence of typical skin involvement.

Prompt administration of epinephrine is essential for treating anaphylaxis. However, awareness about epinephrine uses and accessibility is low among the Indian population. Epinephrine auto-injectors are expensive, making them unaffordable to many, while rural areas face severe shortages.

Patient education is critical. Health practitioners must prioritize educating patients on recognizing early signs of anaphylaxis and administering epinephrine. Patients should be equipped with anaphylaxis action plans, ensuring they and their caregivers understand the importance of immediate medical intervention. Regulatory touchpoints, such as food labeling laws, need enhancement to prevent exposure to hidden allergens in processed foods, thereby reducing the incidence of allergic reactions.

INDICATIONS FOR PRESCRIBING EPINEPHRINE AUTO-INJECTION IN IMMUNOGLOBULIN E-MEDIATED FOOD ALLERGIES

These indications are also similar to cases where there are chances of developing severe symptoms due to food allergy **(Table 3)**.

An anaphylaxis action plan can be given to the patient and the caregiver after an episode of anaphylaxis to understand how to identify and treat anaphylaxis in future.

FOOD DEPENDENT EXERCISE-INDUCED ANAPHYLAXIS

Food-dependent exercise-induced anaphylaxis (FDEIA) is a unique and rare medical condition where an allergic reaction, potentially life-threatening, is triggered by the combination of consuming specific foods and subsequent physical exercise. Unlike typical food allergies, where consuming an allergenic food alone can provoke symptoms, individuals with FDEIA tolerate these foods unless they engage in physical activity shortly after eating. Age at the onset of FDEIA can vary, and they sometimes begin in childhood and adolescence, but onset most commonly occurs during adulthood.

Common food triggers: These include wheat, shellfish, and certain fruits, though this can vary

TABLE 3: Absolute and relative indications for prescribing epinephrine auto-injection in immunoglobulin E (IgE)-mediated food allergies.

Absolute indications	*Relative indications*
Previous episodes of food induced anaphylaxis	Foods likely to cause allergic reactions and to be associated with anaphylaxis
Co-existing severe asthma	Allergic reaction to trace amount of foods
Underlying systemic mastocytosis	Remote from medical help

Flowchart 4: Approach to a patient with food-dependent exercise-induced anaphylaxis (FDEIA).

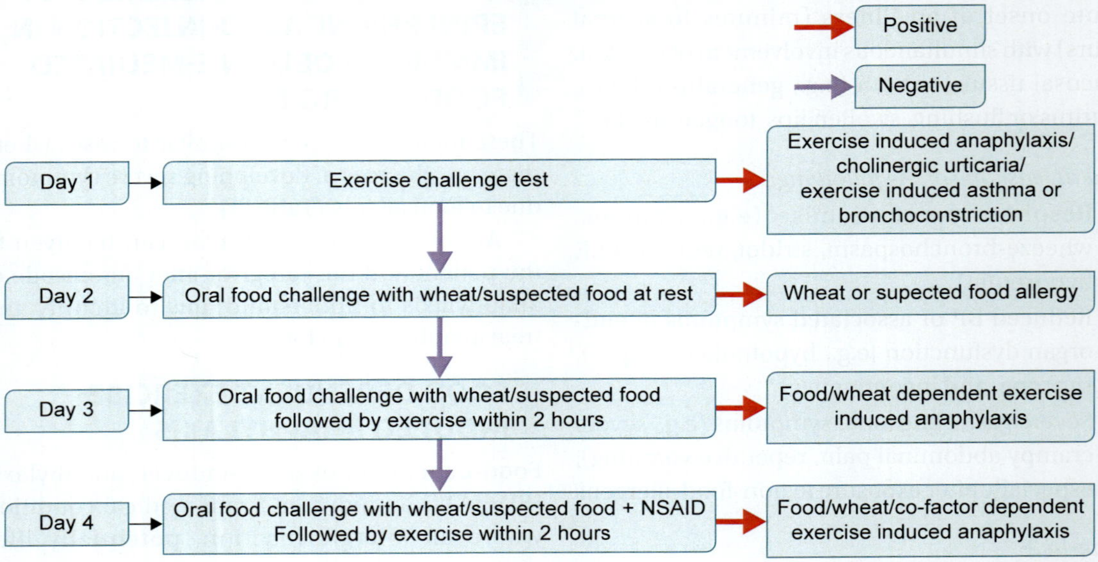

among individuals. In the Indian context, we get rice, lentils, and chickpea as the possible triggers also on rare occasions.

Co-factors: These can exacerbate or trigger episodes of FDEIA and include exercise most commonly, non-steroidal anti-inflammatory drugs (NSAIDs), alcohol, and certain climatic conditions such as high humidity or temperature. Stress and hormonal fluctuations, such as those observed in women during menstruation, can also play a role. These factors can modify immune system outcomes or enhance food absorption increasing the possibility of an anaphylaxis episode. The pathophysiology of FDEIA includes the effects of exercise altering intestinal permeability and blood flow, thereby enhancing the absorption of allergenic proteins into the bloodstream, which then triggers an immune response.

Management of FDEIA primarily involves avoiding identified food triggers, especially before physical activity, and being cautious about co-factors known to exacerbate symptoms. For those diagnosed, carrying emergency medication such as epinephrine is recommended to manage unexpected reactions **(Flowchart 4)**.

ROLE OF COMPONENT RESOLVED DIAGNOSTICS IN FOOD ALLERGY

Using naturally pure or recombinantly generated allergens coated on a solid surface, component-resolved diagnostics (CRD) technology detects specific immunoglobulin E (sIgE) antibodies against the coated components in addition to the patient sample. It helps us to get a detailed evaluation of allergic sensitization of an individual by recognition of specific components which may be clinically relevant to the patient.

Healthcare providers can learn more about the specific allergens causing a patient's allergic reactions by employing CRD. Better diagnosis, enhanced risk assessment, and customized treatment plans are made possible by this information, which improves the management of allergic illnesses.

Indications of Component Resolved Diagnostics in Food Allergy

- Understanding the risk of an allergic reaction
- Initiation of oral immunotherapy in patients with persistent food allergies
- Understanding the cross reactivity between different groups of foods to differentiate primary food allergy
- Predict probability of persistence/outgrow of food allergy

ORAL FOOD CHALLENGE TEST

Oral food challenge (OFC) tests are used to diagnose both IgE-mediated and non-IgE-mediated food allergies. It is used to diagnose, resolve a food allergy, or determine the threshold of reactivity in applicants considering oral immunotherapy (OIT).

Oral food challenge allows for the consumption of the suspected food in a controlled environment, which requires supervision by healthcare experts specialized in conducting oral food challenges.

Indications

- When diagnosing food allergies, OFC can be used to confirm or rule out both IgE-mediated and non-IgE-mediated reactions.
- To know whether tolerability for an allergenic food
- Identification of the threshold of responsiveness in patients with persistent food allergies when undergoing a baseline food challenge
- To test a cross-reactive meal that has never been added to the diet or to test a specific food in sensitized individuals who have never consumed it.

Contraindications

- The oral food challenge should not be administered to children who have experienced recent anaphylaxis or who have measurable levels of IgE specific to a suspected food that are >95% positive predictive value (PPV) of a positive challenge.
- Patients with underlying asthma which is not controlled.

ROLE OF IMMUNOTHERAPY IN FOOD ALLERGY

Immunotherapy is a treatment for IgE-mediated food allergies that involves gradually increasing food dosages to cause desensitization and prevent anaphylaxis in the event of an unintentional exposure.

In allergen immunotherapy for food allergies, three current approaches have been employed—oral, sublingual, and epicutaneous **(Table 4)**.

Types of Immunotherapies for Food

ORAL IMMUNOTHERAPY

In OIT, an allergic individual is given an incremental amount of an allergenic food with the intention of increasing the threshold that triggers a reaction. OIT is the therapeutic approach with the largest body of evidence in clinical trials for food allergy to date. The major hurdle in the success of these studies has been sustained responsiveness which is short-lived.

Despite successfully causing desensitization, high-certainty evidence indicates that available peanut oral immunotherapy regimens significantly increase allergic and anaphylactic responses in patients with peanut allergies when compared to avoidance or placebo. Although further long-term investigation of safety, efficacy, tolerability, and patient-prioritized outcomes is needed, these studies highlight the efficacy of OIT induction of desensitization and treatment-specific immunomodulation.

Although allergy to milk and egg are commonly outgrown by the age of 5–10 years, allergies to

TABLE 4: Comparison of allergen-targeted immunotherapies in clinical trials.

Comparison factors	*OIT*	*SLIT*	*EPIT*
Allergens	Single allergen: Milk, egg, peanut (others: wheat, tree nuts, and fish) Multiallergen	Peanut, milk, hazelnut, and peach	Milk and peanut
Daily maintenance dose	300–4,000 mg	1–10 mg	50–500 µg
Primary side effects	Oral, gastrointestinal (systemic symptoms associated with infection, exercise, and menses)	Oropharyngeal	Skin
Desensitization	Significant effect	Moderate effect	Moderate effect
Sustained unresponsiveness	Effective in subset of patients	Ongoing investigation	Ongoing investigation
Immune modulation	Significant	Present	Present

(EPIT: epicutaneous-immunotherapy; OIT: oral immunotherapy; SLIT: sublingual immunotherapy)

peanut and tree nuts are often lifelong, persisting into adulthood in 80% of cases.

A number of studies and meta-analyses have shown that OIT treatment is effective in raising the threshold of reactivity to peanuts and other foods in addition to producing a measurable serum immune response to such therapy.

In the PALISADE study, patients exposed to peanut protein were able to tolerate relatively small doses of peanut protein (300 mg or roughly one peanut) on a daily basis as a maintenance dose. Increasing the reactivity threshold from 100 mg or less of peanut protein to at least 300 mg reduces the reaction risk to four common food product categories that may contain trace levels of peanut residue by >95%. Further increase in the threshold to 1,000 mg peanut protein has additional quantitative benefit in risk reduction.

Not only are patients able to tolerate maintenance doses of 300–4,000 mg of peanut protein, but they also have been shown to tolerate doses higher than the maintenance dose, as high as 5,000 mg, equivalent to about 16–20 peanuts, or over a tablespoon of peanut butter, after undergoing up-dosing phases of peanut OIT. This has been evidenced by the success rates of patients in what is often the final phase of clinical trials, a double-blind, placebo-controlled, food challenge by Varshney P.

In the Blumchen et al. study, after maintaining peanut OIT with 125 mg of peanut protein, they found that 41.9% of patients tolerated the highest dose of peanut protein offered (4,500 mg) compared to only 3.2% in the placebo group. This ability to tolerate such high doses is particularly noteworthy given that some patients might desire to consume peanut products in larger quantities, particularly if they have not developed the fear associated with food allergies (i.e., toddlers who have undergone desensitization), while others may just wish for protection from accidental ingestion.

Omalizumab treatment has been approved recently for the management of severe multiple food allergies. Many trials have documented the importance of safety of ingestion of baked egg or milk products in IgE-mediated allergy, in an effort to induce tolerance early—mainly by change in conformational epitopes by heating or baking.

Oral Food Pollen Syndrome

Oral allergy syndrome (OAS) or pollen-food allergy syndrome (PFS/PFAS) is a hypersensitivity reaction to specific foods due to prior sensitization to plant inhalant allergens. Oral allergy syndrome is triggered by a cross-reaction between allergens in pollen and allergens in fresh fruits and vegetables. Oral allergy syndrome is distinct from simple food allergies. In food allergies, a reaction develops after direct sensitization to food proteins rather than cross-reactivity between food proteins and inhalant allergens. Approximately 20–70% of patients sensitized to pollen allergens experience OAS symptoms after eating raw fruits, vegetables, nuts, or certain spices. The incidence of sensitization to plant foods is highest in those with birch pollen allergy.

Symptoms of OAS present within a few minutes of ingestion to the offending fruits or vegetables sometimes lasting a few hours also. Symptoms are limited to the oropharynx and are generally mild and transient. The most common symptom is oral-pharyngeal pruritus, especially of the lips and the palate region; although rarely, there may also be oral and perioral angioedema. Patients typically describe itching or tingling in the lips or mouth, oral burning and swelling, or throat tightness after ingestion of fresh fruits or vegetables. The diagnosis of OAS relies on a history of oropharyngeal symptoms associated with ingestion of specific raw fruits or vegetables and pollen-associated allergies. Avoidance of known food triggers is generally the primary treatment for OAS **(Flowchart 5)**.

Flowchart 5: Approach to a patient with oral allergy syndrome (OAS) or pollen-food allergy syndrome (PFS/PFAS).

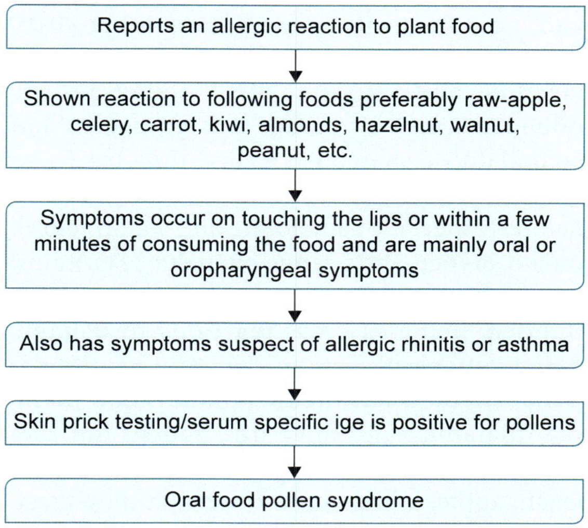

Mugwort and Pollen-Food Allergy Syndrome

Mugwort (*Artemisia vulgaris*) is a common weed in the *Asteraceae* family and a prominent aeroallergen in temperate regions. It is strongly implicated in PFAS, particularly due to cross-reactive plant pan-allergens such as profilins, lipid transfer proteins (LTPs), and pathogenesis-related proteins (e.g., PR-10). One well-characterized variant is the mugwort-spice syndrome, where individuals sensitized to mugwort pollen experience oral allergy symptoms (e.g., itching, tingling, or swelling of the lips, mouth, and throat) upon consuming certain spices. The most common cross-reactive foods include spices such as celery, fennel, coriander, cumin, parsley, paprika, anise, and mustard, due to shared allergenic proteins. Additionally, mugwort cross-reactivity extends to several other foods, notably carrots, apples, peaches, mangoes, nuts (especially hazelnuts), sunflower seeds, and lettuce. The severity of reactions can vary from mild oral symptoms to systemic reactions, particularly with LTP-mediated pathways.

Other Pollen-Food Cross-Reactivity Syndromes

Pollen-food allergy syndrome is not limited to mugwort and encompasses several other well-defined pollen-food syndromes. Birch pollen-related PFAS is the most common in northern Europe and North America, associated with cross-reactivity to foods containing PR-10 proteins such as apple, pear, cherry, carrot, celery, hazelnut, and soybean. Birch pollen-allergic individuals may also react to kiwi, peach, and almond due to shared Bet v 1-like proteins. Grass pollen-associated PFAS involves foods such as melons (especially cantaloupe and watermelon), tomato, orange, and peanut, often due to profilins. Ragweed-related PFAS, more common in North America, includes cross-reactions to banana, melon, zucchini, cucumber, and sunflower seeds. In Mediterranean populations, plane tree (platanus) and olive tree pollens are also significant contributors, linked with reactions to peach, apple, and peanut. Understanding these pollen-food relationships is critical for diagnosis and dietary counseling in allergic individuals.

Alpha-Gal Syndrome

The hypersensitivity to galactose-alpha-1,3-galactose (alpha-gal), a carbohydrate, present in all non-primate mammalian tissues, caused by immunoglobulin E (IgE) is known as alpha-gal syndrome. People become sensitive to alpha-gal in tick saliva after being bitten by a tick. The first onset typically occurs in maturity, following years of consuming mammalian meat. Although anaphylaxis is also common, the majority of patients experience gastrointestinal and/or cutaneous symptoms, such as itching, urticaria, and angioedema. Mammalian meat products (beef, hog, and lamb) cause reactions that are 3–6 hours later and frequently happen at night, in contrast to other food allergies. Patients may occasionally be able to tolerate red meat because intraindividual variability results in uneven reactivity to an exposure. Because of this, the sickness is difficult to diagnose and may be confused with irritable bowel syndrome, recurrent spontaneous urticaria, or unexplained anaphylaxis.

MANAGEMENT OF FOOD ALLERGY

Immunoglobulin E-mediated food allergies have evolved from passive management, which relied on avoiding allergens, the "watch-wait approach", and keeping an eye out for potential spontaneous remission, to more aggressive management. This includes the introduction of allergenic foods as a preventative measure, tailored dietary recommendations (e.g., including baked goods for kids with sensitivities to milk, eggs, or soy), and particular immunomodulatory treatments including biologicals and allergen-specific immunotherapy.

It includes mainly the following:

- *Dietary management:*
  - To identify and eliminate the causative food
  - To advice for safer alternatives
  - Personalized diet plan
- *Treatment plan:*
  - To treat the current episode with pharmacotherapy
  - Giving an anaphylaxis action plan to the patient and training on how to use the adrenaline autoinjector
- *Immunomodulatory treatment:*
  - Allergen-specific immunotherapy
  - Biologicals

FOOD LABELING LAWS IN INDIA WITH RESPECT TO FOOD ALLERGY

In India, food labeling laws are governed under the Food Safety and Standards Authority of India (FSSAI), which mandates comprehensive labeling to ensure consumer safety and informed choices. According to FSSAI regulations, all pre-packaged food products must include crucial information on their labels, such as the product's name, list of ingredients, nutritional information, and the respective vegetarian or non-vegetarian symbol. The labels are also required to disclose the net quantity, manufacturer's name and address,

BOX 1: Common food labeling violations.

- Omission of allergen information: Failing to clearly label common allergens such as peanuts, tree nuts, milk, eggs, wheat, soy, fish, and shellfish
- Cross-contamination warnings: Not providing warnings about possible cross-contamination during processing, which is crucial for those with severe allergies
- Inaccurate allergen claims: Incorrectly labeling products as "allergen-free" or "safe for allergies" without adequate testing or validation
- Non-standardized allergen symbols: Using unclear or unrecognized symbols for allergens, making it difficult for consumers to quickly identify products that might pose a risk
- Misleading descriptions: Using terms such as "natural" or "pure" without clarifying potential allergen risks, misleading consumers into assuming safety without checking detailed ingredients
- Hidden ingredients: Listing allergens under unrecognizable names or as part of other ingredients, such as casein or whey for milk, which can confuse consumers

batch or lot number, date of manufacture, and the best-before or expiry date. Importantly, labeling must comply with prescribed languages and the format designed to ensure clarity and accessibility for consumers.

Additionally, FSSAI mandates specific labeling requirements for genetically modified foods, irradiated foods, and products containing artificial sweeteners or added flavors. The legislation also encompasses guidelines for health, nutrition, and risk-reduction claims, which must be substantiated with scientific evidence. Failure to comply with these rules can result in strict penalties, including fines and prohibitions on product sales. These regulations aim to protect public health, prevent deceptive practices, and promote transparency in the food industry, thereby fostering consumer trust and safety in the national marketplace.

In India, food labeling violations related to food allergies are particularly concerning due to the potential health risks for consumers with specific dietary needs. Some common violations **(Box 1)** include.

Proper and clear labeling is critical for ensuring safety and informed consumption for individuals with allergies.

SUMMARY

The management of food allergies in India faces unique challenges due to cultural dietary habits, cross-reactivity, and limited healthcare infrastructure. Effective diagnosis is often hamstrung by technological and geographical gaps, and emergency protocols require better patient education and regulatory oversight. Food labeling laws are essential to curb hidden allergens and protect consumer safety.

Key Learning Points

- Cultural dietary habits and cross-reactivity complicate food allergy diagnosis in India.
- Cross-reacting allergens add complexity to diagnosis, necessitating careful evaluation.
- Comprehensive emergency protocols and patient education are critical to managing anaphylaxis.
- Strengthened food labeling regulations are necessary to prevent exposure to hidden allergens.
- Enhancing public and healthcare professional awareness can significantly improve outcomes in managing food allergies and anaphylaxis.

SUGGESTED READING

1. Božan M, Vukičević Lazarević V, Marković I, Morović-Vergles J, Mitrović J. Alpha-gal syndrome—Food or drug allergy: A case report. Clin Case Rep. 2023;11:e7830.

2. Cardona V, Ansotegui IJ, Ebisawa M, El-Gamal Y, Fernandez Rivas M, Fineman S, et al. World Allergy Organ J. 2020;13(10):100472.
3. Chinthrajah RS, Cao S, Dunham T, Sampath V, Chandra S, Chen M, et al. Oral immunotherapy for peanut allergy: The pro argument. World Allergy Organ J. 2020;13(8):100455.
4. Dadha P, Nimmagadda S, Venter C, Gupta R, Kumar PU, Warren CM. Reported food-related symptoms and food allergen sensitization in a selected adult population in Hyderabad, India: A hospital-based survey. J Allergy Clin Immunol Glob. 2023;3(2):100204.
5. Francis OL, Wang KY, Kim EH, Moran TP. Common food allergens and cross-reactivity. J Food Allergy. 2020;2(1):17-21.
6. Krishna MT, Mahesh PA, Vedanthan P, Moitra S, Mehta V, Christopher DJ. An appraisal of allergic disorders in India and an urgent call for action. World Allergy Organ J. 2020;13(7):100446.
7. Mahesh PA, Kaleem Ullah M, Parthasarathi A. Allergic sensitization to foods in India and other Low-Middle-income countries. Clin Exp Allergy. 2023;53(7):739-50.
8. Mahesh PA, Ullah MK, Parthasarathi A. Allergic Sensitization to foods in India and other Low-Middle-income Countries. Clin Exp Allergy. 2023;53:739-50.
9. Nagarajan SA, Rao HN. Food allergy: Mechanisms, diagnosis, and management. Karnataka Paediatr J 2020;35(2):100-4.
10. Santos AF, Riggioni C, Agache I, Akdis CA, Akdis M, Alvarez-Perea A, et al. EAACI guidelines on the management of IgE-mediated food allergy. Allergy. 2025;80:14-36.
11. Sehgal S, Gupta N, Dadha P, Nagarajan S, Gupta R, Verma MJ, et al. Understanding the burden of food allergy among urban and rural school children from north India. World Allergy Organ J. 2024;17(6):100916.
12. Sindher SB, Fiocchi A, Zuberbier T, Arasi S, Wood RA, Chinthrajah RS. The Role of Biologics in the Treatment of Food Allergy. J Allergy Clin Immunol Pract. 2024;12(3):562-8.
13. Srisuwatchari W, Kanchanaphoomi K, Nawiboonwong J, Thongngarm T, Sompornrattanaphan M. Food-Dependent Exercise-Induced Anaphylaxis: A Distinct Form of Food Allergy-An Updated Review of Diagnostic Approaches and Treatments. Foods. 2023;12(20):3768.

CHAPTER

10

Skin Allergies

Dipti Pujari
Reviewer: *Nayan Mani Deka*

INTRODUCTION

With modern living and lifestyle changes, allergies in general and skin allergies in particular are on the rise. Atopic dermatitis, chronic persistent or relapsing urticarias, contact dermatitis, and angioedema are some of the allergic skin diseases which could be extremely debilitating and can hamper one's day-to-day activities in a big way. Most of these conditions have highly complex pathophysiology and heterogeneous clinical presentations, imposing a significant burden on patients, families, and healthcare systems. In this chapter I have tried to simplify the common skin allergies and included international standard diagnosis and treatment guidelines, keeping in mind our national and local needs and latest treatment protocols.

ATOPIC DERMATITIS

Atopic dermatitis (AD) is an inflammatory, chronically relapsing, non-contagious, and extremely pruritic skin disease. It affects roughly 20% of the pediatric population worldwide.

The skin barrier impairment in AD applies to the thinner epidermis, with defective lipid and protein composition and function, leading to poor hydration, increased trans-epidermal water loss (TEWL) and increased permeability to microbes, irritants, and allergens.

It is a chronically relapsing-remitting disease with flares triggered by viral, bacterial or fungal infections, food allergens, cosmetics, fragrance, aeroallergens, irritants, weather, contact allergens, and psychosocial factors.

The symptoms may vary, some of them are as follows:

- Dry, scaly, or cracked skin
- Redness and inflammation
- Itching
- Oozing or crusting when scratched
- Thickened or scaly skin
- Darkened or discolored patches of skin

PATHOPHYSIOLOGY

The understanding of pathophysiology is important as it will guide us in the appropriate management of this condition. Various causes of AD can be classified into four groups:

1. *The non-allergic causes:* Especially the barrier dysfunction (commonly due to Filaggrin gene mutation) leads to intense pruritus.

   Pro-filaggrin is converted into filaggrin during keratinization. Filaggrin is then broken down into amino acids in "stratum corneum" layer of the skin. These are the natural moisturizers of the skin as they have water retention property and also maintain the acidic pH of the skin. So filaggrin is important in maintaining moist and acidic barrier of the skin. Intriguingly, decreased filaggrin expression is seen in all patients with atopic dermatitis irrespective of the filaggrin gene defect.
2. *The allergic factors:* These factors such as elevated IgE, infiltration of mast cells, neutrophils, and type 2 inflammation (T2) are also important in causing AD. Type 2 inflammation is the predominant inflammatory pathway in

atopic dermatitis, regardless of the beginning of the first symptoms of the disease, be it in the first 6 months of life to all the way through adulthood. When we compare the development of different cytokines subsets in different ages in AD with those of healthy individuals, there are several differences. Interleukin 13 (IL-13), a type 2 biomarker is increased in the individuals with AD, regardless of their age. Some of the other T2 biomarkers such as IL 4, 25 and 31are also higher in AD.

The expression of filaggrin is down regulated by the presence of these cytokines in AD patients. In addition, IL4 also decreases ceramide, which is important for skin barrier function.

Once the superficial barrier of the skin is disrupted, the sensitizers enter through this skin defect and are captured by the dendrites of Langerhans cells present in the epidermis and by the dendritic cells present in the dermis.

Once this capture occurs, the epithelial keratinocytes release various types of inflammatory mediators namely IL1α, IL4, IL5, TNF-α, TSLP (thymic stromal lymphopoietin), and many more. Of these, TSLP is known to produce dendritic cell mediated type 2 inflammation seen in atopic dermatitis.

T2 is the predominant endotype in AD, but sub-endotypes vary by age, race and ethnicity. In adults, the Th22, Th17, and Th1 pathways are involved, and a weakened epidermal barrier is characteristic.

3. *Immune dysregulation and dysbiosis:* IL4 and IL13 downregulate the expression of antimicrobial peptide leading to repeated skin infections in these individuals. The skin of AD patients shows less microbial diversity, also called "dysbiosis". This in turn leads to decrease in growth of *Staphylococcus* epidermidis and increase colonization of *Staphylococcus aureus (Staph aureus)*.

   As against this, interferon gamma (IFN-γ), the infective biomarker which is type 1 inflammation (T1), is low throughout the life in AD individuals as compared to the healthy individuals.
4. *Repeated hapten exposure:* Low molecular weight (<1,000 MW) substances such as metals (nickel, cobalt, and chromium), urushiol, most of the drugs, preservatives when applied on the broken skin are known to cause contact dermatitis. But it is now known that repeated exposure of these haptens on the broken skin leads to Th2 pathway stimulation leading to atopic dermatitis. This happens due to the suppression of delayed hypersensitivity and shift to immediate hypersensitivity. Biochemically, INF-Y decreases and IL-4 increases in these individuals and eosinophils increase in the skin. This is called "hapten-atopy hypothesis".

Finally, the pathogenesis of pruritus/itch in atopic dermatitis is different when compared to urticarial itch:

- It is mediated by IL-31 secreted from T cells. These cytokines act on the dorsal root ganglion of the peripheral nerves of the skin and produce itch.
- IL4 and IL13 also produce itch by acting on JAK1 (Janus Kinase) signaling by reducing the threshold to other pruritogens and histamine.
- Thymic stromal lymphopoietin acts on peripheral nerves to induce TRPA1 receptors, which are also sensitive to pruritogens and induce itch.

AGEWISE DISTRIBUTION OF ATOPIC DERMATITIS LESIONS

Less than 2 Years

- Commonly starts on face and scalp **(Fig. 1)**
- Progresses to chest and extensor surfaces of limbs **(Fig. 2)**
- Spares genitalia and diaper area

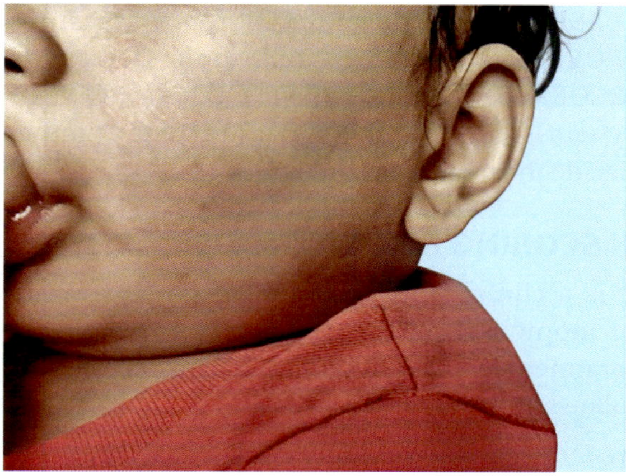

Fig. 1: Dry rash on the face.

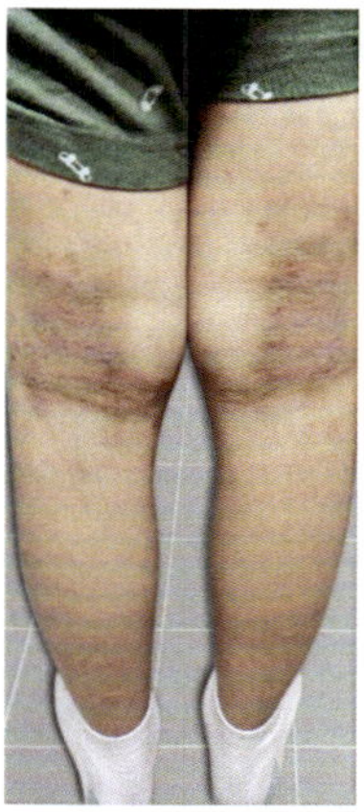

Fig. 3: Atopic dermatitis (AD) rash on popliteal fossa.

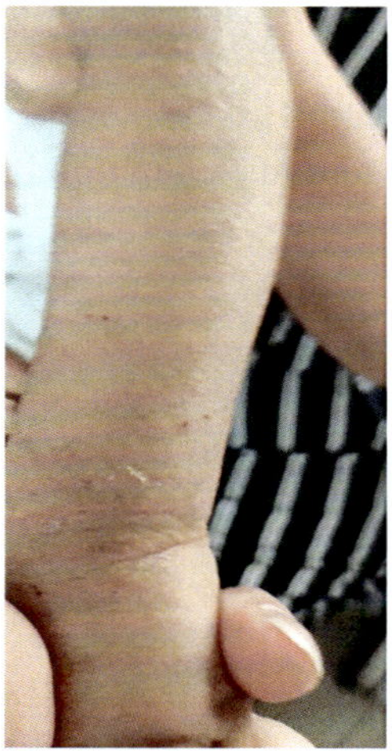

Fig. 2: Rash on the extensor surface of limb.

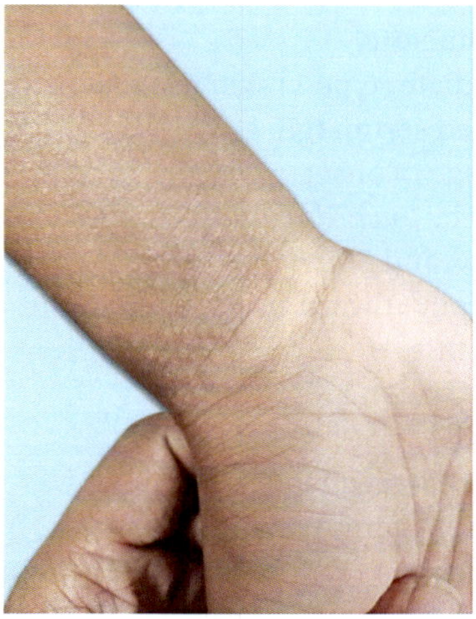

Fig. 4: Atopic dermatitis (AD) rash on volar aspect of wrist.

2 Years—Teenagers

- Mostly involves antecubital fossa and popliteal fossa **(Fig. 3)**
- Also, volar aspect of wrists, ankles, and neck **(Fig. 4)**.

Adults

- It continues on flexor surfaces and also on hands.
- It becomes leathery, rough, and lichenified **(Fig. 5)**.

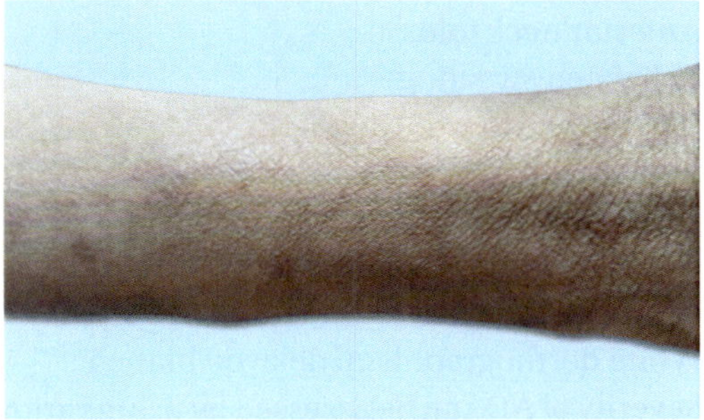

Fig. 5: Lichenified rash in adult.

HANIFIN AND RAJKA DIAGNOSTIC CRITERIA FOR ATOPIC DERMATITIS

Major Criteria: Three or More Required

- Pruritus
- *Typical morphology and distribution:* Facial and extensor involvement in infants and children, flexural lichenification in adults
- Chronic or chronically relapsing dermatitis
- Personal/family history of atopy (asthma, allergic rhinitis, and atopic dermatitis).

Minor Criteria: Three or More Required

- Xerosis
- Ichthyosis, keratosis pilaris, and palmar hyperlinearity
- Immediate (type 1) skin test reactivity
- Elevated serum IgE
- Early age of onset
- *Tendency towards cutaneous infections:* Herpes simplex and *Staph aureus*
- Tendency toward nonspecific hand and foot dermatitis
- Nipple eczema
- Cheilitis
- Dennie-Morgan folds
- Recurrent conjunctivitis
- Keratoconus
- Anterior subcapsular cataract
- Orbital darkening
- Facial pallor
- Pityriasis alba
- Anterior neck folds
- Itch when sweating
- Intolerance to wool and lipid solvents
- Perifollicular accentuation
- Food intolerance
- Course influenced by environmental and emotional factors
- White dermographism, delayed blanch

Severity of AD can be assessed by using various scoring systems. Eczema Area and Severity Score (EASI), Patient Oriented Eczema Measures (POEM), and Scoring for Atopic Dermatitis (SCORAD) are some of them. Of these, SCORAD system is widely used to assess the control (and so decide the treatment) of AD.

SCORING FOR ATOPIC DERMATITIS

It is a clinical tool used to assess the severity of atopic dermatitis and thereby decide the treatment and its outcome. It is calculated as follows:

Area (A): Rule of 9—used to calculate the affected area **(Fig. 6)**.

- Head and neck—9%
- Upper limbs—9% each
- Lower limbs—18% each
- Anterior trunk—18%
- Back—18% genitals, palm and back of hand—1% each

INTENSITY

Based on following signs: Scores are added to give "B" (maximum 18) **(Table 1)**.

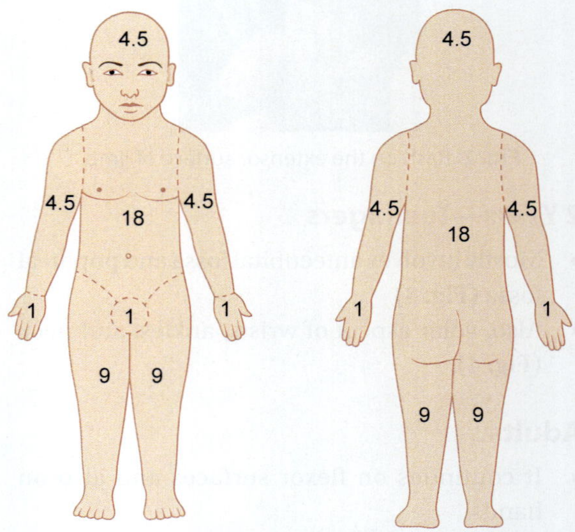

Fig. 6: Rule of "9" to calculate the area affected by atopic dermatitis (AD) rash.

TABLE 1: Scoring of signs in atopic dermatitis (AD) to calculate the intensity of rash.

Criteria	*Absent (0)*	*Mild (1)*	*Moderate (2)*	*Severe (3)*
Erythema (redness)				
Swelling				
Oozing/crusting				
Excoriation (scratch marks)				
Lichenification (skin thickening)				
Dryness				

Subjective symptoms (C): "Itch" and "sleeplessness", scored by the patient:

- 0 is no itch (or sleeplessness)
- 10 is the worst imaginable itch (or sleeplessness).

These scores are added to give "C" (maximum 20). Total score (SCORAD) for any individual is A/5 + 7B/2 + C:

- SCORAD is >50, it indicates severe disease.
- SCORAD 50–25, it indicates moderate disease
- SCORAD is <25, it indicates mild disease.

ENVIRONMENTAL FACTORS AFFECTING ATOPIC DERMATITIS

The Skin Microbiota

- The skin microbiota is crucial to protect from invading pathogens and interact with the immune system.
- It contributes to maintaining the epithelial barrier function and ensures skin homeostasis. Skin microbes secrete proteases involved in the skin renewal process via desquamation; sebum, and fatty acids involved in pH regulation, lipase, and urease enzymes involved in metabolite breakdown.
- Skin diseases, such as AD, psoriasis, acne or rosacea are associated with the disruption of homeostatic skin microbiota rather than the colonization of pathogens.

Lifestyle Factors

Circadian Rhythm

- Circadian rhythms affect skin functions including free radical production and neutralization, DNA damage and repair, keratinocyte and fibroblast proliferation and differentiation, as well as barrier and immune functions.
- At night, the skin has the highest DNA repair, cell proliferation, barrier permeability, and blood flow.

Diet and the Gut-skin Axis

- The gut microbiome is known to modulate the immune response on various organs, including the skin and its residing skin microbiome. This bidirectional interaction plays a crucial role in the development of various skin diseases, including acne vulgaris, psoriasis, and AD among others.
- Understanding the intricate relationship between diet, the gut microbiome and the skin microbiome is essential for maintaining skin homeostasis, preventing the emergence of skin disorders, and exploring potential therapeutic interventions.
- Adequate intake of essential nutrients through diet, for example, vitamin C, supports collagen synthesis, enhances skin barrier function, and protects against oxidative dam age.

Detergent Use/Water Hardness

Detergents and hard water are thought to impair skin barrier functions by increasing skin pH, solubilizing the stratum corneum lipids, altering the protein secondary structure on the skin, reducing a natural moisturizing factor, and upregulating protease activity. These changes may ultimately impact the skin microbiome.

Clothing/Laundry Habits

- Frequent use of detergents and cosmetics and the loss of bacterial diversity on the skin commensals.
- Liquid detergents containing cytotoxic and irritant ingredients remove lipids from the skin, resulting in an impaired skin barrier integrity, thus acting as adjuvants for allergic sensitization.

Environmental Factors (Urban Eczema)

Air pollution, hard water, and modern lifestyle that go hand in gloves with congested city-life, play a big role in triggering eczema and aggravating an already atopic, dry skin. Some of the culprits for "urban eczema" are mentioned below:

- Hard water
- Indoor environment (burning fossil fuel)
- Pollutants (vehicular and industrial smoke)
- Climate
- Ultraviolet (UV)/sunlight

DIAGNOSIS

It is mostly a clinical diagnosis. History, morphology, and distribution of lesions with associated clinical signs help in clinching the diagnosis. No specific biomarkers are recommended for diagnosis and/or assessment of disease severity and monitoring of IgE levels or allergy testing is not recommended routinely. The decision to do allergy tests is purely treating physician's decision (if there is a clear history of aggravation of eczema on exposure to certain foods etc.).

TREATMENT

It can be managed under following headings:

1. Non-pharmacological measures
2. Pharmacological measures
3. Psychological counseling
4. Immunotherapy

Non-pharmacological Measures

These form the backbone of treatment for AD and are the key for good eczema control.

Cleansing and Bathing

- Regular once or twice daily bathing with warm (27–30°C) water is advisable. It should be of short duration (5–10 minutes).
- Non-soap cleansers that are neural to low pH, hypoallergenic, and fragrance free should be used for bathing (syndets) harsh chemicals, fragrant soaps, and bubble baths should be avoided.
- Bleach baths once or twice a week, in a concentration of 0.005% sodium hypochlorite, can be used for prevention of bacterial colonization in moderate-to-severe cases of AD.

Moisturizers

They are the mainstay in the treatment of atopic dermatitis. They decrease the severity and the requirement of other anti-inflammatory treatments for disease control:

- Prompt, frequent, and liberal use of preservative-free and fragrance-free moisturizers should be encouraged.
- *Soak and seal:* Skin should be soaked in warm water for 15 minutes, lightly pat dried, and sealed in moisturizer for best results. Moisturizers should be used at least 2–3 times a day.

Three types of moisturizers are available:

1. *Humectants:* These promote striatum corneum hydration such as urea, glycerol, and lactic acid.

2. *Occludents:* These reduce trans-epidermal water loss, such as petrolatum and liquid paraffin.
3. *Emollients:* They have the ability to instill small droplets of oil into the cracks between the desquamating corneocytes in the dry skin and ultimately improve the appearance of the skin. For examples, linoleic acid, linolenic acid, and oleic acid.

Moisturizers containing intact proteins such as peanuts, colloidal oat meals should be avoided as they may increase the risk of skin sensitization and allergy.

Wet Wrap Therapy

In case of acute flare-ups, first an emollient or a diluted steroid is applied on the inflamed skin. On this, a layer of damp bandage is wrapped, followed by the second dry layer outside it, so that the inner layer can remain wet for a longer duration. This can be used for several hours a day depending on the patient's tolerance.

Clothing

Smooth clothing, which is light weight, loose, and comfortable, like cotton, is recommended. Wool and synthetic clothing should be avoided.

Allergen/Trigger Avoidance

As they increase the skin barrier dysfunction:

- Aeroallergens such as pollens and house dust mites should be avoided in allergen sensitive individuals (proven on skin testing). Rooms should be well ventilated with good sunlight, have comfortable temperature, should be clutter free and with minimal upholstery. Should avoid dry dusting and encourage wet mopping.
- Tobacco smoke avoidance, reduction in exposure to traffic exhaust and volatile organic compounds help in preventing the flare-ups. One should avoid burning wood/essence sticks/mosquito repellents in the house.

Dietary Intervention

Dietary restrictions are recommended in only those individuals with a known food allergy for specific food items.

Pharmacological Measures

These can be divided into two forms—topical medications and systemic medications.

Topical Medications

- *Topical corticosteroids (TCS):* They are very effective, first line of management in controlling inflammation in atopic skin. The choice of topical corticosteroid depends on the severity and extent of the disease, the age of the patient and the area of the body involved and the type of steroid preparation and potency of steroids **(Table 2)**. Correct application with sufficient dose, duration, and strength is important to achieve proper control. The aim should be to taper the steroid to the least potent form, once the acute flare-up is under control.
  - *For acute flare-ups (reactive therapy):* Twice daily application should be done, till active lesions subside. One should review after 2 weeks. If lesions have come under control in 2 weeks, then we need to step down the strength of steroids.
  - *For maintenance (proactive therapy):* Twice weekly application to prevent relapses. (can be used up to 16 weeks) with liberal use of emollients. Steroids should always be applied on well-hydrated skin. Children should be treated with less potent steroids than adults.

Dose: One fingertip unit **(Fig. 7)** is enough to treat an area of skin twice the size of the flat of an adult's hand with the fingers together **(Fig. 8)**.

TABLE 2: Steroids classified according to their potency.

Potency-based classes of topical corticosteroids according to American classification	
Class	***Examples***
Class 1 (superpotent)	Betamethasone dipropionate ointment, cream, 0.05%; clobetasol propionate ointment, cream, 0.05%; halobetasol propionate ointment, cream, 0.05%
Class 2 (potent)	• Mometasone furoate ointment, 0.1%; fluocinonide ointment, cream, gel, 0.05% • Betamethasone dipropionate lotion, 0.05%; halcinonide cream, ointment 0.1%
Class 3 (upper mid-strength)	• Fluocinolone acetonide ointment, 0.025%; fluticasone propionate ointment, 0.005% • Triamcinolone acetonide ointment, 0.1%; halometasone cream, 0.05%
Class 4 (mid-strength)	Mometasone furoate cream, lotion, 0.1%
Class 5 (lower mid-strength)	Betamethasone valerate cream, 0.1%; fluticasone propionate cream, 0.05% hydrocortisone butyrate cream, 0.1%; fluocinolone acetonide cream, 0.025%
Class 6 (mild)	Alclometasone dipropionate ointment, cream, 0.05%; fluocinolone acetonide cream, 0.01%; triamcinolone acetonide cream. 0.025%; desonide cream, 0.05%
Class 7 (least potent)	Hydrocortisone ointment, cream, lotion, 1% or 2.5%; hydrocortisone acetate cream, lotion, 1% or 2.5%

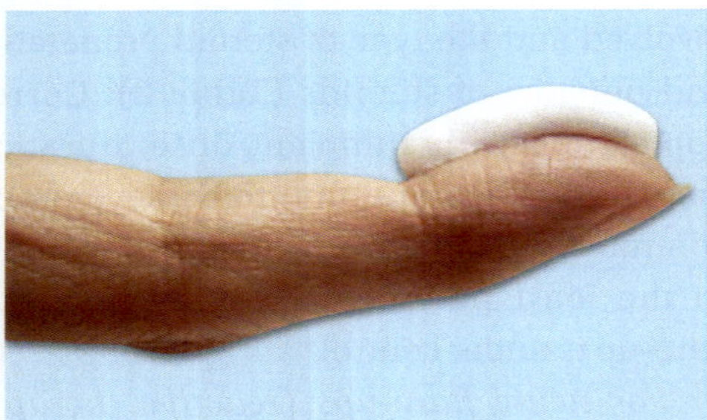

Fig. 7: One fingertip unit of steroid cream.

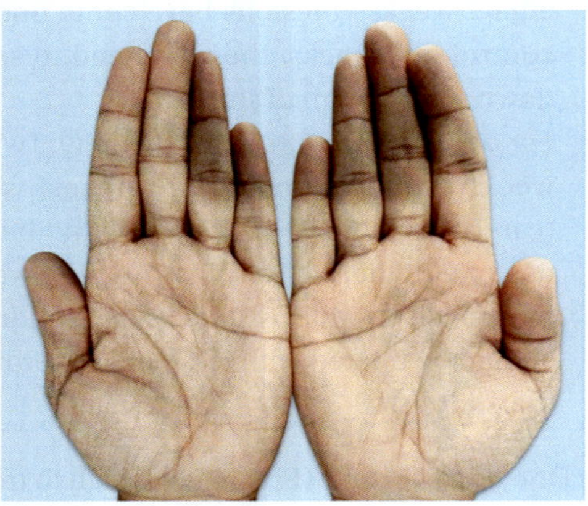

Fig. 8: Two palm size area of skin to be covered by steroid.

Concerns with topical corticosteroids:

- Judicious use is warranted otherwise it can lead to steroid toxicity in the form of thinning of skin with superadded bacterial infections.
- Steroid phobia should be addressed.
- High potency steroids should be avoided on face and flexural areas (as the skin is very thin in these areas).
- To step down to lower potency steroids whenever possible.
- *Topical calcineurin inhibitors (TCI):* They are anti-inflammatory agents that are used in moderate-to-severe AD, when prolonged use of steroids is undesirable. They can be called "steroid-sparing agents". They are very effective especially on face and eyelids, where applying steroids for longer duration is contraindicated.

  They inhibit calcineurin, a protein involved in the activation of immune cells, leading to reduced inflammation in the skin. The two most commonly used molecules are:

  1. *Tacrolimus* 0.03% (for children <15 years) and 0.1% (for > 15 years) ointments
  2. *Pimecrolimus* 1% cream

Their indications for use in AD are as follows:

- *For acute flare-ups (reactive therapy):* Twice daily application (for 2–6 weeks). It is very useful in sensitive skin areas such as face, intertriginous sites, anogenital area as they do not cause skin atrophy, cataract, or glaucoma.
- *For maintenance (proactive therapy):* Twice weekly application has shown to be safe and effective for up to 1 year in reducing flare-ups.

Concerns of TCI: Initial stinging and burning sensation (mostly resolves within a week). Effective sun protection should be recommended when on TCIs:

- *Topical phosphodiesterase-4 inhibitors (PDE4):* AD patients have increased activity of PDE4, leading to an increased production of pro-inflammatory cytokines and chemokines. PDE4 inhibitors antagonize this effect thereby decreasing the production of inflammatory cytokines IL-4, IL-13, and IL-31 in eczematous skin and thus help in controlling the symptoms in mild-to-moderate AD patients:
    - *Crisaborole:* It is a topical phosphodiesterase-4 inhibitor effective in the moderate AD. 2% ointment is approved for use >2 years of age.
- *Janus kinase (JAK) inhibitors:* The Janus kinase pathways are involved in signaling of various AD-related cytokines such as IL-4, IL-13, IL-31, IL-22, and IL-17 mediating barrier alteration and inflammation of the skin. JAK inhibitors decrease AD severity and are found useful in moderate-to-severe atopic dermatitis. They are available in oral and topical forms.
  The topical JAK inhibitors are:
    - *Ruxolitinib:* JAK1 and 2 inhibitors. It is used to treat mild-to-moderate AD in children >12 years.
    - *Delgocitinib:* Pan-JAK inhibitor. It can be used in children and adults.
- *Phototherapy:* Ultraviolet B (UVB), mostly narrow band (NB-UVB) of 311–313 nm and UVA of 340–400 nm has shown marked healing in atopic dermatitis skin due to its anti-inflammatory, immunomodulatory, and anti-microbial properties.

Pharmacological Measures: (Oral/Injectable Therapy)

- *Antibiotics:* Topical and systemic antibiotics/antivirals/antifungals to be used whenever there is skin infection as eczematous skin is very prone for infection.
- *Oral glucocorticoids:* Short course of low dose steroids, 0.5 mg/kg/day up to 1 week can be used for acute flare-ups.
- *Immunosuppressive drugs*:
    - *Cyclosporine A:* For refractory, severe cases of AD, cyclosporin which is a T-cell suppressor, has shown promising results. Given in an initial dose of 5 mg/kg/day in two divided doses. Mostly given for 6–12 weeks in children to treat severe, acute flare-ups. (Serial blood pressure and serum creatinine monitoring to be done.)
    - *Methotrexate (MTX):* There are various dosing schedules available for the use of methotrexate in pediatric patients with AD. The European Taskforce of Atopic Dermatitis (ETFAD) and the International Society of Atopic Dermatitis (ISAD) have put forth the following consensus statements on MTX dosing for patients with AD:

Methotrexate should be administered in a single weekly dose. It should be tried for 8–12 weeks before the effect can be assessed:

- *Azathioprine*
- *Mycophenolate mofetil*

These can be used in severe resistant cases:

- *Janus kinase inhibitors:* Oral JAK inhibitors that have been recently approved for use in atopic dermatitis are:
  - *Baricitinib:* It is an oral JAK inhibitor.
  - *Upadacitinib:* Tablet form can be used >12 years of age in moderate-to-severe AD.
  - *Abrocitinib:* Tablet licensed for adults with severe AD.
  - *Tofacitinib*
  - *Cerdulatinib*
- *Biologicals:* These are a new class of drugs, proving to be game-changers in many serious medical conditions. Because of their precise mode of action, biologicals are ideal for "personalized" or "precision" medicine. Here, we refer to monoclonal antibodies (mAb) as biologicals:
  - *Dupilumab* is a human monoclonal antibody administered subcutaneously to inhibit the interleukin-4 receptor subunit α (IL-4R α). IL-4Rα is a component common to both IL-4 and IL-13 receptor complexes and is ubiquitously expressed in innate and adaptive immune cells to promote the signaling of IL-4 and IL-13.

By blocking this pathway, dupilumab affects three integral disease mechanisms of atopic dermatitis:

- The decrease of skin barrier function
- The class switch to IgE
- The Th2 differentiation

Age approval for atopic dermatitis

- Approved for children aged 6 months to 5 years with moderate-to-severe atopic dermatitis
- Approved for children aged 6 and older with moderate-to-severe atopic dermatitis who are dependent on oral corticosteroids or have an eosinophilic phenotype.

Dosage of dupilumab: Children aged 6 months to 5 years (no loading dose recommended):

- *5 to <15 kg:* 200 mg SC every 4 weeks
- *15 to <30 kg:* 300 mg SC every 4 weeks

TABLE 3: Newer biologicals for the treatment of atopic dermatitis (AD).

Biological	*Target*	*Current phase of clinical trials*
Dupilumab	IL-4/IL-13	Approved for clinical use by EMA
Tralokinumab	IL-13	Approved for clinical use by EMA
Lebrikizumab	IL-13	3, still recruiting
Nemolizumab	IL-31	3, still recruiting
GBR830/IBS830	0X40	2b, finished, results not published
KHK4083	0X40	2a, completed, results not published
Tezepelumab	TSLP	2b, still recruiting
Etokimab	IL-31	2b, still recruiting
Fezakinumab	IL-22	2a, completed

Children aged 6–17 years:

- *≥60 kg:* 600 mg SC once, and then 300 mg SC every other week
- *<60 kg:* 400 mg SC once, and then 200 mg SC every other week

There are numerous biologicals that are in the pipeline for the treatment of AD. Some are approved and some are in clinical trials. Some of them are as follows **(Table 3)**:

Psychosomatic Counseling

- Psychological stress can alter permeability barrier homeostasis and stratum corneum integrity leading to exacerbation of the disease.
- The psychological intervention and behavioral therapy in atopic dermatitis are aimed at breaking itch-scratch cycle, which has a lot of psychological component to it.

Interventions

- Children's hands should be kept busy, and they should be talked to divert attention from scratching. Trimming nails is important.
- Behavioral interventions, such as biofeedback and relaxation techniques, can also be helpful in controlling scratching.

Allergen-specific Immunotherapy

Both subcutaneous immunotherapy (SCIT) and sublingual immunotherapy (SLIT) are effective in reducing the symptoms of AD in selective patients of positive sensitization (mostly with house dust mites). It provides long-term remission and prevents new sensitization. But immunotherapy should only be started if clear one-to-one correlation is established with the inciting allergen and the atopic flare-ups.

STEPWISE MANAGEMENT OF ATOPIC DERMATITIS BASED ON SCORING FOR ATOPIC DERMATITIS

Stepwise management of atopic dermatitis (AD) is guided by clinical severity scores like SCORAD depicted in **Flowchart 1**.

Flowchart 1: Stepwise management of atopic dermatitis based on scoring for atopic dermatitis (SCORAD).

Step 1: Dry skin
- Avoidance of triggers
- Emollients and moisturizers

↓↑

Step 2: Mild AD (SCORAD <25)
- Emollients and moisturizers
- Weak topical steroids/topical calcineurin inhibitors (CNIs)

↓↑

Step 3: Moderate atopic dermatitis (AD) (SCORAD 25–50)
- Emollients and moisturizers
- *Proactive therapy:* Moderate potency topical steroids/topical CNIs

↓↑

Step 4: Severe AD (SCORAD >50)
- Emollients and moisturizers
- *Proactive therapy:* Moderate potency topical steroids/topical CNIs
- *Immunosuppressants:* Cyclosporin A, methotrexate

↓↑

Step 5: Uncontrolled AD
- *Biologicals:* Subcutaneous (S/C) dupilumab in >6 years age

URTICARIA

Definition

Urticaria is a condition characterized by the development of wheals (hives), angioedema, or both:

- *A wheal has three typical features:*
  1. Sharply circumscribed superficial central swelling of variable size and shape, almost invariably surrounded by reflex erythema **(Fig. 9)**.
  2. Itching or sometimes burning sensation.
  3. Fleeting nature, with the skin returning to its normal appearance, usually within 30 minutes to 24 hours.
- *Angioedema is characterized by:*
  - Sudden, pronounced erythematous or skin-colored deep swelling in the lower dermis and subcutis or mucous membranes,
  - Tingling, burning, tightness, and sometimes pain rather than itch,
  - Resolution slower than that of wheals (can take up to 72 hours)

This definition has been taken from the latest published EAACI guidelines on urticaria, the article as mentioned: The international EAACI/ GA^{2}LEN/EuroGuiDerm/APAAACI guideline

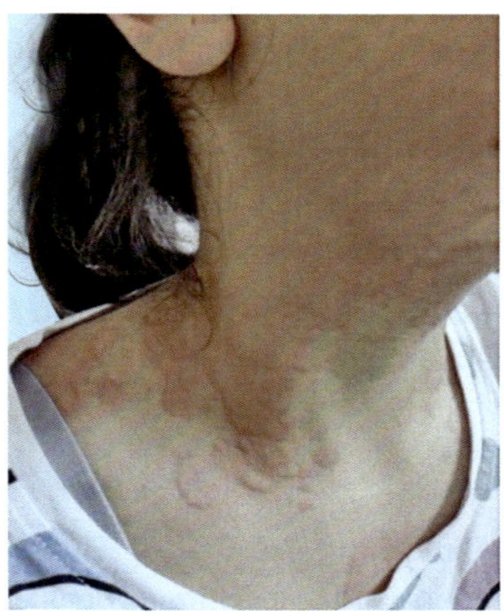

Fig. 9: Well-circumscribed wheals of urticarial rash.

for the definition, classification, diagnosis, and management of urticaria. DOI: 10.1111/all.15090.

Almost 20% of the global population is affected by urticaria at some point in their lifetime and up to 2–3% population suffers from chronic urticaria worldwide. Urticaria can cause severe disruption in a child's day-to-day activities, sleep schedule, schooling, and social life, thereby causing negative impact on learning, cognition, and academic achievement. All this can lead to disruption of family life and lead to a lot of distress in the child and the family. Hence proper understanding of the root cause of urticaria, its treatment, proper counseling regarding the disease and its long-term management should take the priority while dealing with such children. Though acute urticaria is more common in children, chronic urticarias are becoming commoner and can last for even up to 10 years before remission.

MECHANISM OF WHEAL FORMATION

Histamine, leukotrienes, chemokines, prostaglandins, and many other mediators are released from mast cells and basophils due to one of the following mechanisms:

- IgE mediated type 1 hypersensitivity reaction (from allergy to foods/drugs/insects, etc.)
- Complement pathways (antigen-antibody reaction) (serum sickness)
- Direct mast cell activation (from radiocontrast dye injection)
- Extrinsic coagulation pathway (bradykinin-mediated primary angioedema)
- Autoantibodies

Once the mediators are released from the mast cells they cause:

- Sensory nerve stimulation
- Vasodilatation
- Plasma extravasation
- More cell recruitment

These factors lead to swelling, wheal, erythema, and itching seen in urticaria. Histologically, wheals are characterized by edema of the upper and mid dermis, whereas in angioedema, similar changes occur primarily in the lower dermis and the subcutis.

VARIOUS FACTORS CAN SOMETIMES AGGRAVATE URTICARIA

- Fever
- Heat
- Alcohol consumption
- Exercise
- Emotional stress
- Menstruation
- Perimenopausal state
- Hyperthyroidism

This again reiterates the importance of proper history taking and counseling the patient likewise.

Depending on the duration of urticaria and the relevant eliciting factors, it can be classified as **(Flowchart 2)**:

- *Acute urticaria:* Where the occurrence of wheals, angioedema, or both lasts for 6 weeks or less.
- *Chronic urticaria:* It is defined as the occurrence of wheals, angioedema, or both for more than

Flowchart 2: Classification of urticaria.

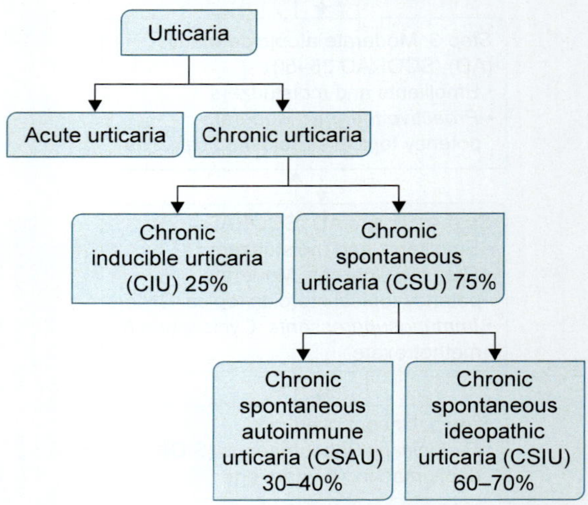

6 weeks. Chronic urticaria can come with daily or almost daily signs and symptoms or an intermittent/recurrent course.

Depending on the triggers, chronic urticaria can be further classified as:

- *Chronic spontaneous urticaria (CSU):* Urticarial rash that comes spontaneously due to some known or unknown causes.
- *Chronic inducible urticaria (CIndU):* Urticarial rash can be produced or induced due to various physical or other forces. This is of two types:
  1. *Physical urticarias:* Symptomatic dermographism, cold urticaria, delayed pressure urticaria (DPU), solar urticaria, heat urticaria, and vibratory angioedema
  2. *Non-physical urticarias:* Cholinergic urticaria, contact urticaria, and aquagenic urticaria.

ACUTE URTICARIA

The most common form of urticaria seen in children is acute urticaria. The various factors that can lead to acute urticarias are:

Allergens

- *Foods:* Eggs, fish, peanuts, tree nuts, shellfish, and lentils are some of the most common food allergens in children.
- Pollens, house dust mites, and pet dander
- Insect stings or bites
- Latex
- Food additives

Medications

Any drug can cause acute urticaria. But the commonly seen reactions are mostly due to:

- Antibiotics (penicillins and sulfa drugs are known to cause acute reactions)
- Non-steroidal anti-inflammatory group of drugs (NSAIDS)
- Angiotensin converting enzyme (ACE) inhibitors

Infections

- Bacterial infections (including dental carries)
- Viral infections
- Parasitic infections

BLOOD TRANSFUSION REACTIONS

Treatment of Acute Urticaria

Identifying the triggers and avoiding them improves acute urticarias most of the times. Symptomatic management should be done according to the symptoms. Short course of oral second-generation antihistamines improves the symptoms. Infections being very common in children, every attempt should be made to rule out any infection, as it is an easily treatable cause to cure acute urticaria.

The **Flowchart 3** shows how to approach chronic spontaneous urticaria (CSU).

Proper history taking becomes an essential part of the work up in CIndU as it provides the clue to the plausible causative mechanical factor leading to the various types of inducible urticaria.

Flowchart 3: Approach to chronic spontaneous urticaria.

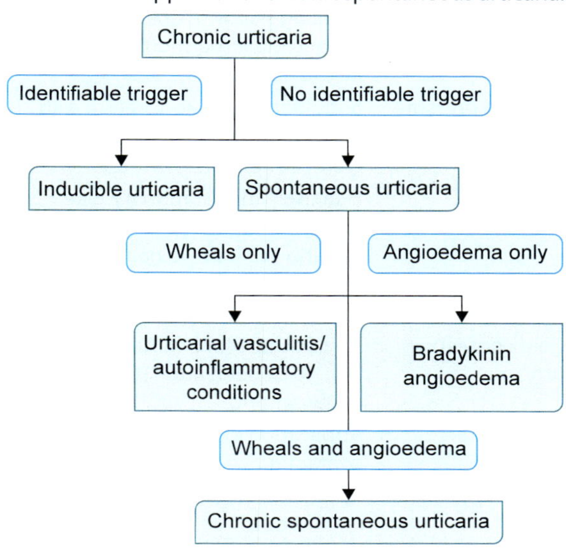

Table 4 shows types of "chronic inducible urticarias".

Table 5 gives an overview of various types of tests, to diagnose inducible urticarias. Each one is further described in detail as we proceed in the chapter.

TABLE 4: Various types of chronic inducible urticarias (CIndU) and their trigger mechanisms.

Types	*Mechanism (triggers)*
Symptomatic dermographism	Mechanical shearing force (stroking and scratching)
Delayed pressure urticaria	Vertical pressure (3–12 hours latency)
Cholinergic urticaria	Increase of body core temperature due exercise, hot baths, and spicy food
Cold urticaria	Cold objects/air/fluids/wind
Heat urticaria	Localized heat contact
Solar urticaria	UV/visible light
Aquagenic urticaria	Contact with water at any temperature
Vibratory angioedema	Vibratory force of any kind

TABLE 5: Tests to diagnose various inducible urticarias.

Disorder	*Test description*
Symptomatic dermographism	Stroking skin with tip of pen/tongue blade/dermographometer at <36 g/mm^2
Delayed pressure urticaria	Shoulder sling 7 kg/forearm 4 kg for 15 minutes. To be seen over next 24 hours
Cholinergic urticaria	Exercise with a stationary bike for 15 minutes beyond onset of sweating or passive heating of one arm to 42°C with water bath or whole-body immersion
Cold contact urticaria	Ice cube test for 5 minutes on arm, to be seen after 10 minutes of rewarming
Heat contact urticaria	Application of test-tube containing warm water at 44°C
Vibratory urticaria	Application of vortex on forearm for 4 minutes

Dermographism (Urticaria Factitia)

- Common physical urticaria 2–5% population
- Wheals at the site of trauma, friction, and scratching **(Fig. 10)**
- Wheal in the shape of applied force
- Mucus membrane unaffected

Treatment: Avoid friction/scratching and wearing loose clothing

Cold Urticaria

- Cold stimulus leads to erythema/angioedema.
- Can be fatal if extensive exposure to cold
- Cryoproteins are thought to be the cause for this phenomenon.

Ice Cube Test (Fig. 11)

- Keep ice for 5 minutes.
- To read after 10 minutes of re-warming. This test can also be performed with a special instrument called "Temptest" **(Fig. 12)** which can adjust the temperature to the desired level and on keeping the forearm on the machine, one can demonstrate cold-induced urticaria.

Delayed Pressure Urticaria

Urticaria/angioedema 3–8 hours after the pressure is applied.

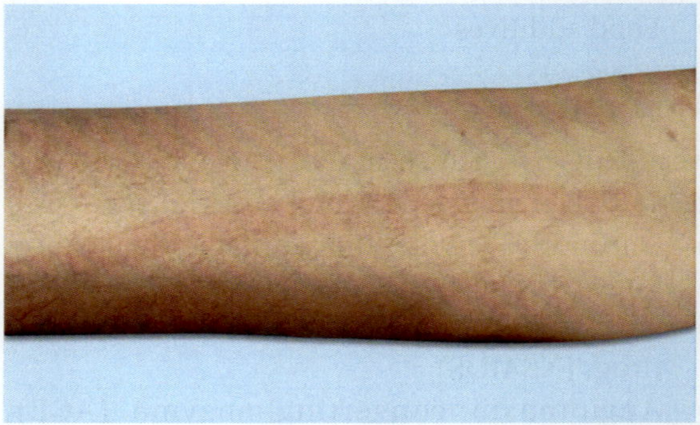

Fig. 10: Dermographism after scratching.

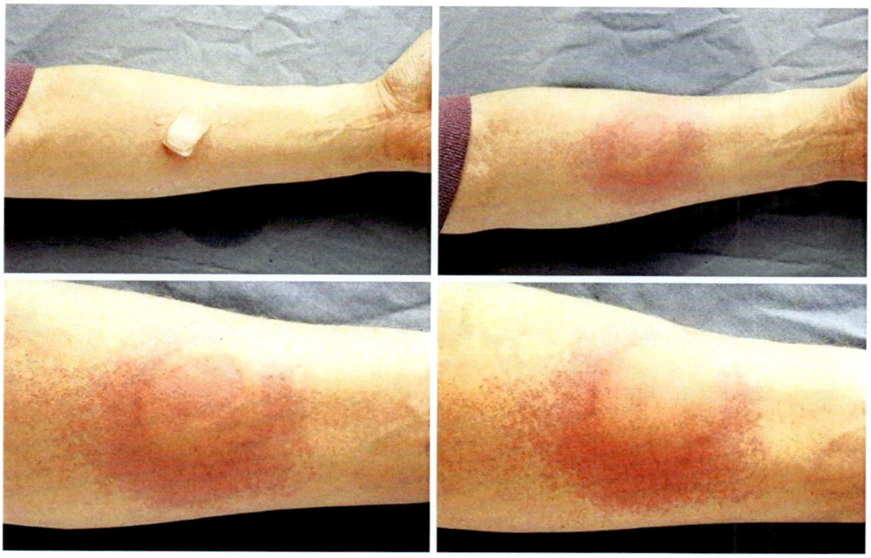

Fig. 11: Demonstration of "ice-cube test".

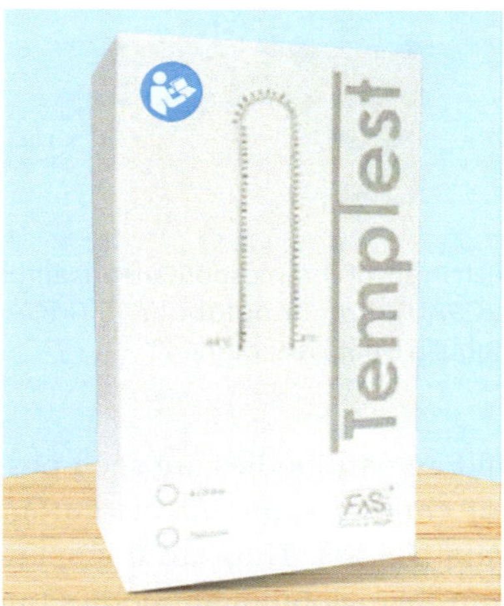

Fig. 12: Temptest.

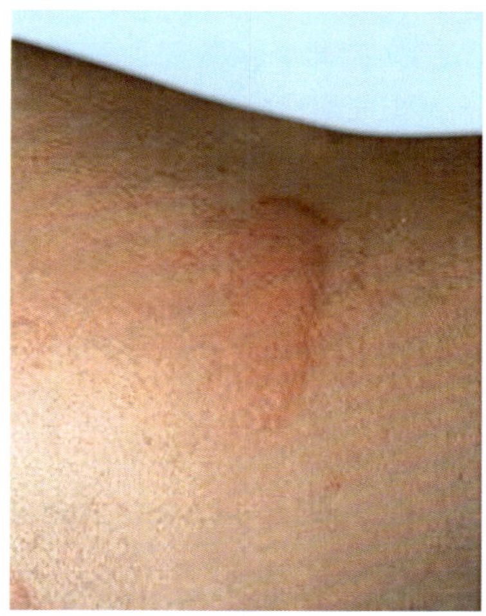

Fig. 13: Delayed pressure urticaria (DPU) due to heavy bag strap.

Causes:

- Tight clothing and belts
- On shoulders, due to heavy school bags **(Fig. 13)**
- On soles after standing for long duration **(Fig. 14)**

Pressure Test to Detect Delayed Pressure Urticaria (Fig. 15)

- Sling attached to 4 kg weight placed on patient's arm for 15 minutes
- Or 7 kg weight sling on shoulder
- To monitor for the next 24 hours

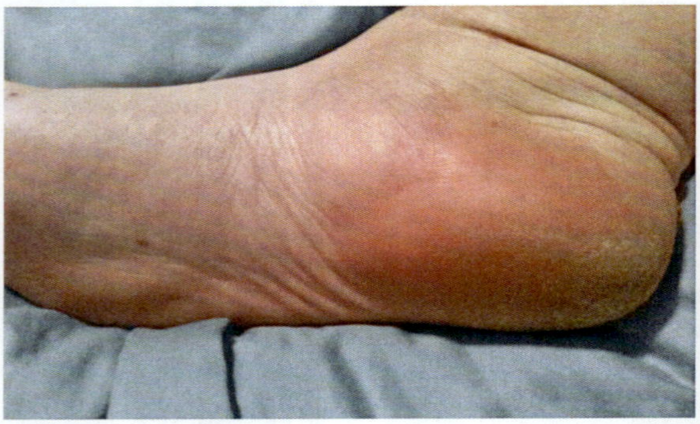

Fig. 14: Delayed pressure urticaria (DPU) on soles due to prolonged standing.

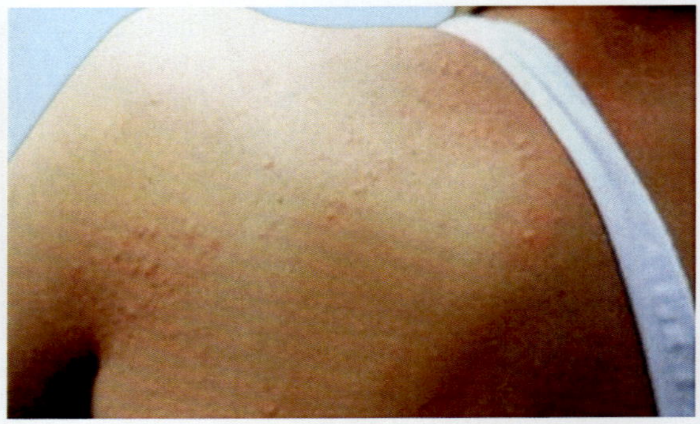

Fig. 16: Papulonodular rash of cholinergic urticaria.

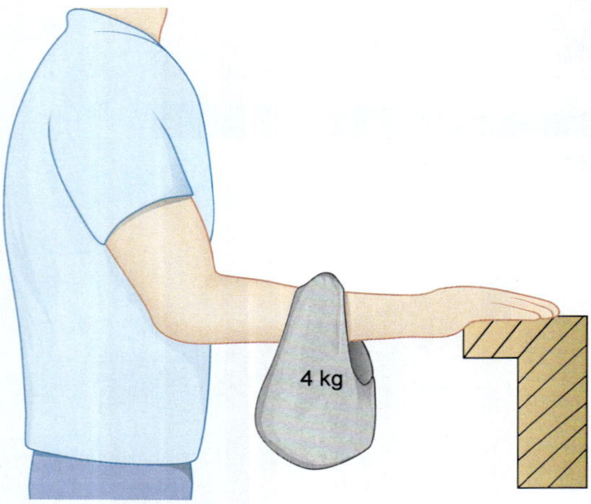

Fig. 15: Pressure test to detect delayed pressure urticaria (DPU).

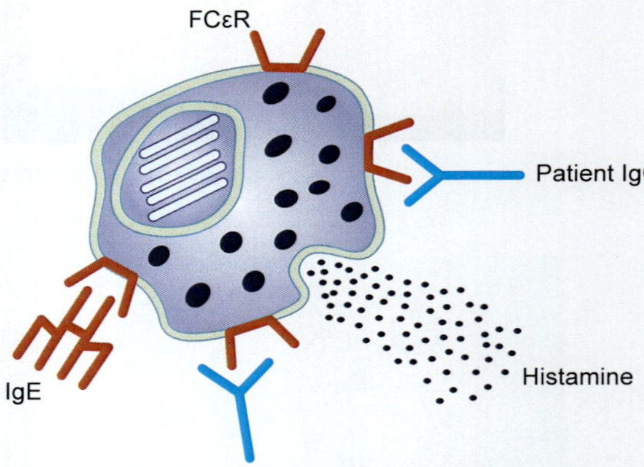

Fig. 17: Mechanism of chronic spontaneous autoimmune urticaria (CSAU), immunoglobulin G (IgG) against immunoglobulin E (IgE) receptor.

Cholinergic Urticaria

- Pruritic, maculopapular, and nodular rash **(Fig. 16)**
- It can occur on trunk, neck, and limbs.
- Triggered by exercise and emotional stress.
- It resolves within 1–2 years.

CHRONIC SPONTANEOUS AUTOIMMUNE URTICARIA

- Autoantibodies (IgG) directed against IgE receptor (FCεR1) or IgE **(Fig. 17)**
- They will crosslink the IgE receptor and degranulate the mast cells
- Thyroid autoantibodies are seen positive in 15% of chronic spontaneous autoimmune urticaria (CSAU). They are thyroperoxidase anti and thyroglobulin antibodies (anti-TPO and anti-TG).

These autoantibodies can be detected by autologous serum skin test (ASST), where patient's own serum is tested on the patient's body. Normal saline is used as a negative control and histamine as a positive control **(Fig. 18)**.

Any wheal on patient's serum, which is >1.5 mm more than the negative control, is considered a positive test for autoantibodies.

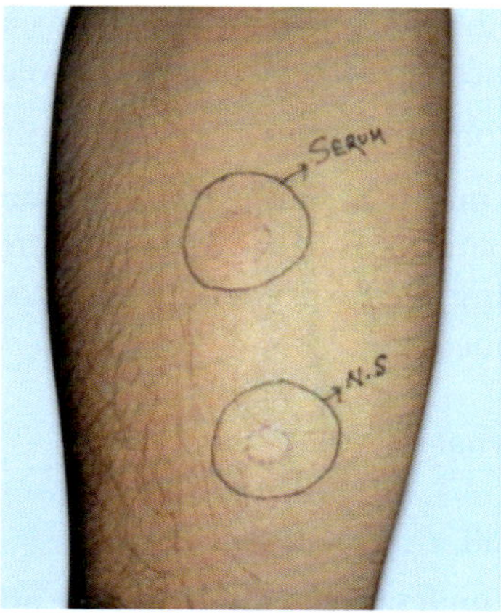

Fig. 18: A positive autologous serum skin test (ASST) with patient's own serum and normal saline as a negative control.

Chronic Spontaneous Idiopathic Urticaria

When in spite of thorough investigation, no cause can be found then it is called chronic spontaneous idiopathic urticaria (CSIU). Some of the underlying conditions associated with this form of urticaria are:

- Psychological stress
- Infections:
  - *Bacterial: Streptococcal pharyngitis*, sinusitis, dental carries, *Helicobacter pylori* (*H. pylori*), urinary tract infections (UTIs)
  - *Viral:* Hepatitis B, C, CMV, coxsackie A and B
  - *Parasitic: Ascaris, Ancylostoma, Echinococcus, Schistosoma, Toxocara,* and *Trichinella*
  - *Fungal:* Dermatophytes and Candida
- *Drugs:* NSAIDS, ACE inhibitors, and antibiotics
- Vasculitis
- Urticaria pigmentosa (cutaneous mastocytosis)
- Rheumatological conditions such as systemic lupus erythematosus SLE, JRA, MCTD, dermatomyositis
- *Neoplastic conditions such as:* Lymphoma and leukemia
- *Food additives:* Coloring agents, artificial sweetens, flavoring agents, preservatives, etc.

Investigations for Chronic Spontaneous Idiopathic Urticaria

- *History:* Onset, shape, size, duration, pain, burning, menstrual history, and joint involvement
- *Infections:* Complete blood count (CBC), urinalysis, stool examination, cultures, and serology
- *Skin prick test:* Food and drugs
- *Patch test:* Drugs
- *Thyroiditis:* TSH, thyroperoxidase (TPO), and thyroglobulin (TGO) antibodies
- *Collagen vascular disease:* ESR, CRP, CH50, C3, C4, ANA, and RF
- *Vasculitis:* Skin biopsy
- *Mastocytosis:* Bone marrow biopsy
- *Urticaria pigmentosa:* Skin biopsy
- Serum tryptase level
- *Angioedema:* C1q and C1 inhibitor level
- *Autoimmune:* ASST

DIFFERENTIAL DIAGNOSIS OF URTICARIAL RASH

- Maculopapular cutaneous mastocytosis (urticaria pigmentosa) and indolent systemic mastocytosis with involvement of the skin
- Mast cell activation syndrome (MCAS)
- Urticarial vasculitis
- Bradykinin-mediated angioedema (e.g., HAE)
- Exercise-induced anaphylaxis
- Cryopyrin-associated periodic syndromes (CAPS; urticarial rash, recurrent fever attacks, arthralgia or arthritis, eye inflammation, fatigue, and headaches), that is, familial cold autoinflammatory syndrome (FCAS), Muckle-Wells syndrome (MWS), or neonatal onset multisystem inflammatory disease (NOMID).
- Schnitzler's syndrome (recurrent urticarial rash and monoclonal gammopathy, recurrent fever attacks, bone and muscle pain, arthralgia or arthritis and lymphadenopathy)
- Gleich's syndrome (episodic angioedema with eosinophilia)

- Well's syndrome (granulomatous dermatitis with eosinophilia/eosinophilic cellulitis)
- Bullous pemphigoid (prebullous stage)
- Adult-onset Still's disease (AOSD)

MONITORING BY URTICARIA ACTIVITY SCORE (UAS7) (TABLE 6)

Sum of score: 0–6 is summarized for each day over 1 week (maximum score 42/week)

Interpretation of Urticaria Activity Score

See **Table 7**.

Urticaria Control Test

The urticaria control test (UCT) was developed and validated to determine the level of disease control in all forms of CU (CSU and CIndU). The UCT is a simple four-item tool with a clearly defined cutoff for patients with "well-controlled" versus "poorly controlled" disease, and it is, thus, suited for the management of patients in routine clinical practice. Its recall period is 4 weeks.

TABLE 6: Monitoring by urticaria activity score (UAS7).

Score	Wheals	Pruritus
0	None	None
1	Mild (<20 wheals/24 hours)	Mild (present but not annoying or troublesome)
2	Moderate (20–50 wheals/24 hours)	Moderate (troublesome but not interfering with daily activity/sleep)
3	Intense (>50 wheals/24 hours or large confluent areas of wheal)	Intense (severe pruritus, interfering with daily activity/sleep)

TABLE 7: Urticarial activity score (UAS) interpretation.

UAS	Disease activity
<6	Well controlled
7–15	Mild
16–27	Moderate
28–42	Severe

Urticaria control test has following questions:

Q1. How much a person has suffered from physical symptoms of the urticaria, (itch, hives, and swelling) in the preceding 4 weeks?

- Very much
- Much
- Somewhat
- Little
- Not at all

Q2. How much was the quality of life affected by urticaria in the preceding 4 weeks?

- Very much
- Much
- Somewhat
- Little
- Not at all

Q3. How often was the treatment of urticaria not enough to control the symptoms of urticaria in the preceding 4 weeks?

- Very often
- Often
- Sometimes
- Seldom
- Not at all

Q4. How well was the urticaria under control in the preceding 4 weeks?

- Not at all
- A little
- Somewhat
- Well
- Very well

The UCT cutoff value for well-controlled disease is 12 out of 16 possible points. (Taken from EAACI guidelines: MOXIE GmbH, Berlin, Germany).

MANAGEMENT OF URTICARIA

Points to consider:

- The goal of treatment is to treat the disease until it is gone.

- Try to find the underlying cause for the urticaria.
- Once the cause is known, avoiding the eliciting factor as much as possible.
- Symptom control with antihistamines and other drugs to give a good life and improve quality of life of patients suffering from this disease.
- We should follow the principle of treating as much as needed and as little as possible for complete disease-free life.
- Regular follow-up to step-up or step-down the treatment whenever needed.

PRINCIPLES TO STEP-UP OR STEP-DOWN THE TREATMENT BASED ON URTICARIA CONTROL TEST SCORE

- *If UCT is 16:* Then the disease is considered completely under control and one can step down on the treatment by either decreasing the dose of the drug or increasing the interval of the drug.
- *If UCT is between 12 and 15:* That means the disease is well under control. One needs to continue the optimal treatment.
- *If UCT is <12:* Then we need to step-up the treatment of either antihistamines or omalizumab.

Avoidance/elimination of eliciting factors is a must. One should try to find the triggers and aggravating factors:

- If in doubt about the trigger factor, then provocation test should be done.
- The autoantibodies in autoimmune urticaria can be reduced by plasmapheresis.
- Drugs such as NSAIDS, ACE inhibitors, sartans etc., if found to be causative agents, should be strictly avoided.
- Triggers of CIndU should be eliminated. For example:
    - One should wear loose fitting clothes in dermographism.
    - Use sunscreens in solar urticaria.
    - Try and broaden the handles of heavy bags in delayed pressure urticaria.
    - Not use very hot/cold water in heat and cold-induced urticaria.
- Infections, if any, should be properly treated with antibiotics, antivirals, or antifungals.
- If chronic inflammatory conditions are associated with urticaria, they should be properly managed.
- Stress, if any, should be addressed and reduced as it can aggravate urticaria.
- Immunoglobulin E-mediated food allergies are extremely rare in chronic urticarias. But if detected should advise strict avoidance. Pseudoallergens (food additives) should be avoided where possible.
- Tolerance induction in some CIndU such as cholinergic urticaria, cold-induced urticaria, solar urticaria can be useful in some cases. The key to this therapy is consistent daily exposure to the stimulus just at threshold level. For example, in the case of cold urticaria where daily cold baths/showers are needed to achieve this.

PHARMACOTHERAPY FOR CHRONIC URTICARIA (FIG. 19)

First-line Treatments

- *Second generation H1-antihistamines* are the first line of therapy.
- Fexofenadine, cetirizine, levocetirizine, desloratadine, loratadine, ebastine, rupatadine, mizolastine, and bilastine
- To be taken regularly, as they are inverse agonist.
- Increase the dose (double) if needed
- Can quadruple the dose of same second generation H1-antihistamine if control is not achieved with double dose in 2–4 weeks.
- First generation antihistamines—to be avoided

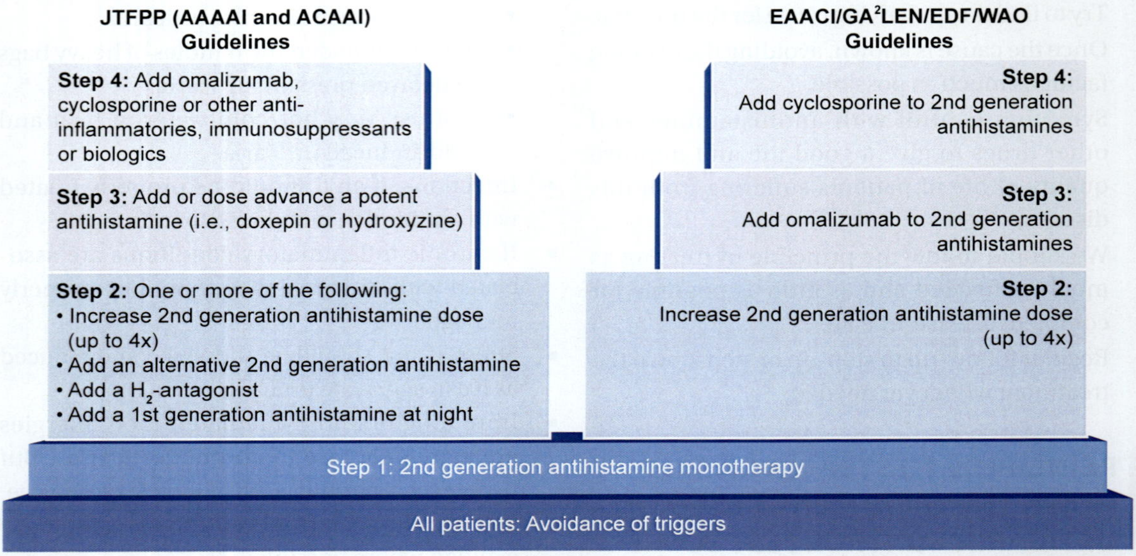

Fig. 19: Comparison of the Joint Task Force on Practice Parameters (JTFPP) guidelines (representing the American Academy of Allergy, Asthma, and Immunology, and the American College of Allergy, Asthma, and Immunology) with the EAACI/GA²LEN/EDF/WAO guidelines. (EAACI: European Academy of Allergology and Clinical Immunology; GA²LEN: Global Allergy and Asthma European Network; JTFPP: Joint Task Force on Practice Parameters; WAO: World Allergy Organization)

Source: Yosipovitch G, Biazus Soares G, Mahmoud O. Current and Emerging Therapies for Chronic Spontaneous Urticaria: A Narrative Review. Dermatol Ther (Heidelb). 2023;13(8):1647-60.

Second-line Treatments

- *Omalizumab (Anti-IgE therapy):* Omalizumab to be added to second generation H1- antihistamine for patients who do not respond adequately to antihistamines. It has been shown to significantly improve symptoms in CSU.
- Dose is 300 mg every 4 weekly. Can be increased to 600 mg every 2 weekly. Subcutaneous injections.

Third-line Treatment

- *Cyclosporin:* To be added to second generation H1-antihistamines if inadequate response with omalizumab even after 6 months of treatment.
- Dose is 3.5–5 mg/kg/day.
- Cyclosporin is immunosuppressive and has a moderate, direct effect on mast cell mediator release.

Corticosteroids: Prednisolone—short course (3–7 days) for acute exacerbation only.

- Dose 0.3–0.5 mg/kg/day
- Not for long term/frequent use
- No role of topical steroids except DPU on soles

H2-antagonists and leukotriene receptor antagonists: These may be used as adjuncts for patients with inadequate responses to antihistamines.

Other Drugs

- *Cyproheptadine:* Cold induced urticaria
- *Montelukast:* NSAIDS, food additives, and DPU
- *H1 + H2:* After max dose of second generation H1 antihistamines

- *PUVA Therapy:* Solar urticaria
- *Doxepin:* DPU
- *Hydroxychloroquine:* Urticarial-vasculitis (UV)
- *Cyclophosphamide:* Autoimmune urticaria, UV
- *Plasmapheresis:* Autoimmune urticaria, UV
- *I/V Ig:* Autoimmune urticaria
- *Treat the cause:* Infections, collagen vascular disease, myelomas, leukemias, and vasculitis

New and Emerging Therapies

- *Bruton's tyrosine kinase inhibitors:* These are in clinical trials and may provide new options for CSU patients, particularly those with autoimmune features.
- *Anti-KIT monoclonal antibodies:* Targeting mast cell activation, these therapies show promise in treating patients with resistant CSU.
- *Janus kinase inhibitors and MRGPRX2 antagonists:* New agents targeting specific pathways in mast cell degranulation are under investigation.

Newer drugs are under research for the treatment of CSU and are in phase 3 trials **(Table 8)**:

TABLE 8: Drugs under research for the treatment of chronic spontaneous urticaria (CSU) and are in phase 3 trials.

Name of the drug	*Mechanism of action*
Dupilumab	Monoclonal antibody against IL-4/13Rα
UB221	Monoclonal antibody against CD23-bound IgE
Remibrutinib	Bruton tyrosine kinase inhibitor
Rilzabrutinib	Bruton tyrosine kinase inhibitor
Mepolizumab	Anti-IL5 monoclonal antibodies
Benralizumab	Anti-IL5 monoclonal antibodies
Tezepelumab	Anti-TSLP monoclonal antibody
Lirentelimab	Anti-Siglec-8 monoclonal antibody
Barzolvolimab	Anti-KIT monoclonal antibody

SUMMARY

This chapter offers an extensive overview of skin allergies, focusing on *atopic dermatitis (AD) and chronic urticaria*, both of which significantly impact pediatric and adolescent quality of life. AD is described as a chronic, relapsing, inflammatory skin disease with complex pathophysiology involving skin barrier dysfunction, type 2 inflammation, immune dysregulation, and microbiome imbalance. The chapter outlines age-specific patterns, diagnostic criteria (Hanifin and Rajka), and severity scoring systems such as SCORAD. Management is structured stepwise, with emphasis on non-pharmacologic care (moisturizers, trigger avoidance, and skin care), topical agents (steroids, calcineurin inhibitors, and JAK inhibitors), systemic therapies (immunosuppressants, biologics such as dupilumab), and emerging pharmacologic strategies. Chronic urticaria is discussed in detail, including classification (acute, chronic spontaneous, and chronic inducible), diagnostic approach, and modern treatment guided by UAS7 and UCT scoring. The chapter bridges global guidelines and Indian-specific nuances, making it a vital resource for practitioners managing pediatric skin allergies.

Key Learning Points

- *Atopic dermatitis is driven by skin barrier defects and type 2 inflammation*, with IL-4, IL-13, and IL-31 playing key roles; filaggrin dysfunction is central to pathogenesis.
- *SCORAD is a validated tool* to assess AD severity and guide treatment steps, from emollients to systemic immunosuppressants or biologics such as dupilumab.
- *Topical corticosteroids and calcineurin inhibitors remain first-line pharmacotherapies*, while newer options such as PDE-4 inhibitors, JAK inhibitors, and phototherapy enhance individualized care.
- *Chronic urticaria is categorized as spontaneous or inducible*, with antihistamines being first-line therapy, and escalation to omalizumab or cyclosporine for refractory cases.
- *Monitoring tools such as UAS7 and UCT* provide practical frameworks to assess control and adjust therapy, reinforcing a treat-to-target approach in urticaria management.

SUGGESTED READING

1. Bracken SJ, Abraham S, MacLeod AS. Autoimmune Theories of Chronic Spontaneous Urticaria. Front Immunol. 2019;10:627.
2. Can P, Salman A, Hosgören-Tekin S, Kocatürk E. Effectiveness of Omalizumab in patients with chronic inducible Urticaria: real-life experience from two UCARE centres. J Eur Acad Dermatol Venereol. 2021;35(10):e679-82.
3. Donnelly J, Ridge K, O'Donovan R, Conlon N, Dunne PJ. Psychosocial factors and chronic spontaneous urticaria: a systematic review. BMC Psychol. 2023;11(1):239.
4. Giavina-Bianchi M, Giavina-Bianchi P. Systemic Treatment for Severe Atopic Dermatitis. Arch Immunol Ther Exp (Warsz). 2019;67(2):69-78.
5. Irvine AD, Mina-Osorio P. Disease trajectories in childhood atopic dermatitis: an update and practitioner's guide. Br J Dermatol. 2019; 181(5):895-906.
6. Kolkhir P, Fok JS, Kocatürk E, Li PH, Okas TL, Marcelino J, et al. Update on the Treatment of Chronic Spontaneous Urticaria. Drugs. 2025;85(4):475-86.
7. Magerl M, Altrichter S, Borzova E, Giménez-Arnau A, Grattan CE, Lawlor F, et al. The definition, diagnostic testing, and management of chronic inducible urticarias - the EAACI/GA2LEN/EDF/UNEV consensus recommendations 2016 update and revision. J Allergy Clin Immunol. 2016; 71(6):780-802.
8. Moreno A, Renert-Yuval Y, Guttman-Yassky E. Shedding light on key pharmacological knowledge and strategies for pediatric atopic dermatitis. Expert Rev Clin Pharmacol. 2023;16(2):119-31.
9. Muñoz M, Kiefer LA, Pereira MP, Bizjak M, Maurer M. New insights into chronic inducible urticaria. Curr Allergy Asthma Rep. 2024;24(8):457-69.
10. Paller AS, Siegfried EC, Simpson EL, Cork MJ, Sidbury R, Chen IH, et al. Dupilumab safety and efficacy up to 1 year in children aged 6 months to 5 years with atopic dermatitis: results from a phase 3 open-label extension study. Am J Clin Dermatol. 2024;14:655-68.
11. Terhorst-Molawi D, Fox L, Siebenhaar F, Metz M, Maurer M. Stepping Down Treatment in Chronic Spontaneous Urticaria: What We Know and What We Don't Know. Am J Clin Dermatol. 2023; 24(3):397-404.
12. Tsai SY, Gaffin JM, Hawryluk EB, Ruran HB, Bartnikas LM, Oyoshi MK, et al. Evaluation of dupilumab on the disease burden in children and adolescents with atopic dermatitis: A population-based cohort study. Allergy. 2024;79(10):2748-58.
13. Weidinger S, Simpson EL, Silverberg JI, Barbarot S, Eckert L, Mina-Osorio P, et al. Burden of atopic dermatitis in pediatric patients: an international cross-sectional study. Br J Dermatol. 2024;190(6):846-57.
14. Wollenberg A, Barbarot S, Bieber T, Christen-Zaech S, Deleuran M, Fink-Wagner A, et al. Consensus-based European guidelines for treatment of atopic eczema (atopic dermatitis) in adults and children: part I. J Eur Acad Dermatol Venereol. 2018;32(5):657-82.
15. Yosipovitch G, Biazus Soares G, Mahmoud O. Current and Emerging Therapies for Chronic Spontaneous Urticaria: A Narrative Review. Dermatol Ther (Heidelb). 2023;13(8):1647-60.
16. Zuberbier T, Abdul Latiff AH, Abuzakouk M, Aquilina S, Asero R, Baker D, et al. The international EAACI/GA2LEN/EuroGuiDerm/APAAACI guideline for the definition, classification, diagnosis, and management of urticaria. Allergy: European. J Allergy Clin Immunol. 2022;77(3):734-66.

CHAPTER

11

Allergy Management in Special Populations

Nandana Bala
Reviewer: *D Rama Rajyam*

INTRODUCTION

Allergic diseases represent a rapidly growing global health burden and special attention is warranted for vulnerable groups such as infants, pregnant women, and the elderly. Each of these populations has distinct immunological and physiological characteristics that complicate allergy care. Infants have immature, rapidly evolving immune systems and may exhibit subtle or atypical allergy symptoms, which can challenge standard diagnostic testing and limit therapeutic options. Pregnant women, who are in a unique immunological state, undergo pronounced Th1/Th2 balance shifts and myriad physiologic adaptations (e.g., expanded blood volume, altered enzyme activity); allergy treatments must, therefore, balance maternal benefit against fetal safety, with adjusted dosing and careful drug selection. Older adults face immunosenescence—age-related immune dysregulation—along with multimorbidity and polypharmacy, all of which can mask allergic manifestations and heighten the risk of adverse drug interactions. These differences underscore the importance of tailored management strategies that account for developmental and age-related immune function, organ system physiology, and pharmacokinetic constraints in order to optimize efficacy and safety for each group. **Table 1** summarizes salient features, special precautions, and important differences in allergy management in the different populations of patients.

PEDIATRICS: DIAGNOSIS AND TREATMENT CHALLENGES IN INFANTS AND TODDLERS

Allergic diseases in infants and toddlers present unique diagnostic and management challenges due to non-specific clinical symptoms and limitations in available diagnostic tools and treatment options. Food allergies, atopic dermatitis, allergic rhinitis, and asthma can manifest differently in young children, complicating early recognition and treatment.

The first years of life are critical for immune system development, during which genetic, environmental, and dietary factors influence allergic disease susceptibility. The "atopic march" describes the progression from atopic dermatitis and food allergy to allergic rhinitis and asthma, with early intervention potentially altering disease trajectory.

Challenges in Diagnosis

Atypical Presentations

Key challenges include:

- *Overlapping symptoms with other conditions like infections:* Food allergy and eosinophilic gastrointestinal disorders (EGIDs) can mimic gastroesophageal reflux disease (GERD) or viral gastroenteritis.
- *Subclinical sensitization:* Infants too may exhibit immunoglobulin E (IgE) sensitization without clinical symptoms, complicating diagnosis.

TABLE 1: Allergy management in special populations—summary of salient points.

Population category	*Infants*	*Adults*	*Elderly*	*Pregnancy*
Common clinical manifestation	• Atopic dermatitis, food allergies (e.g., cow's milk and egg) • GI symptoms common • Wheezing, allergic rhinitis developing later	• Allergic rhinitis, asthma, and atopic dermatitis • Environmental allergies common • More defined symptomatology	• Often non-specific symptoms • Higher incidence of drug allergies and contact dermatitis	• Symptoms may worsen or improve • Asthma may fluctuate • Nasal congestion common due to hormonal changes
Investigation	• Skin prick test (interpret with caution due to reduced skin reactivity) • Serum-specific IgE can be useful adjunct • Food challenge under careful supervision in select cases	• Skin prick test, serum-specific IgE and patch testing • Pulmonary function tests	• Serum IgE may decline with age • Skin tests less reliable • Evaluate for polypharmacy and comorbidities	• Skin tests often avoided • Prefer serum-specific IgE if needed • Lung function testing—spirometry with caution
Diagnosis	• Based on clinical history, elimination diets, and tests • Parental history important	• Clinical history + testing correlation • Clear symptom patterns assist diagnosis	• Diagnosis may be delayed/missed • Consider age-related immune changes and mimic conditions	• Careful history important • Avoid provocative testing unless essential • Diagnosis should guide safe management
Management	• Allergen avoidance • Nutritional support crucial with food allergies • Limited use of medications	• Allergen avoidance, pharmacotherapy (antihistamines and corticosteroids) • Immunotherapy (SCIT/SLIT) options	• Cautious use of medications (drug interactions) • Emphasize topical over systemic treatments • Manage comorbidities	• Avoid teratogenic drugs (e.g., decongestants in first trimester) • Prefer non-pharmacologic options • Inhaled corticosteroids safe • Immunotherapy not to be initiated but maintenance can be continued

(IgE: immunoglobulin E; SCIT: subcutaneous immunotherapy; SLIT: sublingual immunotherapy)

Limitations of Current Diagnostic Tools

Skin prick test and specific immunoglobulin E:

- *Skin prick test (SPT):* Sensitivity is lower in infants due to immature mast cells and reduced histamine reactivity.
- *Specific IgE (sIgE):* High rates of false positives, particularly in children with atopic dermatitis.

Oral food challenge: The gold standard for food allergy diagnosis but is not commonly performed in young children due to risks of anaphylaxis and difficulty interpreting non-verbal distress in infants.

Atopy patch test: Used for non-IgE-mediated allergies (e.g., FPIES, eosinophilic esophagitis) but lacks standardization and reproducibility.

Newer and emerging diagnostics:

- *Component-resolved diagnostics (CRD):* Distinguishes between true allergy and cross-reactivity (e.g., Ara h 2 for peanut allergy).
- *Basophil activation test (BAT):* Measures functional allergen response but is not widely available.
- *Microbiome and metabolomic markers:* Potential early indicators of allergy risk, though still in research phases.

Challenges in Treatment

Early Allergen Introduction versus Avoidance

- *Food allergies:*
  - The LEAP and EAT studies demonstrated that early peanut and egg introduction reduces allergy risk.
  - Implementation remains challenging due to parental concerns and variability in healthcare provider recommendations.
- *Environmental allergens:* Reducing exposure to dust mites, pet dander, and air pollution is advised, but effectiveness remains inconclusive.

Pharmacologic Challenges

- *Antihistamines:* Second-generation options (cetirizine and loratadine) are safer than first-generation agents, but infant safety data are limited. None of the second-generation antihistamines are licensed below the age of 6 months.
- *Corticosteroids:* Topical corticosteroids remain first-line therapy for atopic dermatitis but are underused due to steroid phobia. Inhaled corticosteroids (ICS) for early wheezing may not prevent asthma. Intranasal corticosteroids such as mometasone and fluticasone furoate are only licensed above the age of 2 years.
- *Biologics:* Dupilumab (IL-4/IL-13 inhibitor) is approved for severe atopic dermatitis in infants ≥6 months. Its use is limited by the availability and cost, particularly in India.

Omalizumab and anti-IL-5 biologics are being explored for early asthma and food allergy intervention. Omalizumab is approved by Food and Drug Administration (FDA) for the reduction of allergic reaction including anaphylaxis that may occur with an accidental exposure in one or more foods in adults and children aged 1 year and older with food allergy.

Immunotherapy in Young Children

- *Oral immunotherapy (OIT):* Effective for desensitization but associated with high rates of gastrointestinal side effects.
- *Sublingual immunotherapy (SLIT):* Recent studies suggest that early intervention with allergen immunotherapy (AIT) may alter the natural course of allergic diseases. SLIT has gained attention due to its non-invasive nature and improved safety profile compared to subcutaneous immunotherapy (SCIT). Clinical trials indicate that SLIT can reduce allergic symptoms and medication use in young children, potentially preventing progression to asthma. However, large-scale studies are needed to confirm these findings.

Safety concerns are a primary reason for hesitancy in prescribing AIT to very young children. Although SLIT has a favorable safety profile, minor adverse effects such as oral pruritus and gastrointestinal symptoms are common. SCIT, while effective, poses a higher risk of systemic reactions, making it less suitable for this age group. Careful patient selection and adherence to treatment protocols are crucial to minimizing risks.

The immature immune system of children <5 years may influence AIT outcomes. Early exposure to allergens through AIT may promote immune tolerance, yet the optimal timing remains uncertain. Studies suggest that earlier intervention might prevent allergic march progression, but further research is needed to establish standardized guidelines.

Future Directions and Conclusion

Advances in allergen-specific diagnostics, machine learning-based prediction models, and microbiome-targeted therapies offer promising avenues for improving early allergy identification. Future strategies may include personalized immunotherapy approaches, incorporating biologics, and immune-modulating interventions to prevent disease progression.

A multidisciplinary approach involving professionals such as allergists, pediatricians, and dietitians is essential to optimize outcomes in allergic infants and toddlers. Ongoing research into immune tolerance induction and gut microbiome interventions may further reshape early allergy management.

CLINICAL PROTOCOL SUMMARY: DIAGNOSIS AND MANAGEMENT OF ALLERGIES IN INFANTS AND TODDLERS

Allergic diseases in infants and toddlers, including food allergies, atopic dermatitis, allergic rhinitis, and asthma present diagnostic and therapeutic challenges due to immune system immaturity and non-specific symptomatology. This protocol outlines a systematic approach for evaluating and managing allergic conditions in this age group based on current evidence and clinical guidelines.

Diagnostic Approach

Clinical History and Risk Assessment

- *Family history* of atopy (e.g., asthma, allergic rhinitis, eczema, food allergies).
- *Perinatal factors:* Mode of delivery (C-section vs. vaginal birth), antibiotic exposure, and feeding history (breastfeeding vs. formula)
- *Symptoms and triggers:*
    - *Skin:* Eczema, urticaria, and flushing
    - *Respiratory:* Recurrent wheezing, chronic cough, sneezing, and rhinorrhea
    - *Gastrointestinal:* Vomiting, diarrhea, feeding intolerance, and failure to thrive
    - *Anaphylaxis symptoms:* Acute respiratory distress, hypotonia, and loss of consciousness

Diagnostic Tests

Skin prick testing and specific immunoglobulin E:

- Performed for *suspected IgE-mediated allergies*
- *Interpretation:*
    - Positive SPT (≥3 mm wheal) or elevated sIgE levels suggest sensitization but not necessarily clinical allergy
    - Requires correlation with clinical symptoms.

Oral food challenge:

- *Gold standard* for food allergy diagnosis, particularly for non-IgE-mediated reactions. Done in carefully selected cases. *Not performed if the diagnosis is clinically certain.*
- Conducted in a controlled setting with emergency preparedness.

Emerging tests:

- *Component-resolved diagnostics,* e.g., for peanut, milk, egg allergies
- *Basophil activation test (BAT)* (research use)

Management Strategies

Food Allergy Management

- *Early introduction* of allergenic foods (e.g., peanut, egg) in high-risk infants per LEAP/EAT study guidelines.
- *Avoidance* only if clinically necessary; ensure nutritional adequacy with dietitian support.
    - *Acute reactions:* Epinephrine auto-injector prescription for IgE-mediated food allergy.
- *Chronic management:* Education of the family, allergy action plan. Antihistamines for mild symptoms, oral immunotherapy (OIT) under specialist care in select cases.

Atopic Dermatitis Management

- *First-line:* Regular emollients and topical corticosteroids (low-to-medium potency)
- *Second-line:* Calcineurin inhibitors (tacrolimus, pimecrolimus) for steroid-sparing effect
- *Biologics:* Dupilumab for moderate-severe cases (≥6 months)

Allergic Rhinitis Management

- *Environmental control:* Dust mite, pet dander reduction—specific avoidance advise based on result of allergy test
- *Pharmacotherapy:* Second-generation antihistamines, intranasal corticosteroids if >2 years of age
- *Consider allergen immunotherapy* in selected cases (under expert supervision only)

Asthma and Wheezing Management

- *Early wheezing:* Trial of ICS for up to 3 months if persistent symptoms.
- *Stepwise approach per GINA guidelines:*
    - *Intermittent symptoms:* Short-acting beta-agonists (SABA)
    - *Frequent wheezing:* Low-dose ICS
    - *Severe cases:* Consider biologics (omalizumab and mepolizumab).

Conclusion

This protocol provides a brief summary of an evidence-based approach for diagnosing and managing allergic diseases in infants and toddlers.

ALLERGY PREVENTION IN INFANTS: STRATEGIES AND RECOMMENDATIONS

Allergic diseases, including food allergies, eczema, asthma, and allergic rhinitis are increasing worldwide. Early-life interventions play a crucial role in reducing the risk of allergy development in infants, particularly in those with a family history of atopic diseases.

Key Strategies for Allergy Prevention

Maternal Diet and Pregnancy Considerations

- No evidence supports avoiding allergenic foods (e.g., nuts, eggs, dairy) during pregnancy to prevent allergies.
- A *balanced diet* rich in omega-3 fatty acids, fruits, and vegetables may support a healthy immune system.
- Probiotic supplementation during pregnancy may help reduce the risk of *eczema* in high-risk infants.

Breastfeeding and Infant Nutrition

- Exclusive *breastfeeding for at least 4–6 months* is recommended to support immune system development.
- If breastfeeding is not possible, hydrolyzed formulas may be considered in high-risk infants, though benefits remain uncertain.

- *Early introduction of allergenic foods* (e.g., peanuts, eggs) between *4 and 6 months* can reduce the risk of food allergies, as supported by the *LEAP and EAT studies.*

Microbiome and Gut Health

- A diverse gut microbiome plays a role in immune tolerance.
- *Probiotics and prebiotics* (via diet or supplementation) may help modulate immune responses, particularly in infants with a family history of allergies.

Environmental Considerations

- *Avoidance of smoking* and secondhand smoke exposure is crucial in reducing asthma and allergic sensitization.
- *Pet exposure:* Early exposure to pets may reduce the risk of allergic rhinitis but should be considered on a case-by-case basis.
- *Household allergen control* (e.g., reducing dust mites) may be beneficial for infants at high risk of allergic disease.

Immunomodulation and Future Directions

- Emerging research supports the role of biologics and immune-modulating therapies in high-risk infants.
- Ongoing studies explore the impact of prebiotics and probiotics, early vitamin D supplementation in allergy prevention.

Conclusion

Preventing allergies in infants requires a *multi-faceted approach* that includes proper nutrition, microbiome support, and environmental modifications. Early interventions, particularly *breastfeeding and timely introduction of allergenic foods*, can help reduce the incidence of allergic diseases. Further research continues to refine strategies for personalized allergy prevention.

SPECIAL CONSIDERATIONS IN ALLERGY MANAGEMENT IN GERIATRICS: IMMUNE AGING AND MODIFIED TREATMENT APPROACHES

As the global population ages, allergic diseases in older adults are becoming an increasing concern. While allergies are often considered a condition of childhood and young adulthood, they persist or even develop de novo in geriatric patients. Managing allergies in this population requires a nuanced approach due to age-related changes in the immune system (immunosenescence), polypharmacy, and comorbid conditions.

Immune Aging and Allergy in Older Adults

Aging affects both innate and adaptive immunity, leading to a phenomenon known as immunosenescence. Key aspects of immune aging that impact allergic conditions include:

- *Reduced immune responsiveness:* With age, the immune system becomes less effective at mounting strong allergic reactions, leading to atypical presentations of allergic diseases.
- *Altered T-cell function:* A decline in naive T-cells and a shift toward memory T-cells can modify the response to allergens, often resulting in decreased hypersensitivity but increased susceptibility to chronic inflammation.
- *Increased regulatory T-cell activity:* This can blunt allergic responses, making conditions such as allergic rhinitis less prominent but increasing the risk of non-IgE-mediated hypersensitivity reactions.
- *Changes in mast cells and basophils:* These cells become less responsive in some cases, altering the manifestation of anaphylaxis or urticaria.
- *Reduced mucosal barrier integrity:* Aging compromises the epithelial barriers in the skin, lungs, and gut, increasing susceptibility to allergens and irritants.

Common Allergic Conditions in the Elderly

- *Allergic rhinitis:* Symptoms may be less pronounced due to reduced histamine release but can still cause nasal congestion and postnasal drip.
- *Asthma:* Late-onset asthma is more likely to be non-atopic and difficult to distinguish from chronic obstructive pulmonary disease (COPD).
- *Drug allergies:* Polypharmacy increases the risk of drug hypersensitivity, often presenting as delayed reactions rather than immediate anaphylaxis.
- *Food allergies:* Newly developed food allergies, especially to seafood and nuts, can be severe in older adults.
- *Contact dermatitis:* Due to thinning skin and increased use of topical medications, elderly patients are prone to allergic contact dermatitis.

Diagnostic Challenges

- *Atypical presentations:* Elderly patients may have muted symptoms, leading to underdiagnosis or misdiagnosis.
- *Comorbidities:* Conditions such as COPD, heart disease, and cognitive decline complicate diagnosis.
- *Reduced skin reactivity:* Skin prick tests may yield false-negative results due to decreased skin mast cell activity.

Modified Treatment Approaches

- *Pharmacologic therapy adjustments:*
    - *Antihistamines:* Second-generation antihistamines (e.g., loratadine, cetirizine) are preferred due to a lower risk of sedation and cognitive impairment.
    - *Corticosteroids:* Intranasal and inhaled steroids should be used cautiously to prevent osteoporosis and adrenal suppression.
    - *Leukotriene receptor antagonists:* Can be an add on therapy in asthma and allergic rhinitis in older adults.
- *Immunotherapy:*
    - Allergy shots (SCIT) and SLIT can be effective but require careful consideration due to potential cardiovascular risks.
    - Sublingual immunotherapy may be preferable due to a lower risk of systemic reactions.
- *Lifestyle and environmental modifications:*
    - *Air quality management:* Use of air purifiers and avoidance of smoke exposure to prevent exacerbation of respiratory allergies.
    - *Dietary adjustments:* Identifying and eliminating food allergens with the help of a nutritionist.
    - *Skin care regimen:* Using hypoallergenic and fragrance-free products to reduce contact dermatitis risk.
- *Patient education and monitoring:*
    - Older adults should be educated on recognizing atypical allergy symptoms.
    - Regular medication reviews to avoid drug interactions and polypharmacy-related complications.
    - Close monitoring for adverse effects of long-term corticosteroid or immunotherapy use.

Conclusion

Managing allergies in geriatric patients presents unique challenges due to immune aging, comorbidities, and medication interactions. A tailored approach that includes careful diagnosis, modified pharmacologic therapy, and lifestyle modifications can significantly improve quality of life. As the elderly population grows, further research is needed to refine best practices for allergy management in this vulnerable group.

SPECIAL CONSIDERATIONS IN ALLERGY MANAGEMENT IN PREGNANCY: SAFE MEDICATIONS AND FETAL RISK CONSIDERATIONS

Pregnancy introduces unique challenges in the management of allergic diseases due to physiological changes, potential risks to fetal development, and limited safety data for many medications. Allergic conditions such as asthma, allergic rhinitis, and urticaria must be carefully managed to ensure maternal well-being while minimizing fetal risks. This chapter discusses the special considerations in allergy management during pregnancy, emphasizing safe medications and fetal risk considerations.

Physiological Changes in Pregnancy and Their Impact on Allergic Conditions

Pregnancy alters immune function, respiratory physiology, and hormonal balance, which can influence allergic diseases:

- *Immune modulation:* Pregnancy shifts the immune response toward a Th2-dominant state, potentially exacerbating IgE-mediated allergic diseases such as asthma and allergic rhinitis.
- *Increased mucosal congestion:* Higher estrogen levels contribute to nasal congestion, often mimicking or worsening allergic rhinitis.
- *Respiratory changes:* Reduced functional residual lung capacity and increased oxygen demand can impact asthma control.

Allergy diagnosis during pregnancy requires a careful and individualized approach to ensure both maternal and fetal safety. While the physiological changes of pregnancy can influence immune responses, existing allergic conditions such as asthma, rhinitis, or food allergies often persist or may fluctuate. The diagnostic process primarily relies on a thorough clinical history and physical examination. Specific IgE blood tests may be considered. Skin testing is generally deferred unless essential, due to potential systemic reaction. Overall, non-invasive methods and conservative evaluation are preferred during pregnancy, with the emphasis on avoiding allergen exposure and optimizing symptom control using the safest available treatments. Spirometry can generally be performed safely in pregnancy.

Common Allergic Conditions in Pregnancy and Their Management

Asthma

- Uncontrolled asthma increases the risk of maternal and fetal complications, including preterm birth and low birth weight.
- *Preferred medications:*
  - *Inhaled corticosteroids:* Budesonide is the preferred ICS due to its extensive safety data.
  - *Short-acting beta agonists (SABAs):* Albuterol (salbutamol) is considered safe for quick relief.
  - *Long-acting beta agonists (LABAs):* Used only when necessary and always in combination with ICS.

Allergic Rhinitis

- Symptoms can worsen due to pregnancy-induced nasal congestion.
- *Safe treatments:*
  - *Intranasal corticosteroids:* Budesonide and fluticasone are preferred options.
  - *Antihistamines:* Second-generation antihistamines such as loratadine and cetirizine are preferred due to lower sedative effects and better safety profiles.
  - *Saline nasal irrigation:* A safe non-pharmacologic option to reduce nasal congestion.

Urticaria and Anaphylaxis

- Pregnancy can exacerbate chronic urticaria or lead to increased mast cell activation.
- *Safe treatments:*
    - *Antihistamines:* Loratadine and cetirizine are preferred over first-generation options such as diphenhydramine, which may cause sedation.
    - *Epinephrine:* In cases of anaphylaxis, intramuscular epinephrine remains the treatment of choice as the benefits outweigh the risks.

Fetal Risk Considerations in Allergy Medications

When prescribing medications for allergic conditions in pregnancy, safety categories, and fetal risks should be carefully evaluated:

- *Antihistamines:*
    - *Safe:* Loratadine and cetirizine (Category B)
    - *Use with caution:* Diphenhydramine, chlorpheniramine (Category B but can cause sedation)
- *Inhaled corticosteroids:*
    - *Safe:* Budesonide (Category B, extensive safety data)
    - *Use with caution:* Fluticasone, beclomethasone (Category C, less safety data but generally considered low risk)
- *Decongestants:*
    - *Avoid:* Pseudoephedrine, phenylephrine (associated with fetal malformations and placental insufficiency, especially in the first trimester)
- *Leukotriene receptor antagonists:*
    - *Use with caution:* Montelukast (limited safety data, used when benefits outweigh risks)
- *Epinephrine:*
    - *Essential for anaphylaxis:* No absolute contraindication during pregnancy, as untreated anaphylaxis poses a greater risk to both mother and fetus.

Non-pharmacologic Strategies for Allergy Management in Pregnancy

- *Environmental control:* Reducing allergen exposure by using air purifiers, avoiding pet dander, and practicing dust mite control.
- *Dietary modifications:* Avoiding known food allergens while maintaining proper nutrition.
- *Nasal irrigation:* Using saline sprays or rinses to relieve nasal symptoms naturally.
- *Breathing exercises and yoga:* Can help manage asthma symptoms and stress-related exacerbations.

Allergen Immunotherapy in Pregnancy

Allergen immunotherapy, delivered by either subcutaneous (SCIT) or sublingual (SLIT) routes, is generally considered safe for pregnant patients who have been on a stable maintenance dose before conception. Established AIT in pregnancy may help reduce symptoms of allergic rhinitis and asthma, potentially minimizing the need for systemic medications that carry unknown fetal risks. However, because of the possibility of systemic reactions—including anaphylaxis—even in small numbers, initiating AIT during pregnancy is discouraged. This practice is supported by several guidelines and reviews that emphasize the importance of maintaining a stable regimen rather than starting new therapy during gestation, with careful multidisciplinary oversight involving both allergists and obstetricians.

Use of Biologics in Pregnancy

The use of biologic agents for conditions such as severe allergic asthma or chronic urticaria during pregnancy is an evolving area. Omalizumab, the most extensively studied biologic in this setting, has been evaluated in registries such as the EXPECT study, where observational data have not demonstrated a significant increase in major congenital malformations or adverse pregnancy outcomes. Data on other newer biologics, such as dupilumab, mepolizumab, and benralizumab, are more limited; hence, treatment decisions should be individualized and guided by a careful risk-benefit analysis. In scenarios where disease control is otherwise compromised, and the maternal condition poses its own risks, a multidisciplinary approach is essential to optimize both maternal and fetal outcomes.

CONCLUSION

Managing allergic diseases in pregnancy requires a balance between symptom control and fetal safety. Many medications, including inhaled corticosteroids, second-generation antihistamines, and epinephrine are considered safe and necessary for maternal well-being. Non-pharmacologic interventions should also be emphasized to minimize medication use. Close monitoring and individualized treatment planning are essential to ensuring optimal outcomes for both mother and baby.

SUMMARY

Allergic diseases in special populations—infants, pregnant women, and the elderly—require tailored approaches due to differences in immune function, physiology, and treatment safety. Infants present with atypical symptoms and limited diagnostic accuracy, making early allergen introduction, nutritional support, and selective use of newer therapies important. In pregnancy, management must balance maternal benefit with fetal safety, using well-established safe medications and avoiding initiation of immunotherapy or teratogenic drugs. In the elderly, immunosenescence, comorbidities, and polypharmacy complicate care, requiring cautious pharmacologic choices and lifestyle modifications. Preventive measures and multidisciplinary, individualized care are central to optimizing outcomes across these vulnerable groups.

Key Learning Points

- *Infants and toddlers* present with atypical allergy symptoms, limited diagnostic accuracy, and restricted therapeutic options; early intervention, nutritional support, and emerging therapies like biologics and SLIT hold promise.
- *Pregnant women* require a balance between maternal benefit and fetal safety; inhaled corticosteroids (budesonide), second-generation antihistamines, and epinephrine are generally safe, while teratogenic drugs and new immunotherapy initiation must be avoided.
- *Older adults* face challenges of immunosenescence, multimorbidity, and polypharmacy, necessitating cautious pharmacologic choices, attention to drug interactions, and reliance on safer options like second-generation antihistamines and SLIT.
- *Preventive strategies* in infancy—such as exclusive breastfeeding, early allergen introduction (peanut, egg), maternal probiotics, and environmental control—can reduce the risk of allergic diseases.
- *A multidisciplinary, individualized approach* involving allergists, pediatricians, dietitians, and obstetricians is vital to ensure safe, effective, and patient-centered allergy management in these special populations.

SUGGESTED READING

1. Bakhireva LN, Schatz M, Jones KL, Chambers CD. Asthma medication use in pregnancy and fetal growth. J Allergy Clin Immunol. 2005;116(3):503-9.
2. Cork MJ, Danby SG, Vasilopoulos Y, Hadgraft J, Lane ME, Moustafa M, et al. Epidermal barrier dysfunction in atopic dermatitis. J Invest Dermatol. 2009;129(8):1892-908.
3. Du Toit G, Roberts G, Sayre PH, Bahnson HT, Radulovic S, Santos AF, et al. Randomized trial of peanut consumption in infants at risk for peanut allergy. N Engl J Med. 2015;372(9):803-13.
4. Fiocchi A, Dahdah L, Dupont C, Campoy C, Fierro V, Nieto A. Cow's milk allergy: towards an update of DRACMA guidelines. World Allergy Organ J. 2016;9:35.

5. Fujimura KE, Sitarik AR, Havstad S, Lin DL, Levan S, Fadrosh D, et al. Neonatal gut microbiota associates with childhood multisensitized atopy and T cell differentiation. Nat Med. 2016;22(10):1187-91.
6. Global Initiative for Asthma (GINA) (2024). Global Strategy for Asthma Management and Prevention, 2024 Update. [online] Available from: https://ginasthma.org/2024-gina-report/ [Last accessed August 2025]
7. Hemmings O, Kwok M, McKendry RT, Santos AF. Basophil activation test: old and new applications in allergy. Curr Allergy Asthma Rep. 2018;18(12):77.
8. Hill DJ, Heine RG, Hosking CS. The diagnostic value of skin prick testing in children with food allergy. Pediatr Allergy Immunol. 2004;15(5):435-41.
9. Källén B. Use of antihistamine drugs in early pregnancy and delivery outcome. J Matern Fetal Neonatal Med. 2002;11(3):146-52.
10. Lidholm J, Ballmer-Weber BK, Mari A, Vieths S. Component-resolved diagnostics in food allergy. Curr Opin Allergy Clin Immunol. 2006;6(3):234-40.
11. Murase JE, Heller MM, Butler DC. Safety of dermatologic medications in pregnancy and lactation: Part II. Lactation. J Am Acad Dermatol. 2014;70(3):417.e1-417.e10.
12. Namazy JA, Blais L, Andrews EB, Scheuerle AE, Cabana MD, Thorp JM, et al. Pregnancy outcomes in the omalizumab pregnancy registry and a disease-matched comparator cohort. J Allergy Clin Immunol. 2020;145(2):528-36.e1.
13. Namazy JA, Schatz M. Asthma and pregnancy: Part I. Physiology and risk assessment. J Allergy Clin Immunol Pract. 2014;2(1):1-10.
14. O'Byrne PM, Naji N, Gauvreau GM. Severe asthma: future treatments. Clin Exp Allergy. 2012;42(5):706-11.
15. Oykhman P, Kim HL, Ellis AK. Allergen immunotherapy in pregnancy. Allergy Asthma Clin Immunol. 2015;11:31.
16. Paller AS, Siegfried EC, Thaçi D, Wollenberg A, Cork MJ, Arkwright PD, et al. Efficacy and safety of dupilumab with concomitant topical corticosteroids in children 6 to 11 years old with severe atopic dermatitis. J Am Acad Dermatol. 2020;83(5):1282-93.
17. Perkin MR, Logan K, Tseng A, Raji B, Ayis S, Peacock J, et al. Randomized trial of introduction of allergenic foods in breast-fed infants. N Engl J Med. 2016;374(18):1733-43.
18. Pfaar O, Agache I, de Blay F, Bonini S, Chaker AM, Durham SR, et al. Recommendations for allergen immunotherapy in older adults: an EAACI position paper. Allergy. 2021;76(3):664-78.
19. Pfaller B, Agache I, Yepes-Nuñez JJ, Akdis CA, Bousquet J, Klimek L, et al. Biologicals in atopic disease in pregnancy: an EAACI position paper. Allergy. 2021;76(1):71-89.
20. Platts-Mills TA, Thomas WR, Aalberse RC, Vervloet D, Chapman MD. Dust mite allergens and asthma: report of a second international workshop. J Allergy Clin Immunol. 1992;89(5):1046-60.
21. Prenner BM. Role of long-acting beta2-adrenergic agonists in asthma management. Curr Opin Pulm Med. 2008;14(1):57-63.
22. Saito J, Arakawa H, Suwabe A, Matsui E, Seto Y, Morikawa A. Management of rhinitis and asthma in pregnancy. Curr Opin Pulm Med. 2003;9(1):31-6.
23. Shamji MH, Durham SR. Mechanisms of allergen immunotherapy for inhaled allergens and predictive biomarkers. J Allergy Clin Immunol. 2017;140(6):1485-98.
24. Sicherer SH, Sampson HA. Food allergy: A review and update on epidemiology, pathogenesis, diagnosis, prevention, and management. J Allergy Clin Immunol. 2018;141(1):41-58.
25. Simons FER. Advances in H1-antihistamines. N Engl J Med. 2004;351(21):2203-17.
26. Ventura MT, Scichilone N, Paganelli R, Minciullo PL, Patella V, Bonini M, et al. Allergic diseases in the elderly: biological characteristics and main immunological and non-immunological mechanisms. Clin Mol Allergy. 2017;15:2.
27. Vickery BP, Vereda A, Casale TB, Beyer K, du Toit G, Hourihane JO, et al. AR101 oral immunotherapy for peanut allergy. N Engl J Med. 2018;379(21):1991-2001.

CHAPTER

12

Environmental and Lifestyle Factors Affecting Allergy Management

Shebna A Khader
Reviewer: *Krishna Mohan R*

INTRODUCTION

Allergy is a multifactorial disease having genetic, epigenetic, and environmental factors which affects its phenotypic expression. The cause of rapid increase in allergy over last few years correlate well with the changes in environmental factors like pollution and global warming.

With increasing trend of pediatric allergy, it is essential to look into the environmental factors, its effects, and methods to control environmental triggers.

ENVIRONMENTAL CHANGES AND POLLUTION

Both outdoor and indoor pollution are emerging global issues associated with increased morbidity and mortality related to various illnesses, especially allergy. Global life expectancy, according to WHO, has been reduced by at least 1 year due to the effects of air pollution.

Let us see the indoor and outdoor changes that have contributed to increased environmental pollution. Pollutants can be primary or secondary. Primary pollutants are those emitted directly by human activity, while secondary pollutants are those formed when primary pollutants react in the atmosphere **(Box 1)**.

BOX 1: Changes in indoor and outdoor environment contributing pollutants.

- *Changes in residential environment:*
  - Treated wood for pest control
  - Chemicals in wallpaper
  - Modified paints
  - Adhesives, resin
  - Particle board
  - Cosmetic product
- *Changes in health and sanitation environment:*
  - Increased sanitation (hygiene hypothesis)
  - Increased use of chemicals
  - Pesticides
  - Insect repellents
  - Antimicrobial products
- *Change in food environment:*
  - Additives in food and containers
  - Coloring agent
  - Preservatives
- *Indoor pollutants:*
  - Construction material—Radon
  - Insulation—Asbestos
  - Furniture—CO, NO_2, CO_2, volatile organic compounds (VOC)
  - Air fresheners—Fluorocarbon
  - Cleaning liquid—VOC
  - Wood compounds—Formaldehyde
- *Outdoor pollution:*
  - *Primary pollutants:*
    - CO—Industrial combustion
    - SO_2—Fossil fuel use
  - *Secondary pollutants:*
    - NO_2—Industrial combustion
    - Vehicles
    - Ozone—Photochemical reaction of NO_2,VOC
  - *Primary and secondary pollutants:*
    - *Particulate matter:*
      - Power plant
      - Vehicle
      - Diesel exhaust particle (DEP)

MECHANISMS OF ACTION OF POLLUTANTS ON ALLERGY

Mechanism of action of pollutants is complex but can be divided as direct action on epithelium and immunity and also through indirect actions interfering with other pollutants.

Direct mechanism:

- *Low-to-moderate level exposure:*
  - Oxidative stress to bronchial cells
  - Activate T helper 2 (Th2) pathway
- *High-level exposure:*
  - Disrupt branchial epithelium
  - Trigger neutrophilic inflammation
  - Activate toll-like receptor (TLR), interleukin 1 (IL-1), IL-6, and IL-8

Indirect mechanism: Climate changes can increase the allergenicity of pollens along with prolongation of pollen season thereby increasing the pollen load. Particulate matter (PM) acts as an adjuvant to other allergens. Ozone and nitric oxide facilitate formation of protein dimers of increased allergenic potential.

EFFECTS ON CHILDHOOD ALLERGY

- *Childhood asthma:* Prenatal exposure to PM2.5 has been found to increase the incidence of asthma at 6 years of age. Increased exposure of NO_2, O_3, and PM2.5 at school and home also is associated with high incidence of respiratory allergies especially asthma.
- *Late-onset asthma:* Pollution triggers genetic, epigenetic, and immunologic changes resulting in high incidence of late-onset asthma in adolescents. PM2.5 and O_3 are found to be associated with asthma—COPD overlap. PM2.5, O_3, CO, SO_2, and NO_2 can precipitate asthma exacerbation on high-level exposure.
- *Allergic rhinitis:* Exposure to TRAP (traffic-related air pollution) during intrauterine period and infancy is significantly associated with allergic rhinitis. Short-term exposure to PM2.5, NO_2, and O_3 has increased the emergency visit for allergic rhinitis and chronic exposure is related to disease progression and severity.

  Pollution is having a multifactorial influence on allergic rhinitis by triggering immunoglobulin E (IgE)-mediated hypersensitivity oxidative. Oxidative stress, neurogenic-mediated mechanism, and immunomodulation. It indirectly affects the allergenicity of pollens and pollen load thereby triggering seasonal pollen-related symptoms.
- *Atopic dermatitis (AD):* Air pollution is linked both to the onset and severity of AD, PM, volatile organic compounds (VOC), gaseous compounds and heavy metals, when exposed in prenatal period and infancy are closely related to the disease progression of AD, by disrupting epithelial barrier and immune modulation.
- *Urticaria:* Short-term exposure to NO_2, O_3, PM2.5, and PM10 increases the risk of acute urticaria. Chronic exposure to PM has cumulative effect on chronic urticaria.
- *Food allergy:* Early-life exposure to high level of indoor and outdoor pollution increases the risk of food allergy in children and triggers allergy march. By causing epithelial damage, airway can act as a route of food sensitization.

NITROGEN DIOXIDE POLLUTION

Environmental NO_2 pollution is a potential driver for increased allergen prevalence and allergenicity.

Sources: Fossil fuel combustion:

- Car exhaust
- Power plant
- Fertilizer—Soil and water pollution

Mechanism of Action

- *Airborne:*
  - NO_2 exposure causes acute and chronic changes in lung function by increasing bronchial neutrophilic inflammation and proinflammatory cytokines.
  - Previous exposure to NO_2 increases response to subsequent allergy exposure.
  - It significantly impacts pollen activity by higher airborne pollen load, increasing

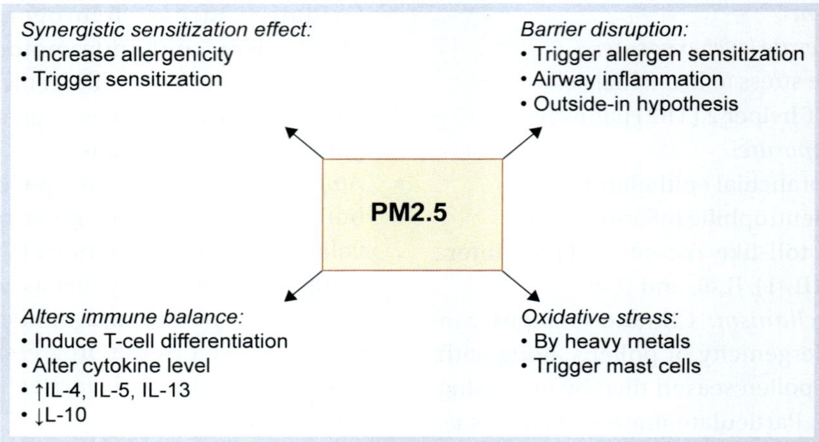

Fig. 1: Actions of PM2.5. (IL: interleukin)

fragmentation of allergenic proteins and promoting the attachment of pollutants on surface.

- *Soil and water pollution:*
    - Increase the pollen allergenicity
    - Wan et al. have observed that it affects composition of omega 5 gliadin which in turn triggers wheat allergy.

Effects

Changes in pollen along with airway mucosal irritation triggers sensitization and clinical symptoms of allergic rhinitis, allergic asthma, allergic conjunctivitis, and urticaria.

PARTICULATE MATTER 2.5

PM2.5, also known as fine particulate matter with aerodynamic diameters <2.5/μm, is characterized by small particulate size and prolonged suspension time. It is a complex mixture of biological components (polyaromatic hydrocarbon, NO_3, sulfate aluminum, and cadmium). Biological components increase the allergen sensitization, and non-biological components cause oxidative stress and immune interference.

Source

- *Outdoor:* Vehicle exhaust
    - Incineration
    - Coal combustion
- *Indoor:* Biomass combustion
    - Gas stoves

Mechanism (Fig. 1)

- Disrupts barrier function
- Increase oxidative stress
- Alters immune balance
- Synergistic sensitization effect

Effects

- High risk of asthma, allergic conjunctivitis urticaria, allergic rhinitis
- Long-term exposure trigger airway inflammation, hyperreactivity, and causes cutaneous inflammation

MEASURES TO MINIMIZE POLLUTION

World Health Organization studies have shown that life expectancy and quality of life is significantly affected by pollution. This stresses on the fact that it is the duty of every citizen to adopt measures that can minimize pollution. Government has to set air quality guideline and waste disposal guidelines for industries to prevent large scale pollution impact.

Some recommendations:

- Use particulate respirators or N95 mark in areas with high ambient air pollution.
- Choose travel route which can reduce pollution—electric vehicle, carpooling, public transport.
- Optimize driving style—drive with windows closed proper maintenance of vehicles.
- Exercise outdoor only with moderate intensity when air quality is poor.
- Maintain cross ventilation at home.
- Avoid usage of firewood, incense sticks, mosquito coils, room fresheners.
- Use air purifiers in areas with poor air quality.
- Proper monitoring of industries and strict adherence to government guidelines

Let us work together to provide clean air and water to our coming generation.

Figure 2 shows the various allergens and their interactions which leads to the clinical spectrum of allergy.

INDOOR ALLERGENS

Indoor allergens play an important role in allergy symptoms along with indoor pollution. Most common indoor allergens are house dust mite (HDM), fungus, and cockroach. This section deals with the preventive strategies for indoor allergen avoidance.

House Dust Mite

House dust mite is the most sensitized allergen across the globe. Dust mites are small arthropods 0.2–0.3 mm size with 72% total body weight being water. Lifespan is around 4–6 weeks. It is the dust mite fecal pellets which is allergenic. Dust mites feed on shed human skin cells. Dust mite fecal pellets contain food, debris, proteolytic enzymes with mucous enclosed in peritrophic membrane. On contact with moisture, peritrophic membrane breaks releasing proteolytic enzymes and allergens.

Favorable Factors	*Clinical Features*
• Warm humid climate • *Temperature:* 18°–27°C • *Relative humidity:* 68–85% • Maximum on mattress, pillow, upholstery, stuffed toys	• Perennial • Indoor • Night, early morning • *Inhalation:* Rhinitis, asthma • *Contact:* Eczema, urticaria • *Ingestion:* Oral allergy syndrome

Preventive Measures

- *Washing sheets:* Wash sheets, pillow covers, twice or once weekly with hot water >60°C. After washing, dry in sun or dryer with hot setting.
- Expose mattress, pillows to sun.
- Vacuum weekly with vacuum cleaner having HEPA filter.
- Remove carpet, soft toys, rugs.
- Maintain cross ventilation.
- Wet mopping and damp dusting preferred.
- Indirect sun exposure.
- Maintain relative humidity <50%.
- Prefer nonfabric upholstery, wood, or plastic furniture.
- *Storage mites:*
  - Store grains in air-tight container.
  - Store in cool dry area.
  - Clean cupboard by damp dusting.
- Dust mite proof encasing is extremely helpful although expensive:
  - Complete encasing of pillow, mattress
  - Tightly woven fabric of pore size <6 µm

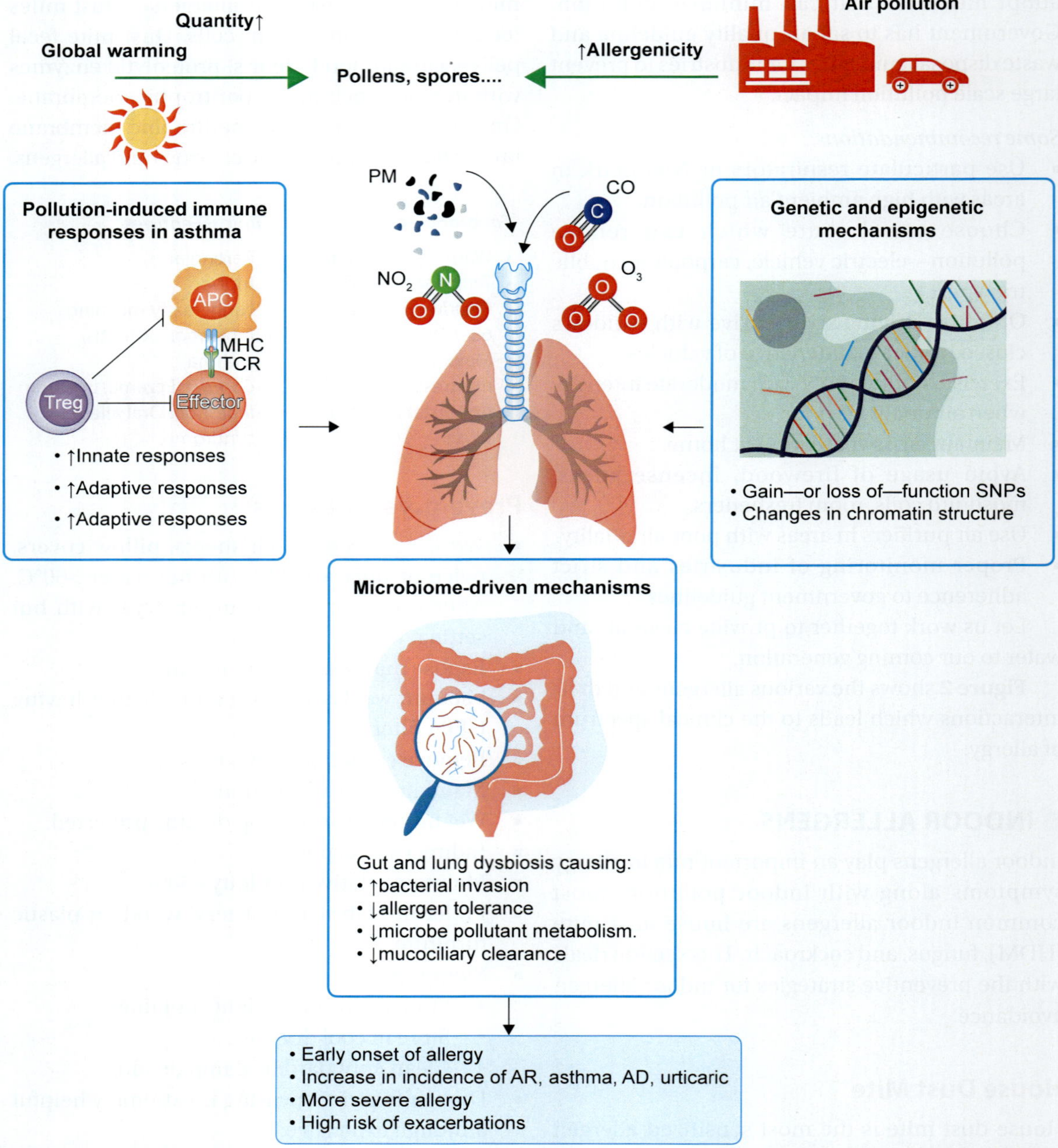

Fig. 2: Allergen interactions resulting in clinical spectrum of allergy. (AD: atopic dermatitis; AR: allergic rhinitis)

Molds

Molds are fungus usually seen in damp areas with its spores suspended in air. Molds can be indoor or outdoor. Indoor being more common. These include *Cladosporium*, *Penicillium*, *Aspergillus*, etc. Outdoor molds include *Alternaria*, *Cladosporium*, etc.

Favorable Factors	*Clinical Features*
• Warm humid environment • *Temperature:* 18°–20°C • Relative humidity >65% • Need organic matter to grow • Indoor mostly on wet ceiling, wallpaper	• Perennial with seasonal variation • Mostly indoor—wallpaper, water leaks • More in bathroom, kitchen, cupboards • Allergic rhinitis, itchy eyes • Cough, wheeze • Allergic fungal sinusitis • Allergic bronchopulmonary aspergillosis (ABPA)

Preventive Measures

- Maintain relative humidity <50%.
- Use of exhaust fan.
- Repair water leak.
- Maintain ventilation.
- Ensure proper maintenance of air conditioners.
- Hypochlorite denatures and kills molds.
- Avoid wallpaper and if severely infested, remove wallpaper, carpet, etc.
- Maintain indoor plants properly.
- Recycle old books and clothes.
- Dehumidifiers
- Antifungal paints

Cockroach

Cockroach allergy is very common in India. Main allergens are the fecal pellets, saliva, and its body parts. Size of the allergenic particle is around 10 μm and hence it is common to cause allergic rhinitis and allergic conjunctivitis symptoms.

Three common cockroach strains are:

1. *German cockroach (Blattella germanica):*
   a. Mainly indoor in urban areas.
2. *American cockroach (Periplanata americana):*
   a. Mainly in basements, godowns
3. *Oriental cockroach (Blatta orientalis):*
   a. Common in India
   b. Body parts are allergenic

Favorable Factors	*Clinical Features*
• Warm humid area • Darkness • Water leaks • Open food particles • Poor drainage system	• Perennial symptoms • Indoor symptoms • Allergic rhinitis • Allergic conjunctivitis • Asthma • Poorly controlled asthma • Symptoms more near drains

Preventive Measures

Integrated pest management:

- *Managing the source:*
  - Seal cracks and holes on exterior.
  - Seal windows and vents.
  - Judicious use of pesticides.
- *Managing favorable factors:*
  - Store food in sealed container.
  - Use closed dustbins.
  - Repair water leaks.
  - Have well-built drainage system.
- *Managing the reservoir:*
  - Cockroach trap on drains
  - Cockroach sticky traps in kitchen cupboards.
  - Remove clutter and cardboard carton.
- *Education and monitoring:* Abovementioned are the preventive measures against common aeroallergens, but as allergy being a multifactorial disease, it is important to look into other preventive measures which can modify the intrinsic factors like gut microbiota and the Th1/Th2 balance.

DIET AND GUT MICROBIOME

Prevalence of food allergy is increasing and has become a significant public health issue. Factors such as alteration in microbiota, lack of contact with microorganism, delayed introduction of foods, and more processed foods have played significant role in its pathogenesis.

Human Gut Microbiome

Our digestive tract is home to complex microbial ecosystem. Human gut microbiome is the most complex and diverse when compared to microbiota in other anatomic locations.

Diversity of microbiome is individual dependent. It is affected by environmental and epigenetic factors. The change in composition of microbiome (dysbiosis) is linked to the development of allergic diseases. The relation between gut microbiota and other organs is explained by lung–gut axis and skin–gut axis hypothesis. Microbial colonization begin in utero with 70% of primary colonization being maternal origin, The composition of gut microbiota changes throughout life with factors like age, diet, antibiotics, lifestyle, and environmental conditions **(Fig. 3)**.

Gut microbiota development during first years of life is related to maturation of immune system. Symbiotic relation of humans and microbes, especially certain strains of *Lactobacillus* and *Bifidobacterium*, provides nutritional benefits by increasing absorption of vitamins and minerals. It also reduces chance of lactose intolerance and increase resistance to infection. Microbiota under normal conditions stimulate thymic stromal lymphopoietin (TSLP) and transforming Growth Factor beta (TGF-beta) which promote tolerogenic antigen-presenting cells (APC) and stimulate T regulatory (Treg) cells.

Alterations in gut microbiota have been found to reduce levels of Treg cells and alter CD4 T cell. This is in turn associated with increased incidence of rhinitis, AD, asthma, and food allergy.

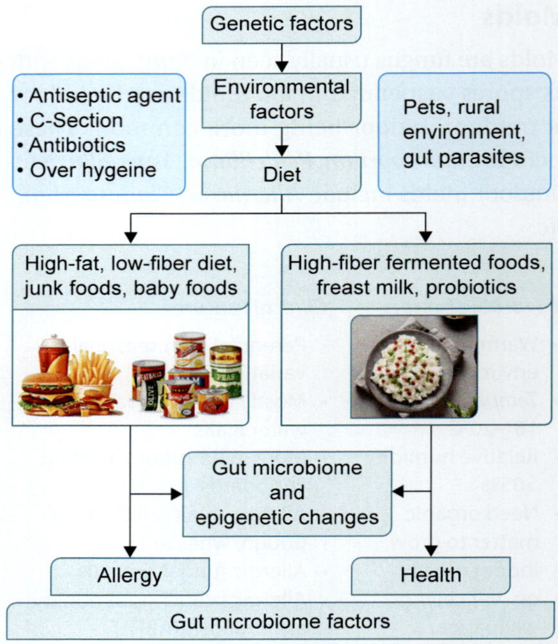

Fig. 3: Factors affecting gut microbiome.

Probiotics

Probiotics or beneficial bacteria are microorganisms which can regulate host's immune system and benefit host if sufficiently administered. Probiotics help to maintain balance between gut microbiota and immune system thereby increasing the chance of preventing allergy.

Mode of Action (Fig. 4)

- Inhibit bacterial adherence to mucosal layer.
- Repair and strengthen intestinal epithelial barrier.
- Maintain diversity of gut microbiota.
- Anti-inflammatory action
- Regulate dendritic cell activity.
- Promote secretion of TGF-beta and induce Treg cells.
- Restore Th1/Th2 cytokine balance.

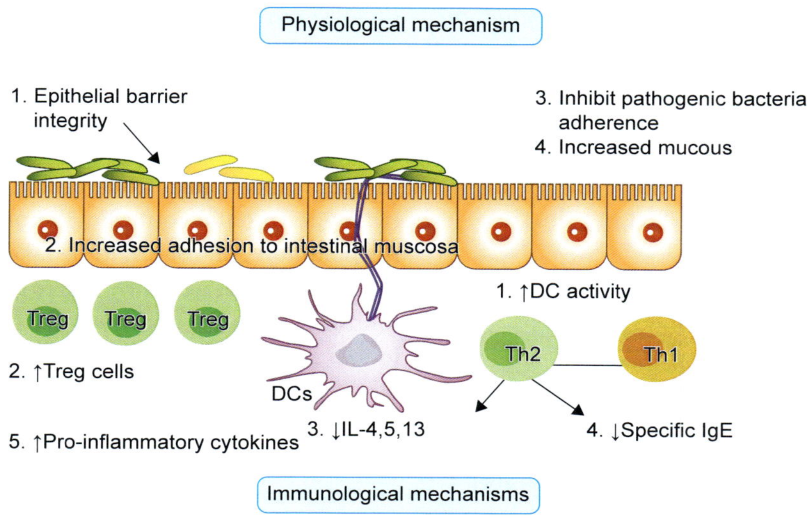

Fig. 4: Role of probiotics. (IL: interleukin; Th: T helper cell; Treg: T regulatory cell)

Clinical Significance

A lot of controlled trials have been conducted aiming on primary prevention of allergy. Role of probiotics have been well documented in some studies.

- Intervention of probiotics during pregnancy reduce the risk of eczema in infancy.
- Prenatal administration changes composition of vaginal microbiota, thereby affecting colonization of gut microbiota in infants.
- Probiotics in infancy reduce the chance of atopic eczema
- Probiotics in infants with milk allergy increase the chance of early oral tolerance to milk

World Allergy Organization has proposed use of probiotics in mothers during pregnancy and lactation, whose infants are prone to allergy and also in infants who are at risk of food allergy.

EARLY FOOD INTRODUCTION

Prevalence of food allergy has been on the rise in developed countries over last few years. The old recommendation of late introduction of possible allergenic foods has been reviewed by various trials.

The landmark LEAP study (Learning Earyl about Peanut), a randomized controlled study comparing early peanut introduction and avoidance until 65 years of age, indicated that 86% reduction in peanut allergy was noted by early introduction. EAT (Enquiring About Tolerance) study examined early introduction of six allergenic foods. Only randomized controlled trial (RCT) to use cooked egg-PETIT study (Prevention of Egg allergy with Tiny amount Intake Trial) in infants with eczema found reduction in egg allergy with early introduction SPADE study (Strategy for Prevention of milk Allergy by Daily ingestion of infant formula in Early infancy) studied introduction of cow's milk formula at 6 months of age and COMEET (Cow's Milk Early Exposure Trial) studies early continuous exposure. Both showed significant reduction in milk allergy.

Immunologically, it is based on "dual allergen exposure hypothesis", which explains need for oral tolerance to predominate before cutaneous sensitization. If early introduction is not followed by regular ingestion, it has been found to trigger allergen sensitization. Hence if regular intake is not feasible, it is better to avoid early introduction. The only adverse event noted on early introduction was increased incidence of FPIES, factors for that are under further study.

Guidelines for Early Introduction of Food in Infancy (AAAAI, ACAAI Guidelines)

Breastfeeding	• Exclusive breastfeeding till 4–6 months • Breastfeeding up to 2 years and beyond
Pregnant and breastfeeding mothers	Maternal exclusion of common allergens not recommended
Introduction of food allergens—All infants	• Peanut and cooked egg around 6 months not before 4 months • Do not delay introduction of allergenic foods beyond 6 months • New foods to be introduced on successive days
Continued intake	Continued intake recommended and is advised to add as regular diet at least few times a week
Cow's milk formula	Not advised [CSACI (Canadian Society of Allergy and Clinical Immunology) advises early introduction around 6 months up to 10 mL/day]

Screening with allergy testing before food introduction is not routinely recommended. Watchful observation of symptoms on introduction of new foods in a child with family history of atopy is recommended.

SUMMARY

With increasing prevalence of allergy over last few years, more focus has been given on primary prevention of allergy by avoidance of allergen triggers. Most important primary prevention measures being pollution control, human microbiota maintenance, and indoor pollution control. Even though new treatment modalities and molecules are being introduced, the pharmacological treatment, if not supported by environmental control, will not be successful. Air pollution control has to be taken as individual responsibility for a healthy newer generation. Early food introduction and lifestyle modification for indoor allergen has proven benefits if individualized based on clinical findings and requirements.

Key Learning Points

- Environmental control measures with trigger avoidance should supplement the pharmacologic management of allergy.
- Pollutants, especially PM2.5, NO_2, O_3 significantly impacts the sensitization, progression, and prognosis of allergy.
- Air pollution has not only direct effect, but also synergistic sensitization effect on respiratory allergies.
- Indoor allergen control measures, e.g., dust mite, cockroach, mold, has to be individualized based on the clinical findings and sensitization pattern.
- Human body microbiome is having a significant role in the prevention of allergy and microbiome maintenance is to be given more importance as primary prevention measurement.
- Early food introduction around 4–6 months of age followed by continued exposure of common allergens is an easy and practical way of inducing tolerance and preventing food allergy.

SUGGESTED READING

1. Abrams EM, Ben-Shoshan M, Protudjer JLP, Lavine E, Chan ES. Early Introduction is not enough: CSACI statement on the importance of ongoing regular ingestion as a means of food allergy prevention. Allergy Asthma Clin Immunol. 2023;19:63.
2. Burbank AJ, Peden DB. Assessing the impact of air pollution on childhood asthma morbidity: How, when and what to do. Curr Opin Allergy Clin Immunol. 2018;18(2):124-31.

3. Chan ES, Abrams EM, Mack DP, Protudjer JLP, Watson W. Primary prevention of food allergy: beyond early introduction. Allergy Asthma Clin Immunol. 2024;20:71.
4. Cipriani F, Calamelli E, Ricci G. Allergen avoidance in allergic asthma. Front Pediatr. 2017;5:103.
5. Kim BE, Hui-Beckman JW, Nevid MZ, Goleva E, Leung DYM. Air pollutants contribute to epithelial barrier dysfunction and allergic diseases. Ann Allergy Asthma Immunol. 2024;132;433-9.
6. Takano H, Inoue KI. Environment pollution and allergies. J Toxicol Pathol. 2017;30:193-9.
7. Wang X, Xu M, Xu M, Jia S, Xu W, Zhang W, et al. Mechanism of PM 2.5 induced/aggravated allergic diseases and its prevention and treatment. Allergy Med. 2004;2:100012.
8. Zubeldia-Varela E, Barker-Tejeda TC, Obeso D, Villaseñor A, Barber D, Pérez-Gordo M. Microbiome and Allergy: New Insights and Perspectives. J Investig Allergol Clin Immunol. 2022;32(5):327-44.
9. Zuiani C, Custovic A. Update on House Dust Mite Allergen Avoidance Measures for Asthma. Curr Allergy Asthma Rep. 2020;20(9):50.

CHAPTER

13

Allergy Prevention Strategies

Hima Mathews P

Reviewer: *Vinay Mehta*

INTRODUCTION

Atopic disease expression is a complex phenomenon influenced by a number of factors in a genetically predisposed individual. The steadily rising prevalence of allergic diseases is a matter of concern which has a great impact on public health as well as the quality of life of the affected individual. In an article by Annesi-Maesano et al. in World Allergy Organization (WAO) Journal stated that every second child born in 2050 will have allergy. Prevention strategies are crucial in reducing the burden of allergic diseases. With the significant rise in the prevalence of allergic diseases in the recent years worldwide, evidence-based prevention strategies are the need of the hour to address the new challenge.

LEVELS OF ALLERGY PREVENTION

Preventive strategies play a crucial role in the management of all diseases, in reducing the incidence, minimizing the impact of the disease and preventing long-term consequences. It has been divided into primordial, primary, secondary, and tertiary level depending on the natural course of the particular disease **(Fig. 1)**.

Pathophysiology of allergy is multifactorial and intervention programs should target every aspect of causative factors **(Fig. 2)**. Allergy prevention should target different groups, like normal population as well as high-risk population and it vary according to the type of allergic disease. Understanding of pathophysiology of allergic diseases are of utmost importance to

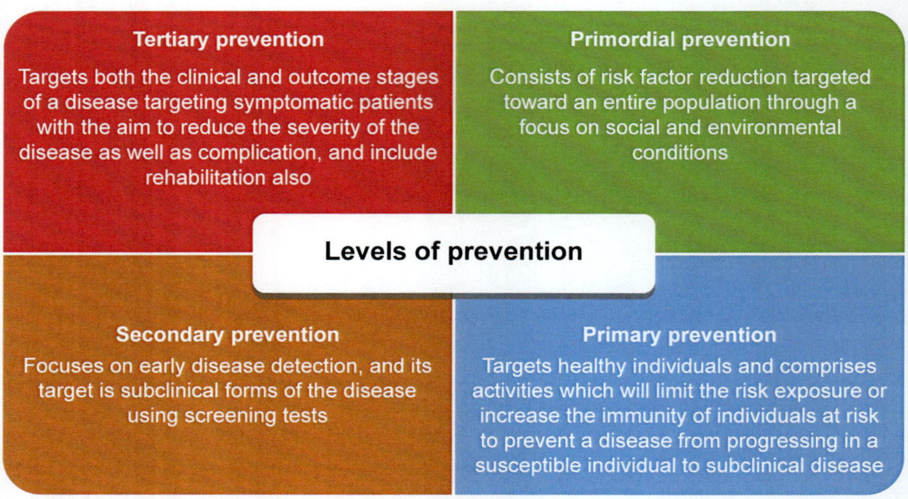

Fig. 1: Levels of prevention.

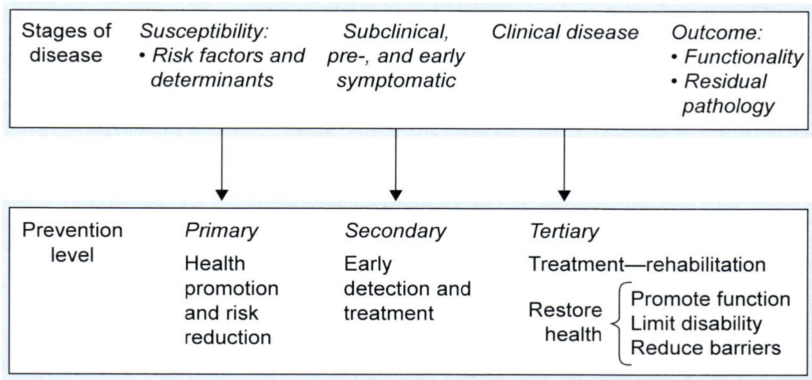

Fig 2: Relation between stage of the disease and preventive strategies.

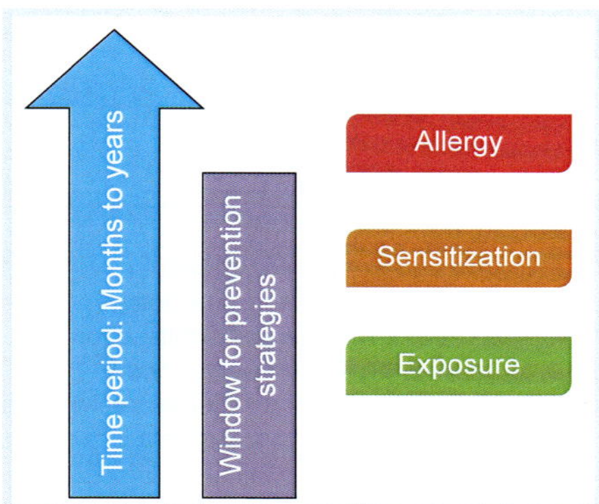

Fig. 3: Window of opportunity in allergy prevention.

decide the prevention measures **(Fig. 3)**. As in all other diseases, preventive strategies should include targeted measures divided into primary, secondary, and tertiary prevention. Only well-designed prospective studies of sufficient duration with well-defined criteria can add evidence-based prevention strategies.

There are numerous modifiable and non-modifiable risk factors associated with increased the risk of developing allergic disorders. Even though we do not have control over the genetic and familial factors, environmental and lifestyle factors can be modified **(Flowchart 1)**.

Early intervention programs in the field of allergy should target:

- Identification of infants having an increased risk of developing allergic disease
- Implementing prevention strategies in the children who are identified as being at high risk of developing allergic disease
- Measures to reduce the development of allergy in general population and hence to reduce the medical, social, and financial burden of the disease

PRIMARY PREVENTION OF ALLERGY

The ideal window of opportunity in allergy prevention strategies extends from the pregnancy period to 2 years of age. Early intervention in allergy depends mainly on the primary prevention strategies.

Pregnancy

Diet during Pregnancy

Avoidance of any particular food item in pregnancy is not recommended for the prevention of allergic disease. There is presently no evidence that avoidance of dietary allergens like egg, milk, and other foods during pregnancy can reduce the risk of allergic diseases. In fact nonnutritious

Flowchart 1: Role of early intervention programs in different aspect of pathophysiology of allergy.

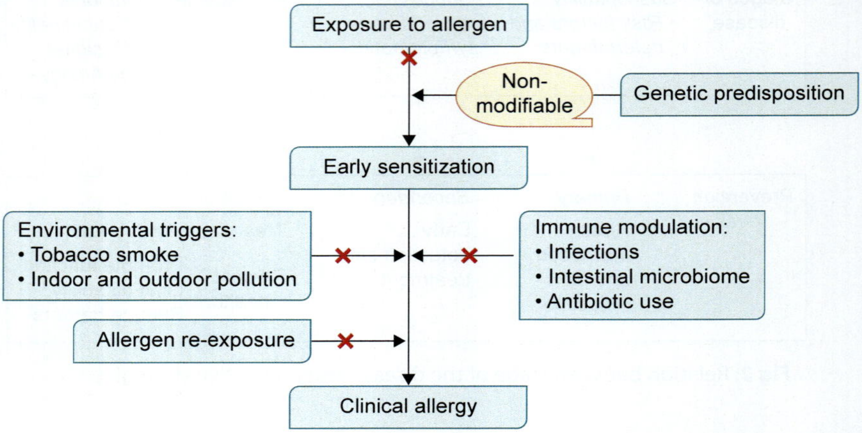

maternal diet carry the risk of preterm birth and result in lower-birth-weight babies. No special diet is recommended or dietary voidance is recommended. Pregnant mothers should consume a diverse and balanced healthy diet.

Smoking and Alcohol Consumption during Pregnancy

Maternal smoking during pregnancy is associated with the development of atopic dermatitis and food allergy in infants. There are studies which has shown association between pre- and postnatal tobacco exposure and recurrent wheezing in childhood as well as asthma. Tobacco exposure during pregnancy could increase the risk of allergy in offspring through multiple mechanisms including transgenerational epigenetic modification affecting fetal T-cell function and DNA methylation. Therefore, mothers should minimize exposure to smoking environment in perinatal time and preferably smoking and alcohol consumption should be avoided.

Vitamin D Supplementation during Pregnancy

The emerging evidences strongly support the multifaceted and complex role of vitamin D in allergy **(Flowchart 2)**.

Flowchart 2: Possible mechanism of action of vitamin D in atopy.

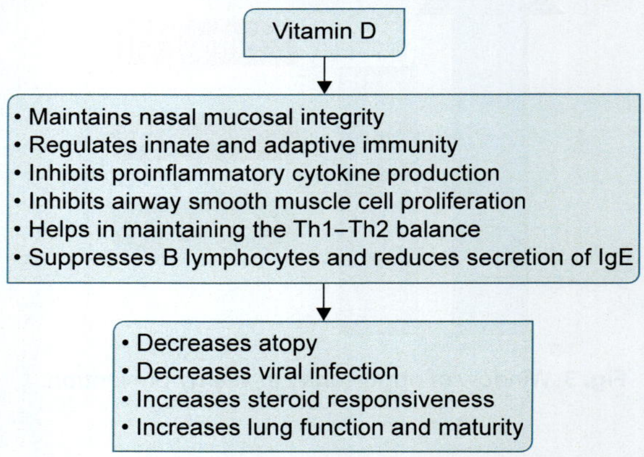

(IgE: immunoglobulin E; Th1: T helper 1)

Even in the absence of strong evidence, supplementation of vitamin D during pregnancy is shown to have an effect in lowering the risk of allergic disease in the newborn. This holds more true for those who have documented low vitamin D levels. In view of the low risk of the intervention, vitamin D supplementation can be considered in mothers who are found to be vitamin D-deficient and more randomized controlled trials (RCTs) without other confounding factors are required to prove the effect.

Supplementation of Pre- and Probiotics in Pregnancy

Supplementation of bacterial products (probiotics, prebiotics, or synbiotics) during the last trimester of pregnancy, mainly *Lactobacillus* species, including *Lactobacillus rhamnosus* GG, and *Lactobacillus reuteri*, has been shown to reduce the risk of atopic dermatitis in high-risk infants. Pregnant women with a personal or strong family history of allergies and atopy can consider taking probiotics during the last trimester of pregnancy. It is currently recommended by WAO for high-risk offspring. More lucidity is yet to be added regarding the choice, dose and duration of the probiotics.

Supplementation of Omega Polyunsaturated Fatty Acids during Pregnancy

There is no recommendation for fish oil supplementation in pregnant women for atopy prevention as per current evidence. Maternal n-3 PUFA (polyunsaturated fatty acid) supplementation with fish oil supplements during pregnancy remains conflicting as per the available studies.

Role of House Dust Mite Exposure Risk Reduction Strategies in Pregnancy

There is no role for HDM reduction strategies in pregnancy based on current evidence to reduce the risk of HDM sensitization in the offspring.

Mode of Delivery

Mode of delivery may interfere with the normal development of the immune system in a newborn. Babies born by cesarean section were found to have a significantly high risk of developing allergy than were those delivered vaginally. The mechanism postulated is gut microbiota can affect host immune maturation, and infants delivered by cesarean section may experience delayed colonization of the gut owing to minimal exposure to the maternal vaginal and fecal microbiota. The infant immune system undergoes rapid development during the neonatal period and this disruption in early life may increase the risk of allergies in later life.

Breastfeeding

Exclusive breastfeeding for 3–4 months and continued breastfeeding beyond that may help prevent eczema and wheezing in early life. There is evidence to support that exclusive breastfeeding during the first 3–4 months reduces the incidence of cow's milk protein allergy (CMPA) and eczema in the first 2 years of life. Breastfeeding should be strongly recommended in all children unless contraindicated, such as with maternal human immunodeficiency virus (HIV) infection. Even though there is no strong evidence supporting protection from breastfeeding against all allergic disease, considering the immunological properties of breast milk and according to the current consensus, it is highly recommended to exclusively breastfeed for at least the first 4–6 months, preferably till 6 months of age.

Maternal Dietary Restriction during Breastfeeding

Maternal dietary restrictions of allergenic food during the period of breastfeeding are not recommended for disease prevention unless there is evidence of a specific food allergy. Infants already having clinical signs of allergy from early life clearly benefit from maternal allergen avoidance and it should be included in the management of allergy.

Role of Formula Feeding in Children <6 Months

If breastfeeding is not possible in high-risk infants, supplementation with a partially hydrolyzed formula containing prebiotics or probiotics can be considered. There is only weak evidence that supplementation with a partially hydrolyzed formula containing prebiotics or probiotics may reduce the incidence of eczema and possibly other types of allergic disease and hence this should be restricted to infants with a risk of atopy. Those children without high atopic heredity may be prescribed normal formula feeds if indicated. Soy formula or other milk such as goat's milk are not recommended for the reduction of food allergy risk.

Maternal Dietary Supplementation during Lactation

Mothers of infants at risk of atopic dermatitis, especially those with history of atopy in first-degree relative, can consider probiotic intake during breastfeeding. Even though there is no strong evidence that maternal probiotic intake while breastfeeding reduces the risk of eczema in the child, various studies has shown that administration of probiotics during the first 6 months of breastfeeding has a role in reduction of allergy in offspring. There is no evidence to advise supplementation of vitamin D or n3 PUFA supplementation during lactation.

Introduction of Complementary Food

Current guidelines by American Academy of Pediatrics (AAP) and European Academy of Allergy and Clinical Immunology (EAACI) recommend introduction of solid foods between the age of 4 and 6 months according to the local standard practice irrespective of genetic risk factors. World Health Organization (WHO) recommends exclusive breast feeding till the age of 6 months considering the health benefits. As oral introduction of allergen is more tolerogenic than cutaneous exposure, leading to Th2 inflammation and allergic sensitization, delayed introduction of allergenic foods increases the risk of developing allergy. There are RCTs which has clearly demonstrated that early introduction of pea nut and egg at 4–6 months reduces the allergic sensitization. Introduction of milk formulas should be delayed for at least 4–6 months unless specifically indicated and this has been shown to have a preventive effect in development of allergy in preterm infants and those children with atopic heredity. The beneficial role of dietary elimination after the age of 4–6 months in preventing allergies needs additional research and is not advised as per the current evidence, and by 1 year dietary diversity is recommended. Those children showing clinical features of allergy, ideally should be assessed by an allergist during the process of initiation of complementary feeding and expert advice on introduction of allergenic foods is highly recommended.

Dietary Supplementation during Early Childhood and Infancy

No evidence to support the benefit of nutritional supplementation in infants and children with vitamin D, omega PUFA, or probiotics in future allergy prevention.

As per the routine supplementation guidelines vitamin D supplementation can be continued till one year of age. There are no recommendations about their immunomodulatory effect of antioxidants or PUFA supplementation in prevention of allergy.

Role of House Dust Mite Avoidance Measures in Infancy and Early Childhood

House dust mite avoidance has been shown to benefit those patients with established disease or sensitization, but whether reduced exposure will protect against the development of new disease remains uncertain. There are a few data suggesting HDM avoidance measures during early infancy may delay the onset of allergic disease, but the results are inconsistent.

Pets

Early exposure, especially in the first year of life to cats and dogs, reduces the risk of developing allergies due to more diverse microbial exposure. Pet removal may be beneficial for those who are sensitized to pet allergens or with established allergy to pets. There is no evidence that avoiding exposure to pets will prevent development of allergy rather early exposure to pet allergen shows a protective effect. It is not required for a family to give up pets in order to prevent allergies, but it is also not advised to acquire additional pets for this reason.

Exposure to Smoking and Environmental Pollutants

Exposure to smoke and air pollutants like ozone, nitrogen dioxide, and particulate matter, causes oxidative stress leading to lung damage, direct irritation and inflammation of the airways, increased airway sensitivity to allergens, immune dysregulation, and epigenetic changes. Air pollution is a significant contributor to the development of respiratory allergies, especially asthma, and hence exposure to cigarette smoke and outdoor air pollutants should be avoided as far as possible.

Infections and Antibiotics

The original hygiene hypothesis focused on an absence of a sufficient viral/bacterial pathogenic burden to educate the immune system in childhood, allowing for the induction of an aberrant Th2 response. Recent evidence suggests that diversity of microbial exposure may be particularly protective and interaction between the immune system and intestinal microbiota in particular has been shown to protect against allergic inflammation in murine models. Nonatopic asthma, providing further evidence that the "narrow" interpretation of the hygiene hypothesis, in which early-life microbial exposure protects against atopic asthma by suppressing Th2 immune responses, is oversimplistic. Even though no evidence-based conclusions are there regarding the role of microbial or viral infection in prevention of allergic disease, literature states that antibiotic usage in early life, especially in the first year of life, is associated with an increased risk of allergic disease due to alteration in the intestinal microbiome. Judicious prescription of antibiotics should be encouraged not only to prevent development of allergy, but to avoid side effects and the emergence of antibiotics resistance. Various studies have shown that recurrent viral infection in childhood acts synergistically with other environmental triggers in the development of asthma.

Skin Barrier Protection

Dysfunctional epithelial barrier is one of the primary defects leading to allergen sensitization. A few RCTs were conducted to demonstrate the effect of use of emollients in allergen sensitizations, but the results were inconclusive. Being a safe action with the significance of epithelial barrier in the pathophysiology of allergy, emollients can be used in high-risk children even with no strong evidence.

SECONDARY PREVENTION

In spite of the existing prevention measures, a significant proportion of "high-risk" children will still develop sensitization or disease. These children should be identified when they have early disease. Preliminary evidence suggests that early interventions in allergic children may modify progression of sensitization patterns and/or the development of new allergic diseases.

- *Early diagnosis:* Identify specific allergens through allergy testing.
- *Allergen avoidance:* Targeted allergen avoidance measures to reduce the exposure

- Early symptom management through effective pharmacotherapy
- *Immunotherapy:* In patients sensitized to aeroallergens, especially HDM should be considered immunotherapy, to arrest the progression of atopic march, reducing the risk of progression to new sensitizations, and to reduce the severity of disease
- *Emergency preparedness:* EpiPen for anaphylaxis/asthma action plan for acute asthma exacerbations
- Parental and patient education

TERTIARY PREVENTION IN ALLERGY

Goal of tertiary prevention is to manage and alleviate the impact of established allergy disease and to tackle the complications. It includes allergy management plans, ensuring proper medication adherence, continuing the allergen avoidance strategies and allergen immunotherapy, adequate emergency management, and thus to improve the quality of life and reduce the healthcare utilization.

PARENTAL COUNSELING

Right parental understanding of allergies, i.e., symptoms, triggers, and treatment options are crucial in long-term management of allergy. Guidance on avoidance of allergens and thus creating a safe environment for children is a key component in allergy prevention. Parents need to understand the treatment plans and emergency management to ensure effective patient outcome.

Parental counseling should address the following:

- *Explaining the diagnosis and providing the accurate information:* Discuss in detail about, symptoms, diagnosis, and available treatment according to the latest evidence-based guidelines. Parents should be counseled in detail regarding medications, recognize the symptom worsening, and emergencies. All levels of allergy prevention strategies and all the current treatment modalities should be explained to them in simple language.
- *Listen to their concerns:* Understanding and addressing their concern in every aspect of the disease is crucial in treatment compliance.
- *Building up a rapport with the parents:* Allergy being a chronic inflammatory state, parental support is inevitable there is a need to allot enough time in the initial visits itself to have a positive relationship with the caretakers.
- *Combined decision-making:* After explaining the allergen avoidance measures and management strategies, active participation of the parents should be encouraged in deciding the treatment modality.
- *Providing written instructions for flare-up:* Clearly written action plans should be provided and explained to the parents in their own language.
- *Ensuring adherence to the treatment:* Try to simplify the medication regimen and encourage to use reminders and monitor the drug compliance regularly.
- *Providing emotional support and forming support groups:* In spite of increasing awareness of allergy diseases, still there is an element of social stigma on long-term inhaled medications and forming support groups can be reassuring.
- *Scheduling regular follow-up:* The need of follow-up visits and readjusting the treatment should be well explained to the parents.

SUMMARY

The high prevalence of allergy along with its substantial impact on economic burden and quality of life necessitates the need of early intervention and primary prevention strategies to reduce allergic diseases. Even with a substantial amount of research work in this aspect, there are only a few evidence-based recommendation on primary preventive strategies on allergy.

Key Learning Points

- Allergy involves interplay of multiple complex factors such as genetic, environmental, and exposure to the allergen triggers.
- Proper implementation of allergy prevention strategies and early intervention can definitely reduce the burden of allergic diseases.
- There are only a few evidence-based prevention strategies in allergic diseases.
- More research is warranted with proper study design with well-defined standards and follow-up for establishing allergy prevention guidelines.
- Effective parental counseling play a crucial role in the long-term management of allergy.

SUGGESTED READING

1. Abrams EM, Shaker M, Stukus D, Mack DP, Greenhawt M. Updates in Food Allergy Prevention in Children. Pediatrics. 2023;152(5):e2023062836.
2. Chu DK, Koplin JJ, Ahmed T, Islam N, Chang CL, Lowe AJ. How to Prevent Atopic Dermatitis (Eczema) in 2024: Theory and Evidence. J Allergy Clin Immunol Pract. 2024;12:1695-704.
3. Cronin C, Salzberg N, Woon Y, Trujillo Wurttele J. Primary, secondary and tertiary prevention of food allergy: current practices and future directions. Allergol Immunopathol (Madr). 2023; 52(2):32-44.
4. de Silva D, Geromi M, Halken S, Host A, Panesar SS, Muraro A, et al.; EAACI Food Allergy and Anaphylaxis Guidelines Group. Primary prevention of food allergy in children and adults: systematic review. Allergy. 2014;69(5):581-9.
5. Halken S. Prevention of allergic disease in childhood: clinical and epidemiological aspects of primary and secondary allergy prevention. Pediatr Allergy Immunol. 2004;15(Suppl 16):9-32.
6. Herman K, Brough HA, Pier J, Venter C, Järvinen KM. Prevention of IgE-Mediated Food Allergy: Emerging Strategies Through Maternal and Neonatal Interventions. J Allergy Clin Immunol Pract. 2024;12(5):1686-94.
7. Iglesia EGA, Fleischer DM, Abrams EM. Health Promotion of Early and Sustained Allergenic Food Introduction for the Prevention of Food Allergy. J Allergy Clin Immunol Pract. 2024;12(7):1670-83.e9.
8. Kim EH, Matsui EC. Allergic Disease Prevention: Current Strategies and a Look Into the Future. J Allergy Clin Immunol Pract. 2024;12:1717-8.
9. Maciag MC, Phipatanakul W. Prevention of Asthma: Targets for Intervention. Chest. 2020;158(3):913-22.
10. Royal C, Gray C. Allergy Prevention: An Overview of Current Evidence. Yale J Biol Med. 2020;93:689-98.
11. Annesi-Maesano I, Fleddermann M, Hornef M, von Mutius E, Pabst O, Schaubeck M, et al. Allergic diseases in infancy: I - Epidemiology and current interpretation. World Allergy Organ J. 2021;14(11):100591.

CHAPTER

14

Standardization of Tests Conducted for Allergies in India

S Narmada Ashok
Reviewer: *Mahesh PA*

INTRODUCTION

India, with its diverse climate, population, and allergen exposure, faces a growing burden of allergic diseases—especially among children. However, the country lacks context-specific standardized protocols for allergy testing, often relying on guidelines extrapolated from Western populations. This chapter aims to bridge that gap by outlining practical, evidence-based protocols for allergy diagnosis and testing tailored for Indian settings, incorporating local aeroallergen patterns, regional food sensitizations, and appropriate in vivo and in vitro diagnostic approaches.

With 1.43 billion people residing in India with great diversity in environment and socioeconomic strata, India has a huge burden of allergic disorders. India has close to about 37.5 million suffering from asthma and also has reported a rise in other allergic disorders. The incidence of asthma in children is about 3.16% among children aged 6–7 years and 3.63% in children aged 13–14 years. The prevalence of allergic rhinitis is substantial with a prevalence of about 20–30% in the general population. Prevalence of atopic eczema also is ranging from 3.6 to 8.9% among children aged 13–14 years which is substantial. With such a high burden of allergic disorders, the current allergy practice in India has centered around focusing on managing symptoms rather than understanding the disease pathology. Recent advancements across the world have targeted the importance of disease modification which is highly dependent on diagnosing the causative allergens and adopting methods to modify the body's response to the same.

The common tests usually adopted by physicians in general practice treating such patients are usually:

- Complete blood count
- Absolute eosinophil count
- Total immunoglobulin E (IgE) levels.

These tests, however, do not give an idea about the specific allergens. It is essential to understand specific allergens to:

- Use avoidance measures and monitoring of the disease process
- Specific treatment like allergen immunotherapy for disease modification
- Early identification of infants at risk for disease progression.

With the growth of several training programs in India, there is an emerging generation of physicians trained in allergy and immunology who are trained to do the specific tests required to detect the specific allergen. The tests adopted generally by physicians in allergy practice for management of allergic disorders are:

- Allergy skin testing
- Serum-specific IgE
- Fractional exhaled nitric oxide (FeNO).

With this scenario, there is now a need to develop management protocols for Indian scenario as most of the current protocols are based on guidelines adapted from data generated from western countries such as Global Initiative for Asthma (GINA) and the British Thoracic Society (BTS) guidelines which may not be appropriate for Indian practice. The prevalence of parasitic infections and infectious diseases like tuberculosis which drive blood eosinophil levels and genetic makeup that drives the production of eosinophilia and serum total IgE we need to look at evidence if these tests are going to be of value in our population. Similarly, though we still have less data on aerobiology from India we are having several studies in recent times that have investigated allergen sensitization pattern for inhalant allergens. This chapter is to develop a standard protocol for allergy testing in Indian scenario among children and will be based on literatures derived from Indian subcontinent as well as taking evidence from well-established international guidelines with modifications suitable for Indian conditions.

TESTS GENERALLY USED BY GENERAL PRACTITIONERS

Complete Blood Count

Asthma being a heterogenous disease with various phenotypes that are classified based on the predominant inflammatory types as eosinophilic, neutrophilic, mixed granulocytic, or paucigranulocytic asthma it may not be completely wrong if practitioners want to use complete blood count as the first test they want to order in their practice. Complete blood count is an inexpensive and precise test that is available widely.

While induced sputum count of the inflammatory phenotypes are considered gold standard, the peripheral blood counts would be a noninvasive procedure to quantify the inflammatory cells and detect the asthma phenotype. Blood eosinophils can be taken as one of the indicators of eosinophilic asthma and studies have shown a good correlation between blood and sputum eosinophils. However, the same cannot be told about neutrophils and neutrophils/lymphocyte ratio (NLR). However, the absence of definite increase in neutrophils count with low blood eosinophil/low neutrophil count could be considered as representing the paucigranulocytic phenotype. But it may not always be accurate. Combined assessment of all clinical features, blood eosinophilia, and assessment of FeNO discussed later could strengthen our assessment.

Blood eosinophils of >4% has been included as one of the criteria in asthma predictive index. Studies done in India by has shown good correlation between severity of asthma and eosinophil counts.

Anemia is also known to be correlated with asthma in children. The possible explanation of underlying association of iron deficiency anemia (IDA) and development of allergic diseases including asthma are low maternal iron levels during pregnancy are negatively associated with increased childhood wheeze and atopic sensitization. The inadequate maternal iron status negatively impacts childhood respiratory health, particularly during critical periods of embryonic and fetal growths. Also, the lifestyle of excessive internet use and television viewing, poor lifestyle habits and fast-food consumption can affect children with asthma and cause anemia. Iron affects the components of immune system and produces Th2 skewness of immune response and favors the development of allergic disease. The above hypothesis has been confirmed by several studies done across India which has shown that asthma in children was associated with IDA in children. However there has also been studies done by Agrawal et al. who showed no possible association between anemia and wheezing in children.

Hence, it can be safely concluded that complete blood count is not a necessary investigation for diagnosis or prognosis of allergic disorders in children. However if done, the presence of anemia should be looked for and higher eosinophil count may indicate the presence of eosinophilic phenotype in asthmatic children after ruling out other causes of the same that may have contributed to rise in eosinophils in Indian scenario like worm infestations.

Role of Absolute Eosinophilic Count and Serum Immunoglobulin E in Children with Allergic Disorders

Immunoglobulin E generally mediates type 1 hypersensitivity reactions and constitutes first line of defense against helminthic infestations. However, in certain conditions there can be an inappropriate IgE-mediated immune response that is capable of mounting an inappropriate immune response to a normally innocuous environmental antigen. The increased production of IgE is mediated through the Th2 immune response. Generally, atopic predisposition is cause of allergic disorders in children. Allergens induce the induction of Th2 immunity. Th2 inflammation induces the production of cytokines and chemokines which mediate inflammation. One of the important cytokines that is produced is IL-4 which is the main reason for production of IgE from B cells. Another important cytokine induced by the Th2 inflammation is IL5 which is capable of inducing eosinophil production.

Level of Immunoglobulin E in Children

Immunoglobulin E contributes to <0.001% of total serum immunoglobulin. It induces the inflammatory cascade and its propagation. The maximum levels vary with age, and it is maximum in the age-group of 8–12 years of age. In India, Indians are also high serum total IgE producers. The mean levels of IgE in adults was 522.19 IU/mL compared to 40.8 IU/mL in the Western population according to a study done in Mysore–Bangalore region in South India. Hence it is essential to interpret the serum IgE levels in the background of the clinical condition of the patients.

Up until the introduction of anti-IgE biologicals, total IgE had not received the attention. Serum total IgE may be used for inclusion and dose determining parameter for omalizumab therapy, diagnostic and monitoring parameter in allergic bronchopulmonary aspergillosis (ABPA) and predict reactivity in food challenge.

Role of Absolute Eosinophil Count

Immunoglobulin E has a strong affinity for basophils and mast cells; IgE has a strong affinity for basophils and mast cells' the FcεRI receptor. IgE cross-linking sets off a series of intracellular processes. This causes a variety of cytokines and interleukins to be produced, which in turn affects the increased eosinophil production. Furthermore, 13% of serum IgE is attributed to epigenetic changes in eosinophils, indicating a connection between them. Blood eosinophils can indicate early wheeze in school age children. Absolute eosinophil count can hence help us to understand the asthma phenotype.

Several studies from India are now being done in children that are looking into the correlation of serum IgE and absolute eosinophil count with allergic disorders in children. Serum IgE levels and asthma severity were found to rise linearly in studies though the total cases were less than 200 in each of the studies.

One another important phenomenon to be considered in an event of uncontrolled symptoms is ABPA. Study done in North India showed significant association between ABPA and poorly controlled asthma and indicated that higher value of total IgE of 1,200 IU/mL should be used for diagnosis. Hence if serum IgE are in higher levels and symptoms appear uncontrolled there is a need to suspect ABPA.

But together, they indicate in contrast to what has been thought earlier levels of serum IgE levels and absolute eosinophil count may have a role in suspecting allergic disorders and there may be a definite role in correlation with severity of the disorders.

TESTS TO BE DONE BY THE SPECIALISTS ONLY

A thorough history and physical examination are essential. History will guide us to identify the allergens and find the temporal relationship of the reaction in relation to eliciting factor which leads to specific confirmatory tests.

Skin Prick Test

Once a child is clinically confirmed to have allergic disorders it is essential to identify the allergens. Skin prick test (SPT) is the most frequently used method for detection of IgE antibodies. It can be done in the clinic and is rapid, simple, and cost is low. When an allergen is introduced into the epicutaneous layer of the skin of allergic individuals, dermal mast cells begin to degranulate due to the cross-linking of allergen-specific IgE bound to their membrane receptors which leads to release of histamine and mediators that leads to wheal (including pseudopods) and erythema that can be measured objectively to assess cutaneous sensitivity. It represents a surrogate indicator of systemic allergic sensitization.

However, SPT must be done by trained allergists with an adequate knowledge of relevant allergens and their clinical correlation with respect to the history and clinical findings in the child. This will then help us to advise on the lifestyle changes as well as plan immunotherapy where indicated. SPT has high sensitivity and good specificity when performed and interpreted correctly.

In SPT we introduce the allergen through a lancet into the epicutaneous layer of skin of allergic individuals. This causes the dermal mast cells to degranulate mainly through the cross-linking of allergen-specific IgE (sIgE) also called as coupling reaction.

The most important steps in performing the SPT are:

1. Knowledge of the allergens
2. What pattern of allergy the patient has—indoor or outdoor, seasonal or perennial, or when specific exposure happens
3. Correlate both and identify the allergens to be tested.
4. Prepare the SPT case sheet or have a printed copy with the names of the allergens selected for testing
5. Test the allergens and interpret it after a second history from the patient to understand the clinical correlation

Clinically important allergens are either found in organisms as a whole or certain structures such as spores of molds, fruit seeds, and fecal pellets of mite and insect. The allergenic protein can also be found in saliva or sweat from several animals like cat or dogs and from the pollens.

Aeroallergens: The common causes of allergic disease are aeroallergens. The sources of the same are from pollens, fungus, insect, mite feces, dust, and animal dander. They may be the cause for perennial symptoms like house dust or seasonal like weed, tree, grass, and shrub pollens. Pollutants and climate influence these exposures. Exposure of exposure to fungal and dust mite allergen can be seasonal because of the reproductive processes and diet.

Food allergens—ingested: 90% of food-induced allergy are accounted by seven most important ingested allergens. These are commonly the egg, peanut, milk, wheat, various nuts, soy, and sea foods especially fish. Animal meat proteins are also important allergenic source.

COMMON AEROALLERGENS IN INDIA

Most common perennial allergens in India according to the study by Indian authors are dust mites (*Dermatophagoides*) and cockroach. Nagaraju et al. in a very detailed study in the dust mite sensitivity pattern in children in India have noticed that among the dust mites *Dermatophagoides pteronyssinus* was found positive in 639 cases (68.2%), *Dermatophagoides farinae* in 626 (66.8%), *Blomia tropicalis* (storage mite) in 304 (32.4%), *Acarus siro* (flour mite) in 302 (32.2%), *Lepidoglyphus destructor* (storage mites) in 268 (28.6%), and *Tyrophagus putrescentiae* (found in food and stored products) in 194 (20.7%) cases. Most of the children were found sensitive to multiple dust mites in SPT. In patients with allergic rhinitis with asthma, *D. pteronyssinus* sensitized children were the most common (72.2%) followed by *D. farinae* (69.5%), and *A. siro* (31.1%). Out of those having perennial rhinitis with seasonal exacerbations (57.7%), most were sensitized to *D. pteronyssinus* (74.7%) followed by *D. farinae* (70%) and *B. tropicalis* (45.8%). However, studies have noted that there is a strong degree of cross-reactivity among the species. The major allergens in *D. pteronyssinus* are 31. Among then Der p1 and p2 have the highest rates of sensitization. Der p 23 is another major allergen. Cross-reactivity has been reported among the species and their fellow crustaceans (shrimp, crab, and lobster) and insects (cockroach, grasshopper) as well as mollusk phylum (snail, oysters, and squid). Der p 10 is the "pan-allergen" responsible for the same. *Hence, it can be safely concluded that for clinical purpose we only test for D. pteronyssinus, D. farinae, and B. tropicalis in India. If for research purposes, we could do a detailed analysis.*

Arthropod-derived aeroallergens: Arthropod-derived aeroallergens are mainly from the species like Insecta and Arachnida. Of these, house dust mites and cockroaches are the most therapeutically significant. Salivary secretions, fecal pellets, and whole bodies are the usual sources of allergenic proteins. In midges, the major allergens are the hemoglobins (chi t1) and the group 1 nitrile-specifier proteins, troponins, and tropomyosin are the major allergens in cockroach. Clinically important species among dust mites belong to Echimyopodidae, Pyroglyphidae, Acaridae, and Glycyphagidae. The major allergens are the enzymes and proteins associated with actin and ligands.

The other significant allergen in India is cockroach. The species are as follows:

- German cockroach (*Blattella germanica*)
- American cockroach (*Periplaneta americana*)
- Oriental cockroach (*Blatta orientalis*)
- Brown-banded cockroach (*Supella longipalpa*)
- Smoky brown cockroach (*Periplaneta fuliginosa*) is known to cause reaction worldwide.

Though there are homologous allergens there may also be a species-specific sensitization. Studies have found *P. americana* and *B. germanica* are the common species in India.

Twelve groups of cockroach allergens are listed worldwide. The groups 1, 2, and 10 are excreted in the feces and is capable of widespread environmental exposure while groups 10, 11, and 12 are digestive enzymes. The rest are predominantly in the bodies. They are numbered from Bla g 1 and the *P. americana* homolog Per a 1 share 70–72% cross-reactivity. Allergens from group 6 and 8 share homology to troponin C and myosin while group 7 includes tropomyosins which is a pan allergen found in many animal species—originally major shrimp allergen. In clinical practice, recombinant cockroach allergens are available in certain countries and have been used for testing. In US the recombinant allergens consist f (Bla g 1, 2, 4, 5 and Per a 7). It is varied in different countries and in India we are using the crude allergen extract where the major allergen is not standardized.

There has also been reports of sensitization to mosquitoes. However, mosquito allergy diagnostic criteria is not affirmative. Salivary allergen has been known to induce cutaneous reaction, however the allergens from the body has been known to induce allergy. 47% of Indian population with asthma or allergic rhinitis in India have shown sensitivity to mosquito allergens. Studies on cross-reactivity from India has been scarce. However, *Aedes aegypti* is very abundant in India. The question of whether mosquito allergens are found in dust or mattresses in quantities enough to cause allergic symptoms is yet to be answered conclusively. The body allergens also cross-react with cockroaches and shrimp. Using whole-body extracts helps us to identify the same. Study done at Vallabhbhai Patel Chest Institute in India, on 200 patients with asthma and/or allergic rhinitis had shown that mosquito-derived aero-allergens may be an important inhalant allergen in India and they identified several important protein from whole body extract. Apart from one study alone, no studies have reported a detailed analysis of the same. Hence, if there is a clinical suspicion we can do the allergen testing. *Hence it can be concluded that cockroach should be tested for sensitization and mosquito sensitization is to be correlated clinically.*

POLLENS TO BE TESTED IN INDIAN SCENARIO

Pollen grains are usually produced during the process of pollination occurring due to wind (anemophilous)—gymnosperms and angiosperms. The source can be either from trees, weeds, or grasses. The exposure depends on the vegetation in the area. The pollen grains sizes range from approximately 5 to greater than 200 μm. 20–100 pollen grains/m^3 of pollen concentration is sufficient to provoke the disease.

Most important issue in testing for pollens is the unavailability of local aerobiological data regarding pollen and fungal spores. Majority of the population in India reside in areas where there has been no aerobiology study. However, we do have region-specific data in India which can be extrapolated to our local area **(Table 1)**. Singh et al. has published an extensive article on aerobiology in India which could be used as a reference.

Clinically important pollens from various parts of India **(Figs. 1 and 2)**.

The main pollen season for:

- *North India:* February to April and September to November
- *West India:* Three pollen seasons reported—March to mid-May, September to November, and December to February
- *East India:* August, March to July
- *South India:* August to November dominated by weeds and grasses, February to April dominated by trees and shrubs

Hence, it is essential that while including pollens in the allergens it is essential to include the common vegetation in the area with representation from trees, shrubs, and grasses. Seasonal variation is to be taken into account.

TABLE 1: Common pollens in India based on regions.

North India	*Central India*	*Eastern India*	*Southern India*	*Western India*
Prosopis	*Argemone*	Poaceae	*Parthenium*	Grasses
Xanthium	*Brassica*	*Chenopodium/Amaranthus*	*Casuarina*	*Parthenium*
Ageratum	*Cannabis*	Asteraceae	*Chenopodium/Amaranthus*	*Chenopodium/ Amaranthus*
Amaranthus spinosus	*Asphodelus*	*Putranjiva*	*Cocos nucifera*	*Cyperus*
Ricinus communis	*Parthenium*	*Mangifera*	*Ricinus communis*	*Cocos*
Chenopodium	*Cassia*	Eucalyptus	Grasses	*Cassia*
Holoptelea	Poaceae	*Cassia*	Poaceae	

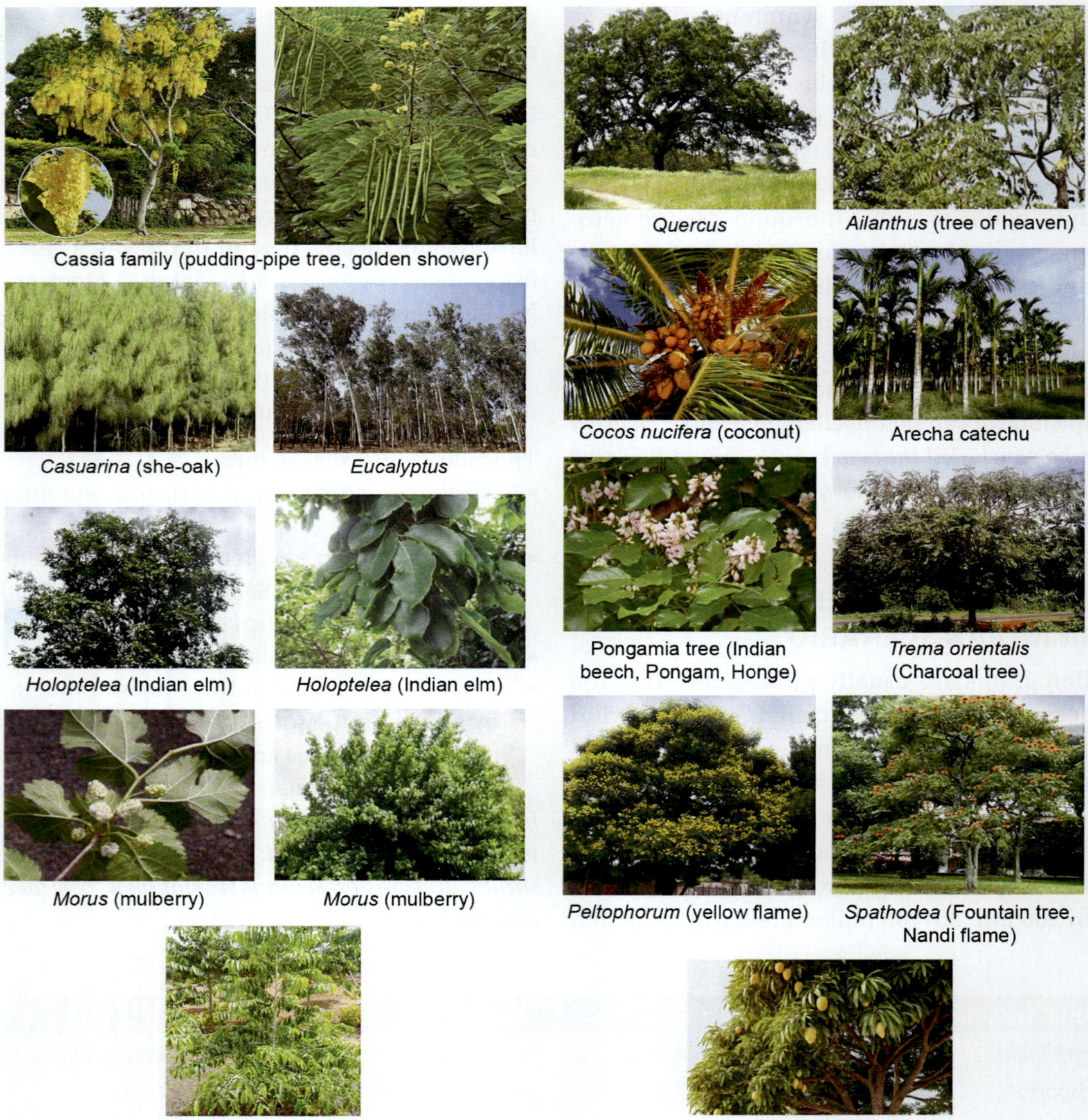
Cassia family (pudding-pipe tree, golden shower)
Quercus
Ailanthus (tree of heaven)
Casuarina (she-oak)
Eucalyptus
Cocos nucifera (coconut)
Arecha catechu
Holoptelea (Indian elm)
Holoptelea (Indian elm)
Pongamia tree (Indian beech, Pongam, Honge)
Trema orientalis (Charcoal tree)
Morus (mulberry)
Morus (mulberry)
Peltophorum (yellow flame)
Spathodea (Fountain tree, Nandi flame)
Putranjiva (child life tree, karuvilai)
Mangifera (mango)

Fig. 1: Common aeroallergens in India—trees.

MOLDS TO TESTED IN INDIAN SCENARIO

Fungi producing allergenic protein are from different sources of allergens. There are more than 180 fungal species. Allergenic proteins are found usually in spores, mycelia, hyphae that becomes fragmented and yeast forms. Most of these allergens are glycoproteins and proteins but can also be mannans. Sensitization occurs when individuals are exposed to fragmented spores or hyphae.

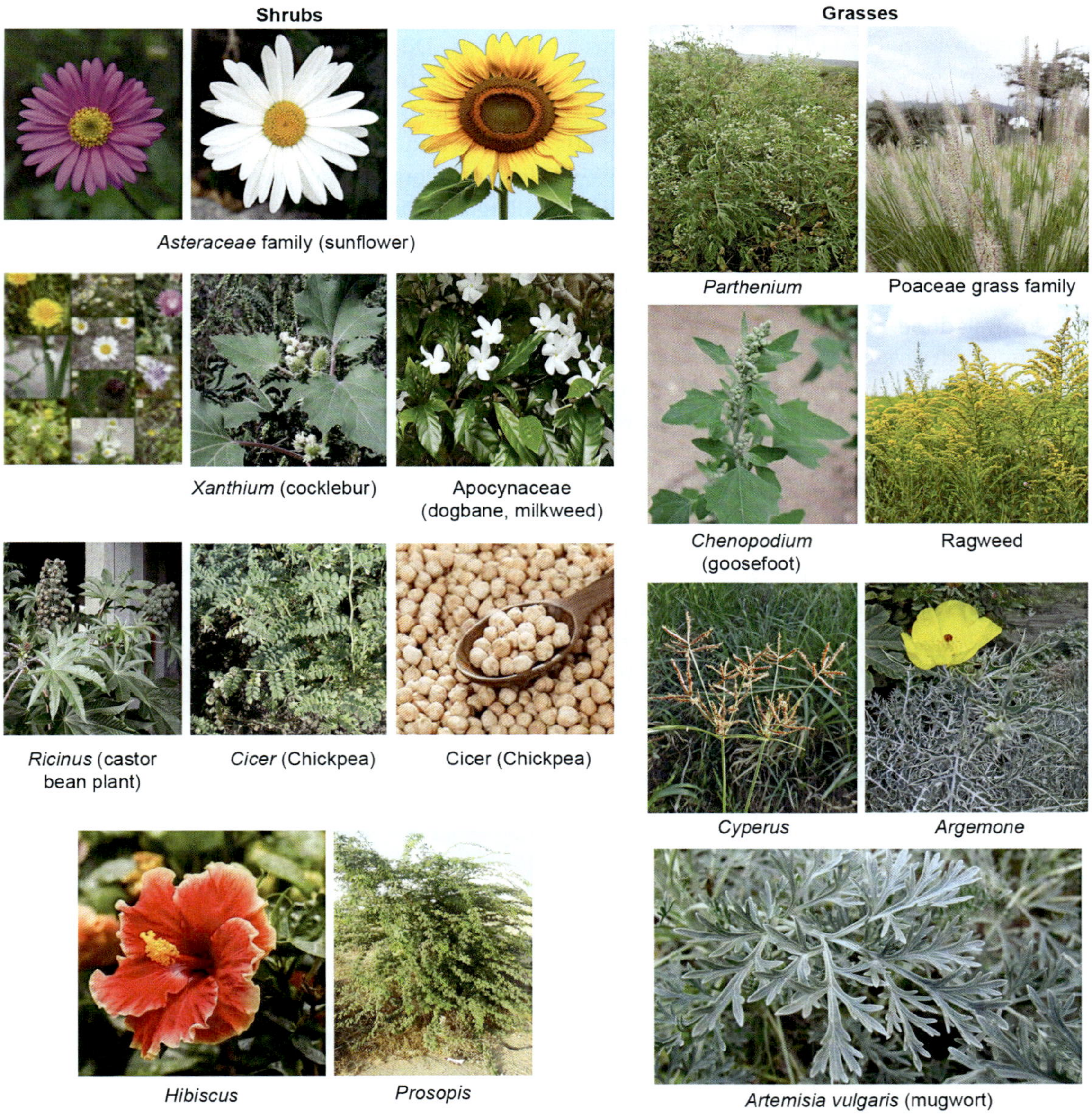

Fig. 2: Common aeroallergens in India—shrubs and weeds.

Allergic sensitization to fungi has been linked to difficult-to-treat asthma and fatal asthma episodes. There are few studies from India to understand the spectrum and concentration of fungal flora in the vicinity of homes. A study done in Delhi homes of asthmatics and non-asthmatics showed *Aspergillus*, *Penicillium*, *Alternaria*, and *Cladosporium* as the prevalent fungal spores. There was also seasonal variation with Alternaria being higher in summer months, *Cladosporium* in winters and *Penicillium* in autumn. *Aspergillus* was the most dominant fungi and was prevalent in autumn and winter. The studies done on fungal sensitization in patients from the similar area showed high degree of sensitization to *Aspergillus* followed by *Fusarium, Rhizopus, Alternaria, Phoma, Candida, Mucor, Helminthosporium,* and *Trichoderma*. Sensitization pattern in Bangalore has shown higher degree of sensitization to fungi in young children from rural areas. They had tested for *Alternaria, Aspergillus, Candida, Curvularia, Helminthosporium,* and *Penicillium*. Meta analysis done to study the ABPA sensitization in children with severe asthma showed high degree of sensitivity to *Aspergillus* in most of the studies from India. In a study done by Kuravi et al. which looked at sensitization pattern of children across India had showed high degree of sensitization to *Aspergillus fumigatus* and *Alternaria alternata*.

Hence, it can be concluded that it is essential to test for molds in all asthmatic children. However, it may be essential to include Aspergillus and Alternaria if done for screening purpose and a detailed analysis involving all species if severe asthma is present.

Animal-derived aeroallergens: Animals like cats, mice, house rats, and dogs are some of the sources of clinically important allergens. However, in rare patients, rabbits, mice, and guinea pigs have also been implicated. It has been discovered that animal dander, epithelium, fur, urine, and saliva are allergens.

Cats and dog dander sensitization: Cats and dogs are the most prevalent household pets. The allergens can cause increased burden to healthcare. Evidence indicates that early exposure to dogs before a year can be protective for prevention of allergic sensitization. The evidence for early cat exposure is contradictory. While there are studies on prevalence of sensitization to cats and dogs from Korea (15.7%), Sri Lanka (12.2% to cats and 8.9% to dogs), and China (34.5% to dogs and 30.8% to cat hair), we do not have any literature on the same for India.

There is a great difficulty to detect sensitization to dogs. Dog component allergens have been identified in serum, dander, pelt, hair, saliva, and urine. Can f 1 is the major allergen from the dander and is considered the preferred source for most commercial dog allergen extract. Seven allergens (Can f 1-7) are identified among which most are found in saliva and dander of the dogs. Can f 5 is from the urine of the dogs. However, contamination is a major problem. The content of the commercial extract has a mixture of dander and hair and hence Can f 1 found in dander may not be adequately represented. There is also no difference in dog breed or to gender. Sometimes even there is apparent difference in same breeds. The self-prepared extracts, where the hair has been used, should be soaked for >24 hours, and dog not been washed for a week was acceptable to detect sensitization.

Detection of sensitization to cats is easier. Fel d1 is the most dominant cat allergen where 96% of all patients react. They cat allergen extract can be easily standardized. It is from the saliva of the cats. More than 96% of patients react to this protein unlike dog proteins where individual species variation exists. *Hence, we may use commercially derived cat dander allergen, however, preferable to use self-prepared extracts for detecting dog sensitization.*

ALLERGENS USED IN SUSPECTED FOOD ALLERGIES

In children sensitization to food can be done under two contexts. One, the child is showing immunologically mediated adverse reaction after ingestion of food which involves the skin or gastrointestinal tract. The second is when it is suspected to be the etiology of asthma or allergic disorders.

We also need to investigate the claims that ingestion of substances like proprietary drinks, chips, crisps, ice and chocolate, and food cooked in oil produce occurrence of wheeze. These cannot be confirmed by using SPTs. Interestingly a study done by Wilson et al. in 1985 showed that these substances were incriminated more by Asian children (all originated from Indian subcontinent) compared to non-Asian children. They found a mean increase in bronchial hyper-responsiveness when compared to a placebo after ingestion of these substances. The mechanism is non-immunological. Hence history from the parents cannot be discredited and requires careful evaluation.

Hence while planning to do SPT using food allergens, we need to clearly understand if it is being done for diagnosing food allergy or for respiratory reactions only. The common foods implicated in food-induced episodes of asthma were peanut, milk, soya, egg, tree nuts, legumes, and beans. Sometimes aerosolized food can also be a cause of asthma when the foods are boiled, fried, or simply exposed to atmosphere. One another important factor to be kept in mind while deciding on the allergens is to look if there is an irritant effect. Chlorogenic acid in banana, histamine, serotonin and others in sea food and brinjal leads to symptoms which are not allergic in nature but appear to be allergic.

Food allergens implicated among patients including adults with respiratory complaints in India are chickpea, black gram, rice, lentils, peas, peanuts, beans, citrus fruits—orange, grapes, fish, mustard, prawn, and egg.

The EuroPrevall-INCO survey, which looked at prevalence of food allergies across several centers in the world including India, had showed while Indian children had a high degree of sensitization (19.1%), the incidence of food allergy was lowest (0.14%). Common food allergens implicated where shrimp, tomato, sesame, buckwheat, wheat, apple, peach, melon, banana, rice, corn, nuts, fish, egg, and milk in decreasing order of prevalence.

The other phenomenon while evaluation of food allergy is pollen-food allergy syndrome (PFAS) which is appearance of itching, numbness, and mucosal edema of lips and mouth within minutes of ingestion of food. It is rarely accompanied by systemic manifestations like wheezing. This phenomenon is IgE-dependent immediate allergy type caused due to cross-reactivity to pollens. PFAS is a subtype of oral allergy food syndrome (OAS) wherein systemic manifestation is also possible in contrast to OAS where symptoms are restricted to oral mucosa. The most common cross-reactivity is noted between birch, mugworts, cedar, and grasses to various fruits and vegetables. Cross-reactivity is due to the similarity of major allergen components present in foods and pollen—the pan allergens. The pan allergens belong to lipid transfer proteins (LTP), profilin, pathogen-related protein (PR 10).

In conclusion, we need to be very careful while selecting and planning the foods to be sensitized for respiratory complaints and for detection of food allergen. Good clinical correlation is essential.

SKIN PRICK TEST: CRITERIA AND STANDARDS

Indications

General clinical conditions where SPT is indicated:

- Asthma
- Rhinitis/rhinoconjunctivitis/rhinosinusitis
- Suspicion of food allergy
- Suspicion of drug allergy
- Insect venom hypersensitivity
- Eczema or atopic dermatitis when there is a suspicion of specific allergens
- Chronic urticaria in cases along with other allergic disorders
- ABPA—test for fungal sensitization

Not Indicated

- Food intolerance
- Chronic urticaria in absence of allergic features

- Food additives/preservants/colorants
- Screening for allergic sensitization in the absence of clinical features

Who can Perform the Tests?

- Clinician who has adequate knowledge and training in the same
- Technician trained in the same can perform only the testing under the supervision of trained clinician who should decide the specific allergens based on history and also interpret.

Figure 3 is an example of a reporting format.

Drugs to be Stopped Before the Skin Test

- H1 antihistamines—preferably 2–6 days for first generation, 3–10 days for second

Clinic name and address

Name *Age* *Gender*

Clinical history:

Drug history:

Antihistamines/beta blockers/Over the counter medications/tricyclic antidepressants

Time in: *Time out*

S.No.	*Allergens*	*Strength*	*Induration (in mms)*	*Remarks (presence of erythema/induration)*
1	*Saline*			
2				
3				
4				
5				
6				
7	*Histamine*			

Result:

(Comment on standardization and then write allergens the patient is sensitized to)

Name of the investigator and signature

Fig. 3: Sample reporting form.

generation, tricyclic antidepressants >10 days, anti-IgE monoclonal antibodies—6 weeks
- No need to stop oral steroids if given for short period but if given in high dose there may be interference
- High-potency topical steroids if locally applied have to be applied 3 weeks before SPT
- Stop antidepressants with antihistamine activity 1 week before the test
- No interference with leukotriene antagonists

SUGGESTED ALLERGEN PANELS IN INDIAN SCENARIO

The allergen panels suggested in Indian scenario are given in the following **Table 2**. This can be individualized based on the region, patient, age, and clinical scenario for which it is done.

Allergens

Allergens should be stored at 2°–8°C to improve stability.

Stability and potency of allergen extracts is important. Indian allergens are stored in saline so shelf life is less than a year. Those preserved with 50% glycerin have long shelf life.

STANDARDIZATION OF ALLERGENS: CURRENT SITUATION IN INDIA

Standardization means the quantity of the major allergens is specified by the manufacturer and is evaluated by a central body and batch to batch variation is low. In US, allergen standardization focuses on ensuring consistent potency and composition of allergen extracts which involves comparing manufactured allergen extracts to US reference standards. They have reference standards for 19 allergens. The reference standards have been prepared by evaluating the erythema induced by intradermal skin tests which are the most sensitive method to determine biologic potency of allergen extract. In Europe, manufacturers have implemented company-specific protocols to standardize the production and quality control of the allergen extracts and to compare to assure batch to batch consistency. In India Drug Controller of India and nodal

TABLE 2: Suggested allergen panels in Indian scenario.

Screening	*Panel for suspected food allergy*	*Fungal panel*
Dust mite—*Dermatophagoides pteronyssinus, Dermatophagoides farinae, Blomia tropicalis*	Chickpea	*Aspergillus* and *Alternaria*
• Cockroach—commercially available • Individual—*Periplaneta, Blattella* if available individually	Bengal gram	*Penicillium*
Mosquito—no evidence but if clinically indicated	Wheat and rice	*Cladosporium*
Pollens—depends on region and season	Peanut and other nuts based on clinical	*Fusarium*
Molds—*Aspergillus and Alternaria*	Fish	*Rhizopus*
Cat dander—commercially available	Shrimp	*Helminthosporium*
Dog dander—self-prepared extracts with the pets without washing pets for a week and soaking in saline for 24 hours	Milk	*Mucor*
Foods—milk, egg, chickpea, Bengal gram, rice, wheat, and nuts; others based on clinical history and correlation is necessary	Egg	*Candida*

officers regulate the allergen manufacture and potency is described as weight/volume (w/v), protein estimation units (pnu in mg/mL), and sodium dodecyl sulfate polyacrylamide gel electrophoresis (SDS-PAGE) protein profile is followed for maintaining/comparing the quality of antigen in different antigens. Government-funded research institutes like National Institute of Biologicals (NIB) and Indian Pharmacopoeia Commission (IPC) have been recognized to ensure quality of commercial allergens. However, we still need to characterize allergens in India as we have several varied allergens from diverse sources.

Procedure

- SPT to be performed on normal skin
- The antecubital fossa is most reactive and wrist is least reactive. Radial portion is less reactive than ulna.
- Saline and histamine are the controls. Saline should be pricked first followed by allergens and then histamine at the last. Histamine reacts quickly. Saline is the negative control and can cause traumatic reactivity induced by skin test device (wheal can approach a diameter of 3 mm with some devices), dermographism or technique of the tester. Saline can be up to maximum 3 mm. Histamine helps to identify presence of medication or disease that interferes with the reaction and the allergen quality.
- Generally, choose the allergens based on geographical location. Testing around 18 allergens is enough for adults. In children, we can test for a smaller number of allergens as they are not likely to be sensitized to many allergens.
- Devices available in India are lancets—3 mm tip **(Fig. 4)** and 1 mm tip **(Fig. 5)**; always use the 1 mm lancet (3 mm tip is a blood lancet and leads to false positives).

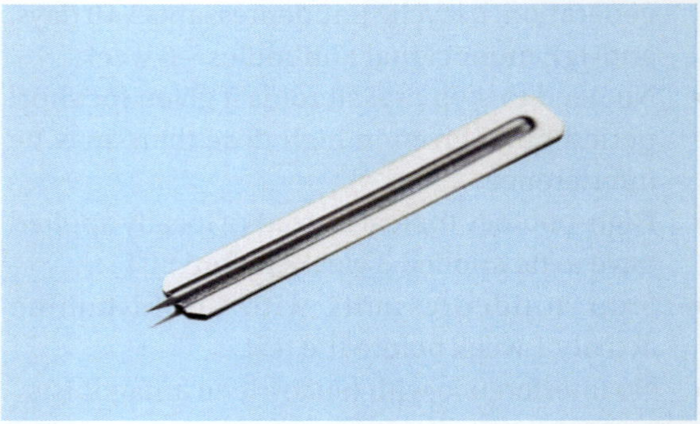

Fig. 4: A 3 mm tip.

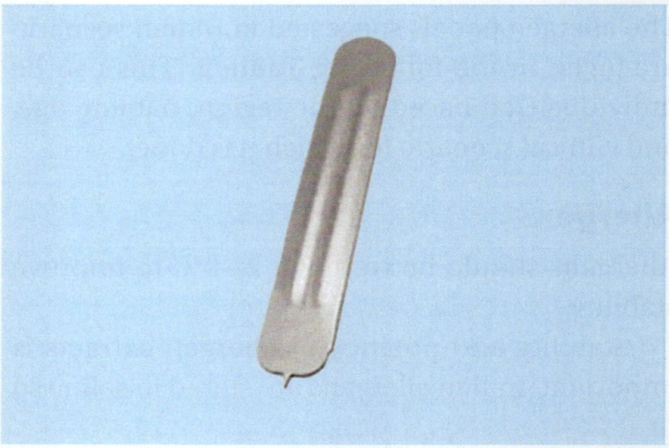

Fig. 5: 1 mm tip.

- SPT to be performed first by cleaning the site with alcohol and allowing it to dry. Need to mark the skin sites to place the extracts with extract coding. The next step is to apply a drop of allergen extract and prick the skin at 45°–60° angle to the skin to allow allergens to reach the epicutaneous layer. Drops to be placed at 2 cm apart and to avoid mixing.
- Information regarding cross-reactivity among allergens is important when interpreting results. Mainly a knowledge on cross-reactivity of important pollens is necessary as there are highly conserved proteins across different species.
- Common errors in SPT are applying it too close, bleeding in the site, insufficient penetration of

skin and spreading of allergen solution when it is wiped away.

- Measurements to be made at 8–10 minutes for histamine and 15–20 minutes for allergens; the reading and evaluation should be done by using a ruler and measuring in millimeters. Pseudopods can be marked separately.
- Consider the SPT to be positive if the wheal diameter is 3 mm greater than negative control and when negative control is <3 mm and has a positive histamine control.

In Vitro Methods of Allergy Testing

In vitro methods of allergy testing involves measuring serum-specific IgE, molecular assays, and basophil activation tests (BATs). Serum-specific IgE assays are the most commonly used in vitro diagnostic methods.

Serum-specific Immunoglobulin E Measurement

The fact that SPT is quicker to do, interprets results in short time, and also can be done with virtually any allergens (prick on prick), there are certain issues like difficulty to do in children, the interference due to drugs and greater reliability on operator training and experience. Hence serum-specific IgE is an alternative to the same giving more quantitative results. However, it measures the free allergens and is next only SPT in top-down strategy of allergy diagnostics.

Principle of Serum-specific Immunoglobulin E

The test involves drawing a blood sample and analyzed using enzyme-linked immunosorbent assay (ELISA). Primarily the serum is incubated along with the test where the allergen has been immobilized on a plate. After the incubation period, the plate is washed to remove unbound IgE and enzyme-linked secondary antibody is added, which binds to IgE allergen complex. An enzyme substrate is then added and the machines then analyze the results.

Changes in the components of testing have increased the reliability and clinical relevance of measurement of specific IgE (sIgE). The reaction site carrying the allergen has changed from agarose and microcrystalline cellulose to development of an encapsulated hydrophilic carrier polymer to which the allergen is covalently coupled. The allergen-containing reagent can be either a solid-phase allegro sorbent or liquid-phase conjugated allergen. This is most complex and variable and confers the specificity to the assay. The introduction of automated assays have helped in reduction of the human sample volumes. Further anti-human IgE Fc detection reagents usually are polyclonal rabbit, sheep, horse, goat, or murine anti-IgE monoclonal antibodies. The labeling techniques initially used were radioallergosorbent test. Nowadays β-galactosidase (β-Gal), alkaline phosphatase (AP), and horseradish peroxidase (HPO) are used.

Enzyme-linked Immunosorbent Assay Reaction—General Scheme

Figure 6 illustrates ELISA reaction.

Various companies use different techniques like chemiluminescence, fluorescence measurements, oxidizing enzymes, or immunoblot techniques. Each of them has its own advantages **(Fig. 7)**.

The commonly used producers are Thermo Fischer, Siemens, Hycor, and Euroimmun. They vary in the type of components discussed above **(Fig. 8)**. There have been comparative studies examining the methodologies had concluded that IgE values obtained are not equivalent between systems and better to use the reference values of the company.

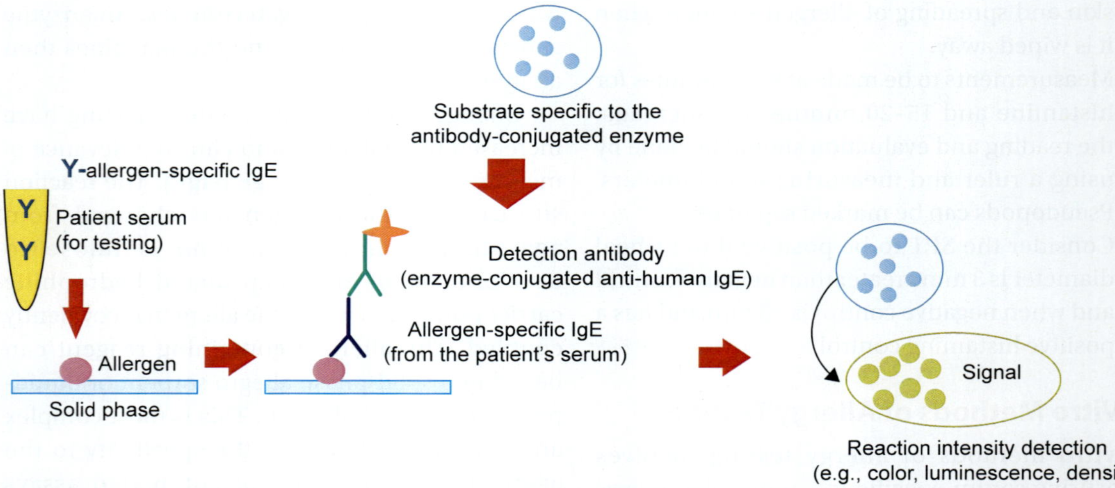

Fig. 6: Steps involved in enzyme-linked immunosorbent assay (ELISA) reaction. (IgE: immunoglobulin E)
Source: Adapted from Lis K, Bartuzi Z. Selected Technical Aspects of Molecular Allergy Diagnostics. Curr Issues Mol Biol. 2023;45(7):5481-93.

MOLECULAR DIAGNOSIS OF ALLERGY

Traditionally in vitro allergy diagnosis is based on allergen extracts and it does not allow for identification of cross-reaction or cross-reactive carbohydrate determinants. Molecular diagnosis of allergy enables us to determine the allergen molecule. It can diagnose single allergen components (molecules) from allergen source. This gives the opportunity to precisely identify a harmful allergen, determine possible cross-reactions, and predict the severity of a possible reaction.

There are various types of molecular diagnosis.

Phadiatop

Phadiatop is also a variant of ImmunoCAP. However, it is essentially a screening test. Phadiatop and Phadiatop Infant blood tests are qualitative screening tests on the same principle and cover a mixture of common aeroallergens.

The proposed algorithm could be to do Phadiatop test **(Flowchart 1)** in screening sensitization to most inhalant allergens in a single test. Zeng et al. had proposed a screening test for using the above tests in sequence. They detected molds and fungal mix together (mfx).

Specific Tests

There are two types of diagnostics are either single component (singleplex) and multicomponent (multiplex) where we measure the concentration of sIgE for many allergenic components in one test for many patients.

Singleplex Assay

What is available in India is Immuno Solid-phase Allergen Chip (ISAC) by Thermo Fisher Scientific. This is a biochip technology-based solid-phase enzyme immunoassays. It is a quantitative test and has a reference standard for in vitro IgE detection for specific allergen. There is a high degree of sensitivity and specificity. Despite the strengths, there is a problem of high costs and volume of serum required is high. When using singleplex we have to be specific about the allergens we want to test just like we do for skin testing.

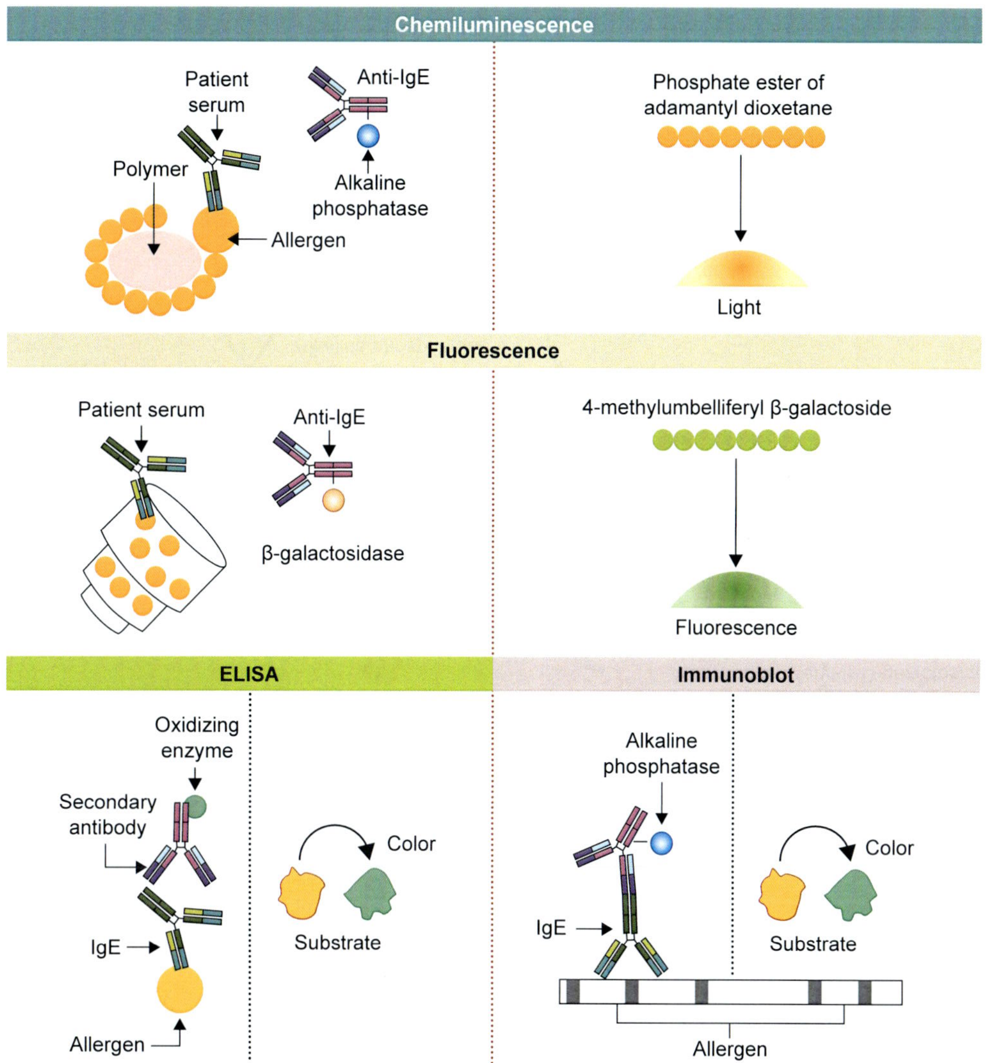

Fig. 7: The different types of components used by various techniques in measuring serum-specific IgE.
Source: Adapted from Velázquez-Soto H, Jimenez Martinez MC. Fundamentals of molecular allergy: From bench to bedside. In: Özdemir Ö (Ed). Allergic Disease - New Developments in Diagnosis and Therapy [Internet]. IntechOpen; 2022. Available from https://www.intechopen.com/chapters/83814.

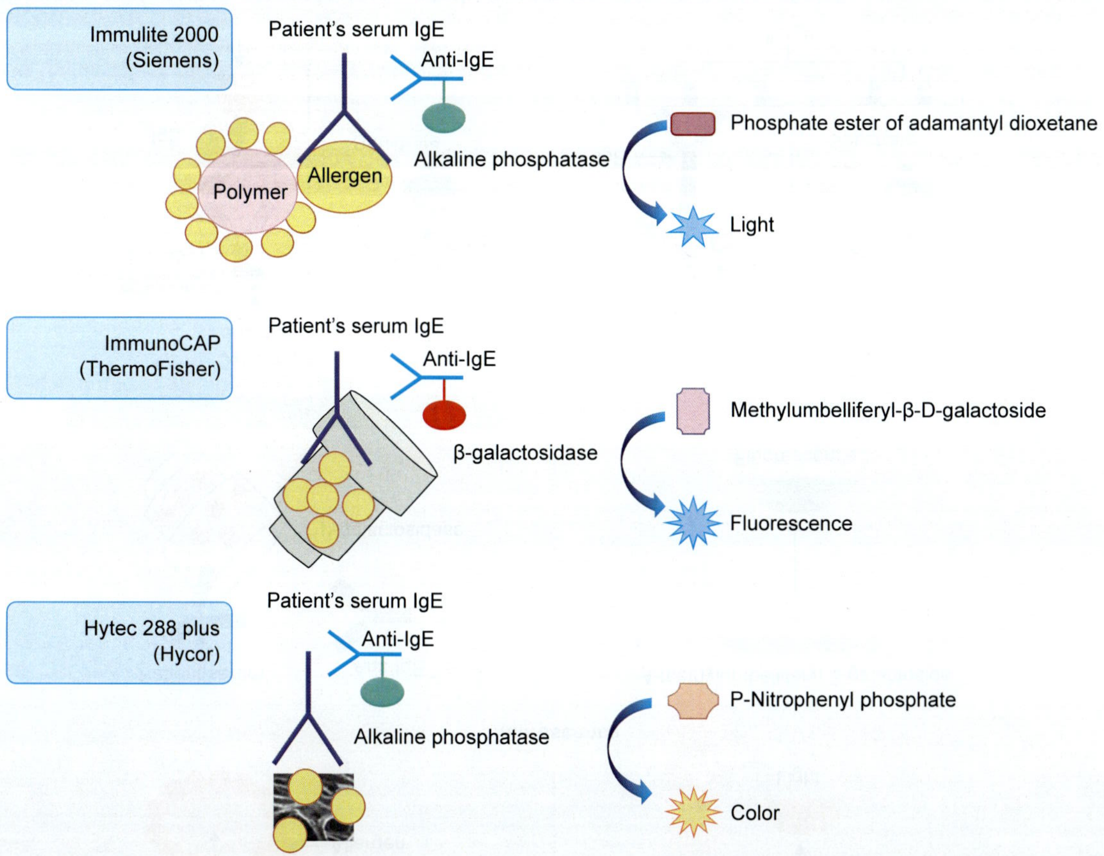

Fig. 8: Methodology of the various IgE detection methods.
Source: Adapted from Goikoetxea MJ, Sanz ML, García BE, Mayorga C, Longo N, Gamboa PM, et al. Recommendations for the Use of In Vitro Methods to Detect Specific Immunoglobulin E: Are They Comparable? J Investig Allergol Clin Immunol. 2013;23(7):448-54; quiz 2 p preceding 455.

Flowchart 1: Proposed algorithm to look for allergen sensitization using Phadiatop.

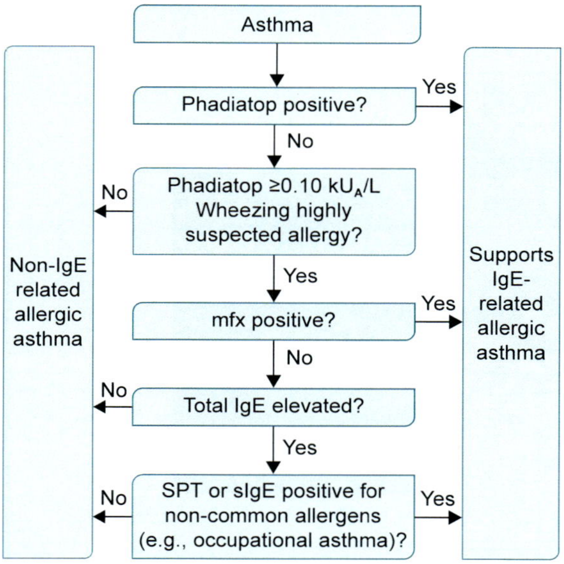

(mfx: molds and fungal mix; sIgE: specific immunoglobulin E; SPT: skin prick test)

The advantages of singleplex systems are:

- Increased test sensitivity
- Increased analytical specificity
- Indicators of cross-reactivity
- Markers of primary, genuine sensitization

Multiplex Assay

Multiplex assays have recently emerged as an alternative method for measuring IgE for a broad array of allergens in a single test. Here several allergens are spotted onto specific sites of a single microchip. The principle is same as that of the singleplex but the results are semi-quantitative and the amount of allergen used is lower than singleplex. This platform allows for simultaneous measurement of 112 allergen components.

The layout and principles of microarray are given in **Figure 9**.

Measurement values are reported not only quantitatively, but also semiquantitatively, divided into four different categories.

- Values <0.3 ISU-E are defined as negative
- Values between 0.3 and 1.0 ISU-E as low-level positive
- Values between 1.0 and 15.0 ISU-E as moderately high
- Values ≥15.0 ISU-E as very high

Source: Adapted from Jakob T, Forstenlechner P, Matricardi P, Kleine-Tebbe J. Molecular allergy diagnostics using multiplex assays: methodological and practical considerations for use in research and clinical routine: Part 21 of the Series Molecular Allergology. Allergo J Int. 2015;24:320-32.

Difference between singleplex and multiplex assays: There are key differences between singleplex and multiplex assays with each having its specific indications and uses **(Table 3)**.

Advantages of the multiplex assay:

- Differentiation between genuine sensitization and cross-reactivity with inhalant allergens
- We can find the sensitization profile of an individual
- Guide in immunotherapy
- Use of tailored allergen chips in research

PRECISION ALLERGY MOLECULAR DIAGNOSTICS APPLICATIONS

The new terminology for component-resolved diagnostics (CRD) is molecular-based allergy diagnostics (MBAD). While the above singleplex and multiplex systems measure IgE against allergens, the CRD looks at allergenic components within an allergen. The main use of precision allergy molecular diagnostics (PAMD) has been in food allergy where knowing the allergenic molecules can help us to understand the likelihood of local versus systemic reactions and predict persistence of clinical symptoms. Some allergenic molecule like storage proteins (e.g., Ara h2) and

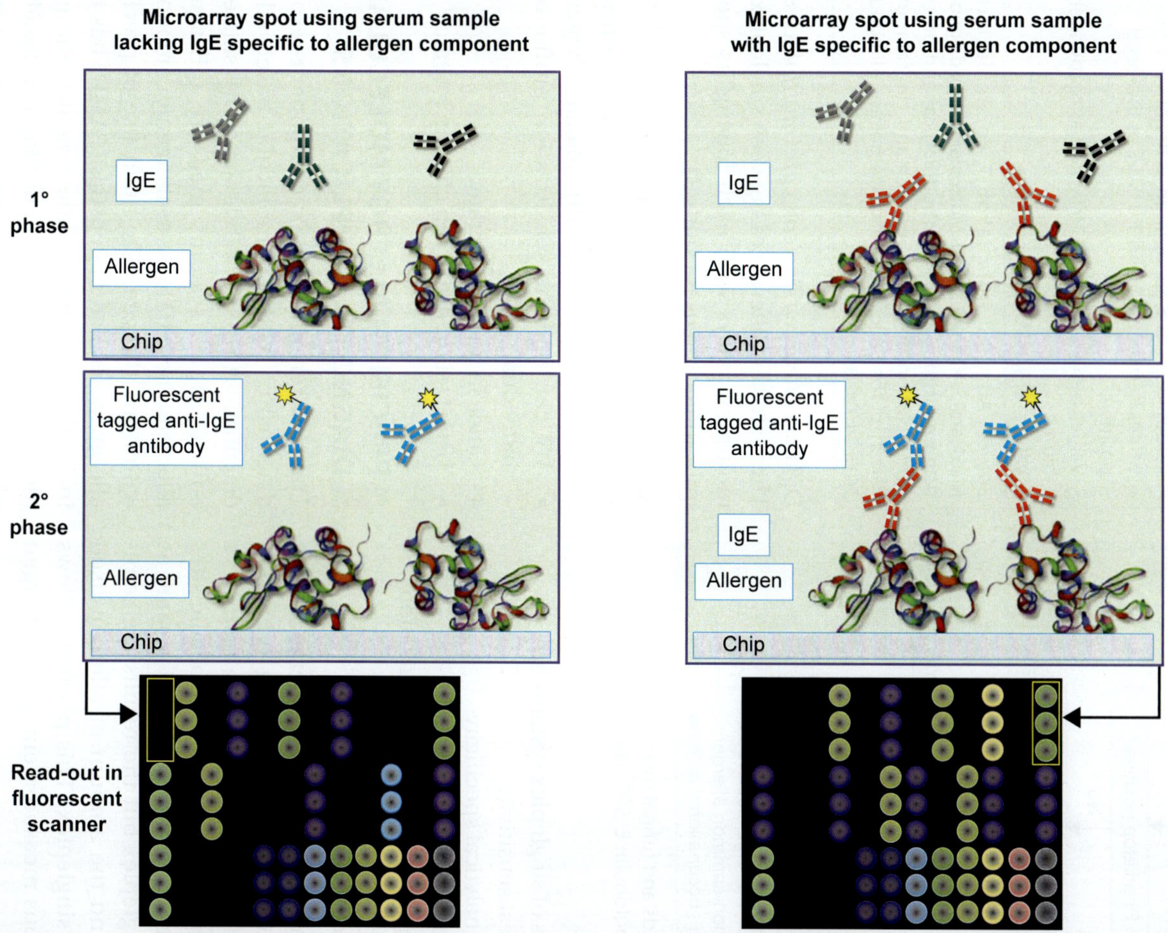

Fig. 9: Technique of various microarray technique.
Source: Adapted from Keshavarz B, Platts-Mills TAE, Wilson JM. The use of microarray and other multiplex technologies in the diagnosis of allergy. Ann Allergy Asthma Immunol. 2021;127(1):10-18.

TABLE 3: Difference between singleplex and multiplex assays.

<table>
<tr><th></th><th>Singleplex extract</th><th>Singleplex component</th><th>Multiplex components</th></tr>
<tr><td></td><td colspan="2">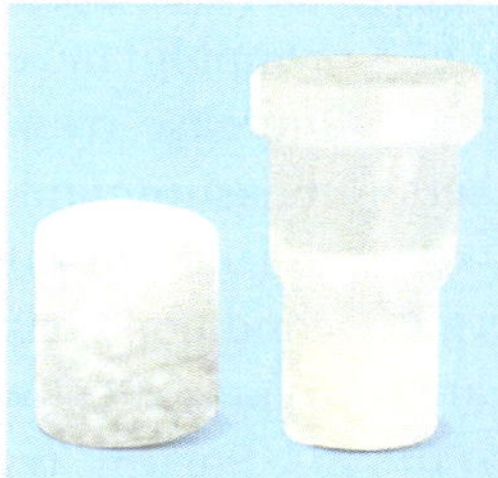</td><td>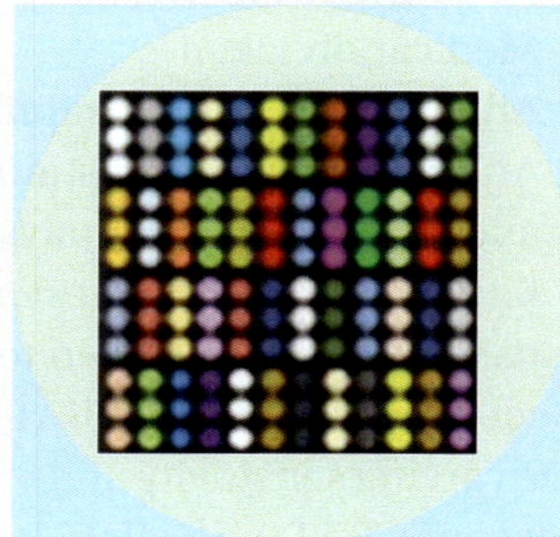</td></tr>
<tr><td>Commercial assay</td><td colspan="2">ImmunoCAP</td><td>ISAC</td></tr>
<tr><td>Materials</td><td colspan="2">Cellulose matrix/resin</td><td>Polymer-coated glass slide</td></tr>
<tr><td>Amount of allergen</td><td colspan="2">~1–2 μg/ImmunoCAP</td><td>~100 pg/spot</td></tr>
<tr><td>Number of allergens</td><td>Mixture</td><td>1/ImmunoCAP</td><td>112/chip</td></tr>
<tr><td>Amount of serum</td><td colspan="2">40 μL/ImmunoCAP</td><td>30 μL/chip</td></tr>
<tr><td>Sensitivity</td><td colspan="2">0.1 kU_A/L</td><td>0.3 ISU</td></tr>
<tr><td>Interference from IgG</td><td colspan="2">No</td><td>Yes</td></tr>
<tr><td>Read-out</td><td colspan="2">Quantitative</td><td>Semiquantitative</td></tr>
<tr><td>Assays unit and scale</td><td colspan="2">Class 0: <0.1 kU_A/L
Class 0/1: 0.1–0.34 kU_AL
Class 1: 0.35–0.70 kU_A/L
Class 2: >0.70–3.5 kU_A/L
Class 3: >3.5–17.5 kU_A/L
Class 4: >17.5–50 kU_A/L
Class 5: >50–100 kU_A/L
Class 6: >100 kU_A/L</td><td>Low: 0.3–1.0 ISU/mL
Moderate: >1.0–15 ISU/mL
High: >15 ISU mL</td></tr>
</table>

Source: Adapted from Keshavarz B, Platts-Mills TAE, Wilson JM. The use of microarray and other multiplex technologies in the diagnosis of allergy. Ann Allergy Asthma Immunol. 2021;127(1):10-18.

in nuts (e.g., Cor a9) are associated with severe reactions. In case of food-dependent, exercise-induced anaphylaxis, it is possible to identify the allergic sensitization to individual component like omega-5-gliadin and nsLTP. PAMD may also be helpful in assessment of idiopathic anaphylaxis. The most important point is molecular allergen IgE assays are not alternative to allergen extract-based assays but complementary to the same.

OTHER IN VITRO TESTS

Basophil Activation Tests

Basophil activation test is a functional assay and measures the degree of degranulation of basophils that have already been stimulated by allergens or control by flow cytometry. Activation of basophils is detected through upregulation of CD63 protein on its surface through flow cytometry.

The factors affecting results of the BAT are:

- Time between blood collection and the performance of BAT
- Medication taken
- Allergens used for basophil stimulation
- Antibodies used for staining of key markers and flow cytometry analyses

Basophil activation test reflects the allergic status of patients sensitized to food, inhalant, and insect venom allergens. BAT has been shown to have varying sensitivity and specificity to different allergens. BAT can also be used to monitor treatment by omalizumab and to allergen-specific immunotherapy.

Indications to consider BAT in clinical settings:

- If the allergen can produce false-positive results in skin testing
- If there is no allergen source to use for skin testing or serum-specific IgE
- There is a discordance between patient history and sIgE/skin tests
- If history suggests that skin testing will results in systemic response
- Before provocation testing to confirm causative allergen

The position of BAT is still in the primitive stage and is offered by certain companies like Thermo Fisher. With the advent of allergy specially we should probably be using more of the tests.

Serum Tryptase

Tryptase is the most abundant mediator found in mast cells. Mast cell tryptase has an important role in inflammation and it is found in increased anaphylaxis and anaphylactoid reactions. A substantial increase in the blood levels above what is measured when a patient is asymptomatic (in ng/mL). This is to rule out if the patient has hereditary alpha tryptasemia (HaT), which is three times higher in those with allergic conditions. It can also be elevated in mastocytosis. Generally, the normal levels are >11.4 ng/mL.

The current approach to confirm increased tryptase levels is to apply a formula termed the *"20 + 2 rule"* where the tryptase level during a symptomatic episode must equal or exceed a 20% increase over a baseline serum tryptase (BST) measurement plus 2 ng/mL. This formula helps to rule out differences due to gender and other conditions. It is also possible to look at ratio of acute tryptase/BST which should be more than 1.685.

Serum tryptase to be measured within 15 minutes to 4 hours during an anaphylaxis episodes. Generally acute elevation will gradually return to normal within 24 hours.

In conclusion recommendations to do serum tryptase after a suspected anaphylactic reaction either due to venom-related, drug-related, or idiopathic are to take a sample ideally within 1–2 hours (but no later than 4 hours) from onset of symptoms and second to understand the baseline levels either on follow-up with the specialist or at least after 24 hours of the incident.

In summary, the following algorithms can be used for testing in Indian scenario under different scenarios **(Figs. 10 to 13)**.

SUMMARY

This comprehensive chapter explores the nuanced approach to diagnosing and managing allergic diseases in special populations—*infants and toddlers, pregnant women,* and the *elderly*. In infants, the immature immune system and nonspecific symptoms complicate diagnosis and management. The chapter underscores emerging diagnostic tools like CRD and the evolving role of oral immunotherapy and biologics such as dupilumab in early childhood. In pregnant women, physiological changes and immunomodulation necessitate careful medication choices, emphasizing safety for both mother and fetus. Conditions like asthma, rhinitis, and urticaria require tailored strategies, often favoring non-pharmacologic interventions

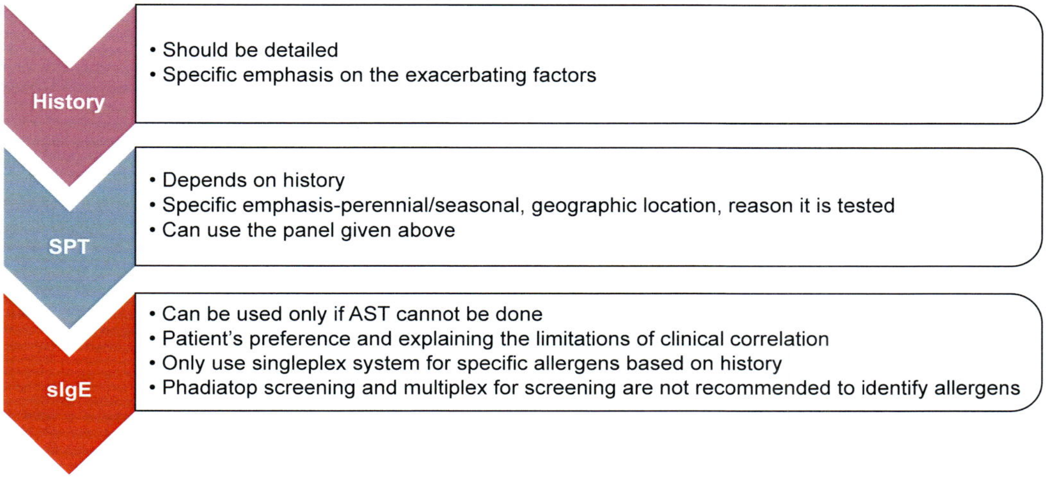

Fig. 10: Tests suggested in respiratory condition.

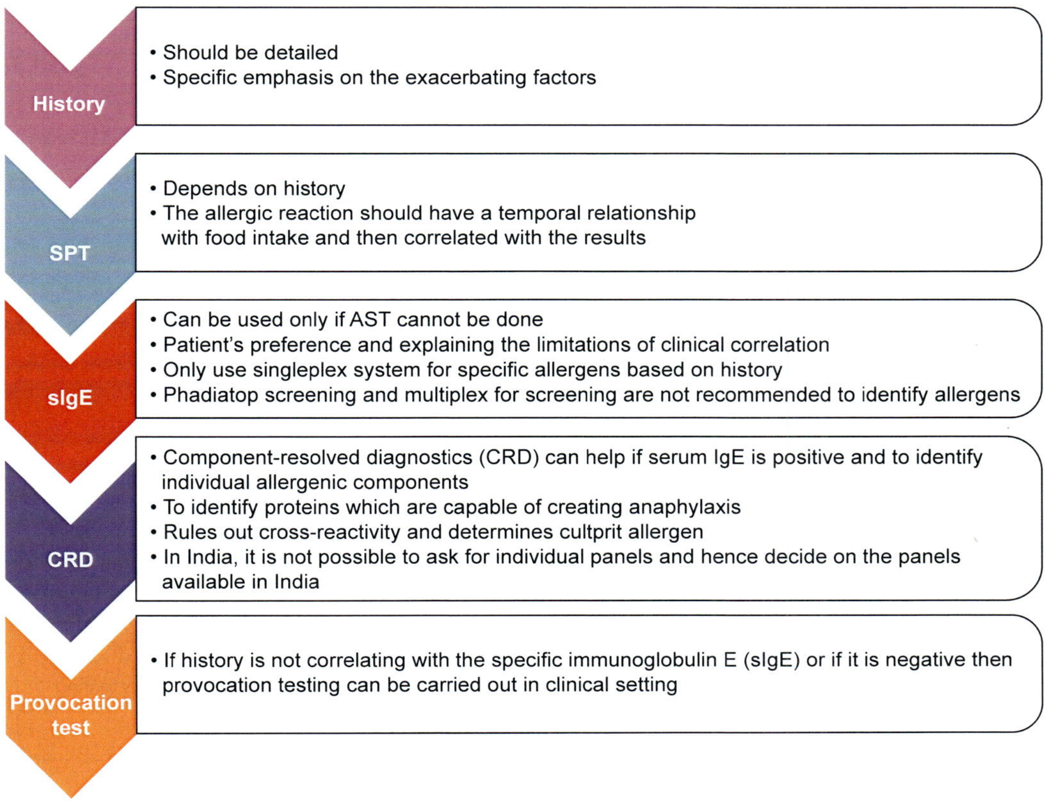

Fig. 11: Tests suggested in food allergy. (SPT: skin prick test)

History
- Should be detailed
- Specific emphasis on identifying the causative insects

SPT
- Depends on history
- Start using the specific allergens present for insect venoms in India
- Start from 1:1,000 dilution to 1:1 dilution

Intradermal
- To be done if history is highly suggestive and skin prick test (SPT) is negative
- To be done in clinical conditions where facility for management of anaphylaxis is there
- Start from 1:100 to 1:1 dilution

sIgE
- Can be used only if AST cannot be done
- Clinical correlation is less

CRD
- Component-resolved diagnostics (CRD) to be used after AST/intradermal is positive to rule out cross-reactivity and cross-reactive carbohydrate determinants (CCD)
- In India, it is not possible to ask for individual panels and hence decide on the insect venom panels available in India

Fig. 12: Suspected insect venom hypersensitivity. (AST: allergy skin testing; sIgE: specific immunoglobulin E)

History
- Should be detailed
- Specific emphasis on identifying the causative drugs and ruling our possible confounders like coexistent viral illness, other preservatives, symptoms due to non-immunological reasons

SPT
- Depends on history
- Start using the specific culprit drugs
- Start from 1:1,000 dilution to 1:1 dilution
- Use a control person to know the irritant concentration as in India we do not have the standard concentration of the drugs

Intradermal
- To be done if history is highly suggestive and skin prick test (SPT) is negative
- To be done in clinical conditions where facility for management of anaphylaxis is there
- Start from 1:100 to 1:1 dilution

Provocation testing
- If history is not correlating with the specific IgE or if it is negative then provocation testing can be carried out in clinical setting

Fig. 13: Suspected drug allergy.

and the cautious use of safe medications like budesonide and loratadine. In the elderly, immunosenescence, polypharmacy, and atypical symptom presentations pose unique diagnostic and therapeutic challenges. The chapter offers guidance on optimizing pharmacotherapy, adjusting immunotherapy strategies, and managing comorbidities. Overall, it promotes individualized care and a multidisciplinary approach for allergy management across the lifespan.

Key Learning Points

- *Infants and toddlers often present with atypical or overlapping allergy symptoms*, and conventional tests like SPT have limited sensitivity; early allergen introduction (e.g., peanuts, eggs) can reduce food allergy risk.
- *Pregnancy alters immune responses*, making allergic diseases unpredictable. Safe medications include second-generation antihistamines (loratadine, cetirizine) and budesonide for asthma; skin testing is generally avoided.
- *Older adults may develop new allergies or show muted symptoms*, requiring cautious pharmacotherapy due to comorbidities and polypharmacy. Diagnosis is often delayed due to immunosenescence.
- *Immunotherapy [subcutaneous immunotherapy (SCIT)/sublingual immunotherapy (SLIT)]* can be continued in pregnancy if already initiated and may be considered in elderly with appropriate monitoring; SLIT is often safer than SCIT in special populations.
- *Multidisciplinary care and individualized treatment plans*—involving allergists, pediatricians, obstetricians, and geriatricians—are essential to optimize outcomes and minimize risks across vulnerable age-groups.

SUGGESTED READING

1. Agarwal MK, Chaudhry S, Jhamb S, Gaur SN, Chauhan UP, Agarwal HC. Etiologic significance of mosquito (Anopheles stephensi) in respiratory allergy in India. Ann Allergy. 1991;67(6):598-602.
2. Agarwal R, Muthu V, Sehgal IS, Dhooria S, Prasad KT, Soundappan K, et al. Aspergillus Sensitization and Allergic Bronchopulmonary Aspergillosis in Asthmatic Children: A Systematic Review and Meta-Analysis. Diagnostics (Basel). 2023;13(5):922.
3. Agrawal A, Gupta R, Sodhi K, Raghav V. Is Iron Deficiency Anaemia, a risk Factor For Wheeze Associated Respiratory Tract Infection in Children? J Nepal Paedtr Soc. 2015;34(3):195-9.
4. Ansotegui IJ, Melioli G, Canonica GW, Caraballo L, Villa E, Ebisawa M, et al. IgE allergy diagnostics and other relevant tests in allergy, a World Allergy Organization position paper. World Allergy Organ J. 2020;13(2):100080.
5. Ansotegui IJ, Melioli G, Canonica GW, Gómez RM, Jensen-Jarolim E, Ebisawa M, et al. A WAO—ARIA—GA2LEN consensus document on molecular-based allergy diagnosis (PAMD@): Update 2020. World Allergy Organ J. 2020;13(2):100091.
6. Bener A, Ehlayel M, Hamid Q. The impact of anemia and hemoglobin level as a risk factor for asthma and allergic diseases. Indian J Allergy Asthma Immunol. 2015;29(2):72.
7. Bhattacharya K, Sircar G, Dasgupta A, Gupta Bhattacharya S. Spectrum of Allergens and Allergen Biology in India. Int Arch Allergy Immunol. 2018;177(3):219-37.
8. Cantillo JF, Puerta L. Mosquitoes: Important Sources of Allergens in the Tropics. Front Allergy. 2021;2:690406.
9. Chan SK, Leung DYM. Dog and Cat Allergies: Current State of Diagnostic Approaches and Challenges. Allergy Asthma Immunol Res. 2018; 10(2):97-105.
10. Chaudhary GS, Kumar A, Shashtri M, Chaudhary V. Comparison of total serum immunoglobulin E and absolute eosinophil count levels among asthmatic and non-asthmatic children. Indian J Child Health. 2017;4(3):345-7.
11. Chauhan K, Srivastava S, Prasad R. Sensitization to indoor allergens in children with bronchial asthma. Indian J Allergy Asthma Immunol. 2020;34:39.
12. Dey D, Mondal P, Laha A, Sarkar T, Moitra S, Bhattacharyya S, et al. Sensitization to Common Aeroallergens in the Atopic Population of West Bengal, India: An Investigation by Skin Prick Test. Int Arch Allergy Immunol. 2019;178(1):60-5.
13. Dey D, Saha G, Podder S. A review of house dust mite allergy in India. Exp Appl Acarol. 2019; 78:1-14.

14. Eigenmann PA, Atanaskovic-Markovic M, O'B Hourihane J, Lack G, Lau S, Matricardi PM, et al.; European Academy of Allergy and Clinical Immunology Section on Pediatrics; European Academy of Allergy and Clinical Immunology-Clemens von Pirquet Foundation. Testing children for allergies: why, how, who and when: an updated statement of the European Academy of Allergy and Clinical Immunology (EAACI) Section on Pediatrics and the EAACI-Clemens von Pirquet Foundation. Pediatr Allergy Immunol. 2013;24(2):195-209.
15. Froidure A, Mouthuy J, Durham SR, Chanez P, Sibille Y, Pilette C. Asthma phenotypes and IgE responses. Eur Respir J. 2016;47(1):304-19.
16. Goikoetxea MJ, Sanz ML, García BE, Mayorga C, Longo N, Gamboa PM, et al. Recommendations for the Use of In Vitro Methods to Detect Specific Immunoglobulin E: Are They Comparable? J Investig Allergol Clin Immunol. 2013;23(7):448-54; quiz 2 p preceding 455.
17. Gupta N, Bang A, Mishra NR; IAP Standard Treatment Guidelines Committee. Standard Treatment Guidelines 2022. [online] Available from https://iapindia.org/pdf/gepAz6wsH5c3B2r_Standard-Treatment-Guidelines-Anaphylaxis.pdf [Last accessed August, 2025].
18. Heutelbeck ARR, Schulz T, Bergmann KC, Hallier E. Environmental Exposure to Allergens of Different Dog Breeds and Relevance in Allergological Diagnostics. J Toxicol Environ Health A. 2008;71(11-12):751-8.
19. Jain AK, Kumar A. Fungal sensitization and its impact on asthma control – A prospective study at allergy clinic. Indian J Allergy Asthma Immunol. 2023;37(1):17.
20. Jakob T, Forstenlechner P, Matricardi P, Kleine-Tebbe J. Molecular allergy diagnostics using multiplex assays: methodological and practical considerations for use in research and clinical routine: Part 21 of the Series Molecular Allergology. Allergo J Int. 2015;24:320-32.
21. Jat KR, Khairwa A. Vitamin D and asthma in children: A systematic review and meta-analysis of observational studies. Lung India. 2017; 34(4):355-63.
22. Kamfar HZ, Koshak EE, Milaat WA. Is there a role for automated eosinophil count in asthma severity assessment? J Asthma. 1999; 36(2):153-8.
23. Kato Y, Morikawa T, Fujieda S. Comprehensive review of pollen-food allergy syndrome: Pathogenesis, epidemiology, and treatment approaches. Allergol Int. 2025;74(1):42-50.
24. Kausar MA, Vijayan VK, Bansal SK, Menon BK, Vermani M, Agarwal MK. Mosquitoes as sources of inhalant allergens: Clinicoimmunologic and biochemical studies. J Allergy Clin Immunol. 2007;120(5):1219-21.
25. Keshavarz B, Platts-Mills TAE, Wilson JM. The use of microarray and other multiplex technologies in the diagnosis of allergy. Ann Allergy Asthma Immunol. 2021;127(1):10-18.
26. Krishna MT, Mahesh PA, Vedanthan P, Moitra S, Mehta V, Christopher DJ. An appraisal of allergic disorders in India and an urgent call for action. World Allergy Organ J. 2020;13(7):100446.
27. Kumar R, Singh BP, Srivastava P, Sridhara S, Arora N, Gaur SN. Relevance of serum IgE estimation in allergic bronchial asthma with special reference to food allergy. Asian Pac J Allergy Immunol. 2006;24(4):191-9.
28. Kumar R, Srivastava P, Kumari D, Fakhr H, Sridhara S, Arora N, et al. Rice (Oryza sativa) allergy in rhinitis and asthma patients: a clinico-immunological study. Immunobiology. 2007;212(2):141-7.
29. Kumari D, Kumar R, Sridhara S, Arora N, Gaur SN, Singh BP. Sensitization to blackgram in patients with bronchial asthma and rhinitis: clinical evaluation and characterization of allergens. Allergy. 2006;61(1):104-10.
30. Kunoor A, PT J, Rakesh P. Allergen profile of patients from central Kerala, India. Int J Pharm Bio Sci. 2017;8:588.
31. Kuravi N, Swaminathan P, Nagaraju K, Mishra NR, Nayak BK. Sensitization Patterns in Immunoglobulin E-mediated Allergic Diseases by Skin Prick Testing Using Standardized Allergens: A Study from Tertiary Care Allergy Center. Clin Rhinol. 2021;12(1):6-15.
32. Lama M, Chatterjee M, Chaudhuri TK. Total Serum Immunoglobulin E in Children with Asthma. Indian J Clin Biochem. 2013;28(2):197-200.
33. Leishangthem A, Venkatesh DP, Kanni P, Komarla NP. Cockroach Allergy, Allergen Based Immuno

Diagnostic and Specific Immunotherapy: Present Status and Future Trends. RGUHS J Med Sci. 2021;11(3).

34. Li J, Ogorodova LM, Mahesh PA, Wang MH, Fedorova OS, Leung TF, et al. Comparative Study of Food Allergies in Children from China, India, and Russia: The EuroPrevall-INCO Surveys. J Allergy Clin Immunol Pract. 2020;8(4):1349-1358.e16.
35. Lis K, Bartuzi Z. Selected Technical Aspects of Molecular Allergy Diagnostics. Curr Issues Mol Biol. 2023;45(7):5481-93.
36. Mahesh PA, Kummeling I, Amrutha DH, Vedanthan PK. Effect of Area of Residence on Patterns of Aeroallergen Sensitization in Atopic Patients. Am J Rhinol Allergy. 2010;24(5):e98-103.
37. Mandal J, Das M, Roy I, Chatterjee S, Barui NC, Gupta-Bhattacharya S. Immediate hypersensitivity to common food allergens: an investigation on food sensitization in respiratory allergic patients of Calcutta, India. World Allergy Organ J. 2009;2(1):9-12.
38. Mateja A, Wang Q, Chovanec J, Kim J, Wilson KJ, Schwartz LB, et al. Defining baseline variability of serum tryptase levels improves accuracy in identifying anaphylaxis. J Allergy Clin Immunol. 2022;149(3):1010-1017.e10.
39. Miller JD. The Role of Dust Mites in Allergy. Clinic Rev Allerg Immunol. 2019;57(3):312-29.
40. Nagaraju K, Swaminathan P, Karthik N, Ranjan N, Kasyapi VV, Srivatsav NS. Demographic Profile of Dust Mite Sensitization among Indian Children using Standardized Allergens: An Observational Study. Ann Rom Soc Cell Biol. 2021;25(4):5832-47.
41. Nam YH, Jin HJ, Lee SK. Clinical significance of serum tryptase. J Allergy Clin Immunol. 2018;141(2):AB162.
42. Nathan MV, Patil SP, Nautiyal K, Janardhanan J, Parween S, V A. A Study of Iron Deficiency Anemia in Children with Bronchial Asthma. J Med Sci Clin Res. 2021;9(7).
43. National Clinical Guideline Centre (UK). Measuring serum tryptase after suspected anaphylaxis. Drug Allergy: Diagnosis and Management of Drug Allergy in Adults, Children and Young People. London: National Institute for Health and Care Excellence (NICE); 2014. Available from https://www.ncbi.nlm.nih.gov/books/NBK274147/
44. Papaioannou AI, Loukides S, Bakakos P. Identification of asthma phenotypes using blood cell count. EBioMedicine. 2022;77:103907.
45. Patil SP, Niphadkar PV, Bapat MM. Chickpea: a major food allergen in the Indian subcontinent and its clinical and immunochemical correlation. Ann Allergy Asthma Immunol. 2001;87(2):140-5.
46. Pomés A, Mueller GA, Randall TA, Chapman MD, Arruda LK. New insights into cockroach allergens. Curr Allergy Asthma Rep. 2017;17(4):25.
47. Ramakrishnan K, Borade A. Anemia as a risk factor for childhood asthma. Lung India. 2010;27(2):51-3.
48. Rathoria E, Bansal U, Gupta A, Gupta NB, Ahuja R, Rathoria R. Study of serum IgE levels in childhood asthma in Barabanki region, India. Int J Contemp Pediatr. 2018;5(5):1755.
49. Roberts G, Lack G. Food allergy and asthma—what is the link? Paediatr Respir Rev. 2003;4(3):205-12.
50. Samajdar SS, Moitra S. Present and Future of Allergy Practice in India. J Pediatr Pulmonol. 2023;2(Suppl 2):S87.
51. Santos AF, Alpan O, Hoffmann HJ. Basophil activation test: Mechanisms and considerations for use in clinical trials and clinical practice. Allergy. 2021;76(8):2420-32.
52. Sharma R, Gaur SN, Singh VP, Singh AB. Association between indoor fungi in Delhi homes and sensitization in children with respiratory allergy. Med Mycol. 2012;50(3):281-90.
53. Singh AB. Allergen Preparation and Standardization: An Update. Glob J Otolaryngol. 2018;17(4):555968.
54. Singh AB. Glimpse of Clinical Aerobiology in India: An Overview. Glob J Otolaryngol. 2017;12(3):60-8.
55. Singh M, Das S, Chauhan A, Paul N, Sodhi KS, Mathew J, et al. The diagnostic criteria for allergic bronchopulmonary aspergillosis in children with poorly controlled asthma need to be re-evaluated. Acta Paediatr. 2015;104(5).
56. Singh S, Salvi S, Mangal DK, Singh M, Awasthi S, Mahesh PA, et al. Prevalence, time trends and treatment practices of asthma in India: the Global Asthma Network study. ERJ Open Res. 2022;8(2):00528-2021.
57. Snehalatha G, Begum A, Raju N, Kumar R. A study on correlation of serum IgE levels with diagnosis and severity of asthma in children. Int J Contemp Pediatr. 2018;5(6):2240-3.

58. Trivedi PP, Patel AH. Serum immunoglobulin E and absolute eosinophil count as markers of severity in childhood asthma. Int J Contemp Pediatr. 2020;7(2):413.
59. Velázquez-Soto H, Jimenez Martinez MC. Fundamentals of molecular allergy: From bench to bedside. In: Özdemir Ö (Ed). Allergic Disease - New Developments in Diagnosis and Therapy [Internet]. IntechOpen; 2022. Available from https://www.intechopen.com/chapters/83814
60. Vidal C, Gude F, Boquete O, Fernández-Merino MC, Meijide LM, Rey J, et al. Evaluation of the phadiatop test in the diagnosis of allergic sensitization in a general adult population. J Investig Allergol Clin Immunol. 2005; 15(2):124-30.
61. Wangorsch A, Jamin A, Eichhorn S, Pablos I, Sharma S, Schweidler B, et al. Component-Resolved Diagnosis of American Cockroach (*Periplaneta americana*) Allergy in Patients From Different Geographical Areas. Front Allergy. 2021;2:691627.
62. Wilson N, Silverman M. Diagnosis of food sensitivity in childhood asthma. J R Soc Med. 1985;78 Suppl 5(Suppl 5):11-6.
63. Wu LC, Zarrin AA. The production and regulation of IgE by the immune system. Nat Rev Immunol. 2014;14(4):247-59.
64. Zakzuk J, Kilimajer J, Lockey RF; World Allergy Organization. [2019]. Allergen Standardization and Characterization. [online] Available from https://www.worldallergy.org/component/content/article/allergen-standardization-and-characterization-josefina-zakzuk-md-phd-jonathan-kilimajer-md-enrique-fernandez-caldas-phd-richard-f-lockey-md-updated-2019?catid=16&Itemid=101 [Last accessed August, 2025].
65. Zeng G, Hu H, Zheng P, Wu G, Wei N, Liang X, et al. The practical benefit of Phadiatop test as the first-line in vitro allergen-specific immunoglobulin E (sIgE) screening of aeroallergens among Chinese asthmatics: a validation study. Ann Transl Med. 2018;6(8):151.
66. Zhang XY., Simpson JL, Powell H, Yang IA, Upham JW, Reynolds PN, et al. Full blood count parameters for the detection of asthma inflammatory phenotypes. Clin Exp Allergy. 2014;44(9):1137-45.

CHAPTER

15

Ethical, Legal, and Practical Considerations

Dhanesh Volvoikar

Reviewer: *Uppin Narayan Reddy*

INTRODUCTION

Allergy is a completely new subject both from the learning point of view and from the point of practicing it in India. The National Medical Commission (NMC) recognized postgraduate qualifications as not being available. One needs to practice without standardized skin prick testing (SPT) antigens and adrenaline autoinjectors. Allergic conditions are increasing at an alarming rate. But silver lining is standardized, imported sublingual immunotherapy (SLIT) tablet, now approved by Drug Controller General of India (DCGI) and is freely available in India. Of late, interest generated among medical practitioners in learning this subject is high. And in such a scenario, how we are going to increase our knowledge and use available testing and treating products for the betterment of patients in relieving their symptoms within the ambit of the existing legal and ethical framework is what we are going to learn in this chapter.

ROLE OF NATIONAL MEDICAL COMMISSION AND MEDICAL ETHICS IN ALLERGY PRACTICE

Medical ethics, for all practical purposes, may be defined as a code of conduct accepted voluntarily by medical practitioners within the profession. Medical ethics implies the obligations of the physician toward the patient as well as the same obligations toward physicians.

Each and every practicing doctor in any field of modern medicine should have complete knowledge of the *professional code of ethics* given by the Medical Council of India (MCI)/NMC. One signs a declaration at the time of registration that he has read and has agreed to abide by this code. If one is found violating the same, the person can be punished by the state council or NMC after a thorough investigation. The aggrieved person can appeal to the High Court. The *code of ethics* is being reviewed by the NMC which has now replaced the erstwhile MCI. The newer version of it "The National Medical Commission Registered Medical Practitioner (Professional Conduct) Regulation, 2023" was published in the Gazette of Government of India on August 2, 2023. But it was subsequently withdrawn with a gazette notification dated August 23, 2024. Once revised and published, these new regulations will be applicable.

Existing Ethical Code No 7.20 of MCI says that a physician shall not claim to be a specialist unless he has special qualifications in that branch (The caveat in this code is not mentioning of word "recognized" before the special qualification.).

If someone has an NMC-recognized qualification in allergy, then there is no issue. MCI had started a process to give recognition to Allergy and Clinical Immunology as a specialized qualification. A diploma in allergy and clinical immunology was listed, but since no medical college or any other recognized institute had taken up this diploma, it has now withdrawn it.

Now, in the absence of this, we need to look into the following:

A specialist is defined as one who learns more about less and less. The Supreme Court, in its various other judgments, has made it clear that medical practitioners should practice within the scope of their qualifications and skills. So, one needs to have proof of having learned about allergy and has acquired skills in various tests and treatment procedures.

What is available today in India for increasing skill and understanding allergy subject is a 1-year part-time diploma and fellowship, which are special qualifications. Authenticity of the same is based on the curriculum, teachers, institute, and Director of Program. One will also need to keep all other proof of obtaining special knowledge of allergy through all other courses, workshops, trainings, etc. Medical Council-accredited programs will give more weightage. Even after the NMC-recognized postgraduate degree and diploma holders come out in clinical practice, all other abovementioned courses will still hold good since they were achieved before such recognized PG qualifications were available in India. In case asked by any authorities or court for proof, it is better to keep records of all of your credentials, including paper presentations, articles in journals, etc. As of now, no foreign qualification is recognized by the NMC in allergy. And the same abovementioned clarification applies to them if the authenticity of training and knowledge is questioned.

The MCI code of ethics No: 1.4.2, which states that "Physician shall display to their names only recognized medical degrees or such certificates/diplomas and membership/honors, which confer professional knowledge or recognize any exemplary qualification/achievements.

The definition of the word recognized is not specified anywhere in the draft of the code of ethics. But code belongs to MCI and recognized qualification is defined in its act, and they are mentioned in different schedules of the MCI Act 1956. Hence, it is advisable not to add any unrecognized qualification immediately after your main qualifications like MBBS, MD, DCH, or DNB. One can add in a separate line all of your other credentials in full form, and from which institute or university one has obtained them.

In the absence of an NMC-recognized qualification, you cannot label yourself as an allergist or allergologist. It will be best to write on the prescription as "XYZ" Allergy Clinic or Allergy and Immunotherapy Clinic, etc. An expert's name can be included as director or consultant.

ROLE OF GUIDELINES AND STANDARD RECOMMENDATIONS IN ROUTINE ALLERGY PRACTICE

It is always advisable to practice within the broad ambit of known guidelines. In India, two guidelines have been framed.

1. Guidelines for Practice of Allergen Immunotherapy in India 2017: Indian Journal of Allergy, Asthma and Immunology, volume 31, issue 1; developed by the Indian College of Allergy, Asthma & Applied Immunology (ICAAI). Since now standardized SLIT tablet is available and is permitted by DGCA for above 11 years of age, the phrase written in this guideline that SLIT is not permissible in India is now nullified. However, all other Indian companies manufacture SLIT drops which will still remain under off-label use.
2. Indian Guidelines on Allergic Rhinitis formulated by The Association of Otolaryngologists of India (AOI)

Allergy chapter of IAP is expected to publish similar practice guidelines this year in 2025. All other important international guidelines and recommendations like those of the World Allergy Organization (WAO), European Academy of Allergy and Clinical Immunology (EAACI), etc., should be considered as a guide to your clinical practice. Wherever there is a gray zone in management, always keep proof by keeping a copy of the guidelines or position paper or any other proof of authentic backing.

The MCI code of ethics 1.2.1 is self-explanatory and states that "Physicians should try continuously to improve medical knowledge and skills and should make available to their patients and colleagues the benefits of their professional attainments. Physicians should practice a method of healing founded on the scientific basis and should not associate professionally with anyone who violates this principle."

Keep your knowledge updated with the latest consensus statement, position papers, or guidelines.

STANDARDIZED ANTIGENS FOR TESTING AND IMMUNOTHERAPY

Standardized allergens are ones where you know the content of major and minor allergens. There is no batch-to-batch variation, and one can get consistent results with the SPT. The result of both the SPT and the effect of immunotherapy is excellent with standardized antigens. It is advisable to use standardized allergen extracts of known potency with good shelf-life for immunotherapy to ensure consistency and reproducibility of the efficacy and safety of the product in the management of allergic diseases. Such authentic standardized imported allergens are now available in India since April, 2025 as SLIT tablet and licensed for 12–65 years of age-group. If used below this age, it will be an off-label use. But standardized antigens for SPT are not yet available in India.

Although they do not match the quality of imported American or European products, indigenously produced antigen products in India for testing and immunotherapy are manufactured and licensed for human use as per pharmacopoeia guidelines. Such products are manufactured and available in India (Indian Pharmacopoeia 2018, volume III). In recent years, a lot of knowledge has been generated in India on the characterization of major/minor allergens of pollen, fungi, food, and insect sources. However, the purified proteins (major allergens) and monoclonal/polyclonal antibodies are not available for characterization based on major allergen content. Under these circumstances, allergen extracts are standardized based on weight/volume and protein estimation by modified Lowry's bicinchoninic acid assay, or micro-Kjeldahl method. In India, as of the date, manufactured and available antigens are labeled as weight/volume (weight in grams per volume in milliliters) or PNU (protein nitrogen unit). Such extracts have a legal basis for usage, but may have a wide variability of biological potency, and final results will be variable. Such allergen extracts vary from one manufacturer to another; hence, it is suggested that diagnostic and therapeutic allergen extracts should be procured from the same allergen manufacturer. The drug controller of India/state units regulates the allergen manufacture in the country. Currently, the emphasis is on good manufacturing practices to be implemented in these drug antigen units. However, the coordinated efforts of authorities are required to upgrade the quality control of allergen extracts following standard WHO/IUIS/EMA (World Health Organization/International Union of Immunological Societies/European Medicines Agency) protocols. There is a need to develop allergen certification centers in the country, such as the Food and Drug Administration (FDA) and the Centre for Biologics Evaluation and Research in the USA and Paul Ehrlich in Europe.

Diagnostic and therapeutic allergens should be used on patients under the supervision of medical professionals trained in allergy and immunotherapy. The manufacturer should dispense therapeutic vaccines only after obtaining the SPT results of the patient (as mentioned in the Indian Pharmacopoeia). These indigenous allergens are licensed for SPT and subcutaneous immunotherapy (SCIT). But their role in SLIT comes under off-label use. Immunotherapy is tailor-made for individual patients. And from available immunotherapy material from authorized licensed Indian manufacturer allergy consultants can use it for their patients as SLIT based on their expertise and competency as off-label medication taking due precaution and appropriate consent. Indian Drug rules permit a doctor to prescribe, compound, dispense, or dilute FDA-approved products for his patients, but cannot sell or commercialize.

Sublingual immunotherapy is approved by Karnataka State Food and Drug Administration for one center in Bengaluru that manufactures and uses it for their patients. Such approval by the State FDA is enough to use that medication across India.

Some centers in India are procuring standardized allergens for their patients from the USA or Europe under import licenses, both for testing and immunotherapy.

OFF-LABEL USE OF A DRUG

Off-label use refers to the prescription of approved (permitted) medicines for an unapproved indication (age/route of administration/duration/different disease/condition/etc.). Absence of labeling for a specific age-group or a specific disorder does not necessarily mean that the drug's use is improper for that age or disorder. It may be due to a lack of sufficient evidence. No law also prohibits off-label drug use in the United States and Canada and many other developed countries.

There is no direct clause regarding this in the Drugs and Cosmetics Act of India, 1940 or the rules of 1945 that bans such off-label use by a registered medical practitioner, but there are important caveats:

1. *Section 104 A of the Drugs and Cosmetics Rules, 1945 (added via amendments):* Promotional claims for unapproved uses are restricted.

   Manufacturers cannot market or advertise a drug for any off-label use unless approved by the CDSCO (Central Drug Standard Control Organisation).

   So, doctors can prescribe off-label, but pharma companies cannot promote off-label use.

2. Indian Medical Council (Professional Conduct, Etiquette and Ethics) Regulations, 2002

   Rule 1.9: Every doctor should practice evidence-based medicine.

   Rule 7.20: Prohibits any "violation of human rights" or "unethical experimentation".

   Off-label use must be backed by credible literature or consensus, and informed consent is highly recommended.

   Hence, SLIT from an Indian Manufacturer can be used by taking above-mentioned precautions.

INSURANCE COVERAGE IN IMMUNOTHERAPY

While specific insurance companies and their coverage for SLIT can vary, several health insurance policies in India offer coverage for allergy treatments, which may include SLIT. Some policies specifically mention covering hospitalization due to allergies. It is crucial to review the specific terms and conditions of your health insurance policy to confirm coverage for SLIT or other allergy treatments. SLIT is a relatively new treatment, and some insurance companies may not have fully established coverage due to the lack of FDA approval for all SLIT products.

To ensure coverage for SLIT, it's recommended to directly contact your insurance provider and ask about the specific details of your policy and whether it covers SLIT or other allergy treatments.

COST-EFFECTIVENESS OF ALLERGEN IMMUNOTHERAPY

There is strong evidence in the collective literature, which includes individual studies and systematic reviews, that allergen immunotherapy (AIT) is cost-effective in the management of allergic rhinitis and asthma as compared with standard drug treatment alone. The magnitude of AIT's cost-effectiveness is likely underestimated because most of the studies considered during-treatment costs and not the long-term benefits or preventive or prophylactic effects of AIT.

UNAVAILABILITY OF ADRENALINE AUTOINJECTOR

There is no other option other than to keep a prefilled syringe (preferably a glass one), ideally in a spectacle case or any other cover to prevent exposure to sunlight. Efficacy and potency of such a technique are not known and have never been tested. It does not have any legal basis, and treatment becomes off-label.

CONSENT FOR ALLERGY TEST AND IMMUNOTHERAPY

Proper informed consent is a must for every procedure which carries some risk. Hence, written consent is required to be taken in every procedure of testing, from SPT, drug test or food challenge test, mentioning the type of procedure and risk involved. The risk involved may be negligible in routine SPTs, to very high in drug provocation or food challenge tests. Also, separate consent is required before initiating immunotherapy. SLIT may have minimal risk compared to SCIT. More important is to equip your clinic to tackle any untoward reaction which can happen on rare occasions. Also, mention that utmost care should be taken during the concerned procedure and if at all in rare occasions any untoward reaction does occur clinic or hospital is well equipped to tackle it. All other routine matter concerned with consent has to be followed, like using the same pen, taking the signature of the witness along with the patient or guardian, etc. And avoid taking blanket consent which has no legal validity, as they do not mention any specific procedure or its possible complications.

GENERAL PRECAUTIONS

Do not venture into a new field without acquiring proper knowledge and training. Just attending a half-day workshop may not be enough to start immunotherapy. Understand the subject, get well-trained and then practice it. This holds good especially when no authentic NMC-recognized curriculum is available in this subject. Stepping into the field of drug testing and desensitization, or oral food challenge, should be done carefully after much experience in basic allergy practice and taking all required precautions. Ideally should be done in a hospital setup where all emergency facilities like the intensive care unit are available. Evolving modes of therapy like oral immunotherapy for certain foods like milk should be attempted as per available protocols only, and if done under therapeutic trials, ethical clearance will be required.

SUMMARY

Every medical practitioner practicing medicine in today's world should be aware of their limitations. And should practice his subject within the ambit of what is permissible. It is always better to regularly update your knowledge, and proof of the same should be produced if asked for. Always take separate written consent for different procedures and treatments, and do not forget to take all required precautions and keep your clinic well equipped to tackle any emergency.

Key Learning Points

- *Practicing allergy within ethical and legal boundaries:* Physicians must follow the *MCI/NMC Code of Ethics*, which prohibits claiming a specialist title (e.g., "Allergist") without an NMC-recognized qualification. However, documented training through accredited diploma/fellowship programs, workshops, and certifications is essential and legally defensible when practicing allergy care.

- *Importance of standardized guidelines and documentation:* It is advisable to follow national (e.g., IAP, ICAAI, AOI) or international (e.g., WAO, EAACI) guidelines for allergy testing and immunotherapy. Keeping printed evidence of practice standards, updated knowledge, and protocols helps justify care decisions, especially in medicolegal scenarios.
- *Understanding off-label use and legal safeguards:* Off-label use (e.g., SLIT drops from Indian manufacturers, adrenaline in prefilled syringes) is legally permissible for doctors in India but not promotable by companies. Such use must be *evidence-based*, accompanied by *informed consent*, and documented carefully to minimize legal risk.
- *Consent and emergency preparedness are mandatory:* Written, specific informed consent is essential for allergy testing and immunotherapy (SCIT/SLIT). Clinics must be equipped for emergency care and follow proper documentation (not blanket consent) with witness signatures.
- *Limitations of current resources and pathways for legitimacy:* Since India lacks widespread availability of standardized SPT antigens and adrenaline autoinjectors, practitioners must use legally permitted indigenous products or approved imports. Training and meticulous recordkeeping of one's credentials (courses, publications, and workshops) enhance legitimacy until formal NMC-recognized qualifications become available.

SUGGESTED READING

1. American Cancer Society. Is off-label drug use legal? [online] Available from http://www.cancer.org/treatment/treatmentsandsideeffects/treatmenttypes/chemotherapy/off-label-drug-use [Last accessed, August, 2025].
2. Baba SM, Rasool R, Gull A, Qureshi TA, Beigh AH, Qadri Q, et al. Effectiveness of sublingual immunotherapy in the treatment of HDM-induced nasobronchial allergies: a 3-year randomized case-control study from Kashmir. Front Immunol. 2021;12:723814.
3. Bijli KM, Singh BP, Sridhara S, Gaur SN, Arora N. Effects of various stabilizing agents on Imperata cylindrica grass pollen allergen extract. Clin Exp Allergy. 2003;33:65-71.
4. Cox LS, Murphey A, Hankin C. The Cost-Effectiveness of allergen immunotherapy compared with pharmacotherapy for treatment of allergic rhinitis and asthma. Immunol Allergy Clin North Am. 2020;40(1):69-85.
5. Frattarelli DA, Galinkin JL, Green TP, Johnson TD, Neville KA, Paul IM, et al.; American Academy of Pediatrics Committee on Drugs. Off-label use of drugs in children. Pediatrics. 2014;133(3):563-7.
6. Gaur SN, Kumar RS, Agarwal MK, Arora N. Guidelines for practice of allergen immunotherapy in India: 2017—An update. Indian J Allergy Asthma Immunol. 2017;31(1):3-33.
7. Gupta R, Singh BP, Sridgara S, Gaur SN, Chaudhary VK, Arora N. Allergens of curvularia lunata during cultivation in different media. J Allergy Clin Immunol. 1999;104:857-62.
8. Medical Council of India. (2016). Code of Medical Ethics Regulations, 2002. (Amended up to 8th October 2016). [online] Available from https://www.nmc.org.in/wp-content/uploads/2017/10/Ethics-Regulations-2002.pdf [Last accessed, August, 2025].
9. Park K. Park's Textbook of Preventive and Social Medicine, 18th edition. Jabalpur: Banarsidas Bhanot; pp. 508-11.
10. Singh BP, Gangal SV. Defined allergen extracts; need for efficient diagnosis of allergy and immunotherapy. Indian J Allergy Appl Immunol. 2001;15:67-72.
11. Singh BP, Kukreja N, Arora N. Clinically relevant allergens from fungi imperfecti and yeast. In: Kurup VP (Ed). Mold Allergy, Biology and Pathogenesis. Trivendrum: Research Signpost; 2005. pp. 77-92.
12. Singh BP, Sridhara S, Arora N, Gangal SV. Evaluation of protein assay method for pollen and fungal spore extracts. Biochem Int. 1992; 27;477-84.
13. Singh BP, Verma J, Arora N, Sridhara S. Status of allergen standardization in India. Arbeiten aus dem Paul Ehrlich Institute Band 93, 9th International Paul-Ehrlich Seminar (1999), GIT Verlag, Darmstadt, FRG; 2000. pp. 41-5.
14. Standing Senate Committee on Social Affairs, Science and Technology. Prescription Pharmaceuticals in Canada: Off-Label Use.

[online] Available from http://www.parl.gc.ca/Content/SEN/Committee/412/soci/rep/rep05jan14-e.pdf [Last accessed, August, 2025].

15. Thangam Sudha V, Arora N, Sridhara S, Gaur SN, Singh BP. Biopotency and identification of allergenic proteins in Periplaneta Americana extract for clinical aplications. Biologicals. 2007;35:131-7.
16. The Association of Otolaryngologists of India. Indian Guidelines on Allergic Rhinitis. [online] Available from https://www.aoiho.org/wp-content/uploads/AOI-AR-Guidelines.pdf [Last accessed, August, 2025].
17. Tiwari S, Baldwa M, Tiwari M, Kuthe A. Textbook on Medicolegal Issues: Related to Various Medical Specialties. New Delhi: Jaypee Brothers Medical Publishers; p. 162.
18. Unni JC, Joseph RB. Off-label medications in pediatrics. Indian J Pharmacy Pharmacol. 2022;9(1):18-23.

APPENDICIES: CONSENT FORMS

Appendix A: Consent Form for Immunotherapy

(Specific changes to be done if SLIT Tablet is used)

Name of Patient: ______________________________ Age: ________ Sex: ________

Address: ______________________________ Date: ________ Time: ________

I, undersigned Mr/Mrs/Ms ______________, father/mother of ________, age ________ years, from ________ have been explained about immunotherapy in detail in a language understood by me. I have been advised to stay in the clinic for 30 minutes after the dose. I have been informed that the antigen to which the patient is sensitive is being given in diluted form and gradually increasing the strength over a long period. The positive effect may take up to 6 months to 1 year, and further, it has to be continued for 3 to 5 years. Chances of improvement of medical condition and untoward effects, if any, are also explained. I have been advised to get medical help instantly if any untoward effects arise. I will take all the precautions explained by my doctor during immunotherapy. I/we have been advised to stay in the clinic/hospital for 30 minutes after every dose of injectable immunotherapy or during 1st dose of sublingual immunotherapy for observation. The chances of adverse effects are extremely rare, and in case they occur, this clinic/hospital is well equipped to handle the emergency. I have opted for Sublingual Immunotherapy as against Subcutaneous or Injectable immunotherapy, given all the pros and cons, like a visit to the doctor's clinic for each dose and lesser chances of severe reaction. I have understood the aforesaid and I am giving my consent willingly with a sound mental state without any coercion, undue influence, fraud, misrepresentation or mistake of facts.

______________________	______________________
Patient/Guardian	Doctor
______________________	______________________
Witness 1	Witness 2

Appendix B: Consent for Skin Prick Test

Name of Patient: ______________________________ Age: ________ Sex: ________

Address: ______________________________ Date: ________ Time: ________

I, undersigned Mr/Mrs/Ms ______________, father/mother/guardian of ________, age ________ years, from ________ give my consent for myself/my ward to conduct allergy testing by various antigens through skin prick testing. The allergen will be placed as drops on the forearm or the back. These drops will be introduced just below the upper layer of skin by a needle/lancet. Allergic response will be noted by red raised itchy hives within 15 to 20 minutes. I/We have been advised to stay in the clinic for 30 minutes after the last prick. I have been explained the procedure and risks involved, if any, in a language understood by me. The chances of adverse effects or risk are extremely rare. But this clinic/hospital is well equipped to handle the emergency. I have understood the aforesaid and I am giving my consent willingly with a sound mental state without any coercion, undue influence, fraud, misrepresentation or mistake of facts.

______________________	______________________
Patient/Guardian	Doctor
______________________	______________________
Witness 1	Witness 2

CHAPTER

16

Building an Allergy Care Network in India

Vikram Patra
Reviewer: *Neeraj Gupta*

INTRODUCTION

India faces a rising tide of allergic diseases, including asthma, allergic rhinitis, eczema, food and drug allergies, and anaphylaxis. Despite the high disease burden—affecting up to 30% of the population—*allergy* and *immunology* remains under-recognized and under-resourced in the Indian healthcare landscape. The lack of trained specialists, standardized diagnostics, and accessible treatments highlights the urgent need for a structured and collaborative approach. This chapter outlines the strategic framework needed to establish a robust and scalable Allergy Care Network (ACN) in India that is inclusive, evidence-based, and tailored to the country's unique challenges.

India is currently seeing a fast rise in allergic diseases. These include asthma, allergic rhinitis, eczema, food allergies, drug allergies, and anaphylaxis. Studies show that 20–30% of people in India may have one or more allergic conditions. Despite the growing burden, allergy remains a relatively neglected discipline within Indian healthcare. There are many barriers for delivery of high-quality allergy healthcare in India. Few important ones are mentioned in the following text.

BARRIERS FOR DELIVERY OF HIGH-QUALITY ALLERGY HEALTHCARE IN INDIA

Economic and Regulatory Factors

- Low national gross domestic product (GDP) and unavailability of essential medicines free of cost or at subsidized prices for patients from lower socioeconomic group:
  - Inhalers
  - Adrenaline autoinjectors
  - *Biologics:* Omalizumab, mepolizumab
- *Lack of access to good-quality allergy diagnostics and treatments:*
  - Nonavailability of standardized allergen-specific immunotherapy products [sublingual immunotherapy (SLIT) and subcutaneous immunotherapy (SCIT)]
  - Nonavailability of standardized allergen extracts for skin tests
  - Limited access and expensive in vitro immunodiagnostic tests
  - Nonavailability of penicillin allergy skin testing kits
- Lack of healthcare insurance for a majority of population
- Lack of area-specific meteorological data on pollen and fungal spores
- Lack of legislation on precautionary allergen labeling
- Lack of infrastructure for drug allergy recording in healthcare system
- Poor reporting of adverse drug reactions

Education and Training

- Lack of specialists in allergy and immunology
- Lack of training in allergy and immunology for organ-based specialists and family physicians delivering allergy care
- Lack of specialist asthma and allergy nurses in healthcare system
- Lack of education tools for patients, carers and parents

Clinical Practice and Research

- Guidelines from high-income countries not "fit for purpose" for Indian population
- Need for phenotypic characterization of allergic diseases in Indian population

Adverse Environmental Factors

- *Outdoor air pollution:* The air is polluted by traffic, burning biomass, and fossil fuels, which leads to high PM2.5 levels.
- *Indoor air pollution:* Indoor air can be polluted by things like incense sticks, dhoop sticks, tobacco smoke, and mosquito coils.
- Cockroach exposure

A well-organized *Allergy Care Network* can bring major improvements in how allergies are diagnosed and treated in India.

- It can help provide care that is standardized and based on the latest evidence.
- It can support early diagnosis and help prevent allergies from getting worse.
- It encourages doctors from different specialties to work together.
- It can improve training for healthcare workers in allergy and immunology.
- It also supports research that fits India's unique population and environment.

This chapter focuses on three key building blocks needed to set-up an effective allergy network:

1. A team-based approach involving experts from different fields
2. Structured programs for training and education
3. The setup of specialized allergy centers across the country

MULTIDISCIPLINARY TEAM APPROACH

Importance of Multidisciplinary Collaboration

Allergic diseases frequently involve multiple systems, such as the respiratory tract, skin, and gastrointestinal system, and they may mimic or overlap with other chronic conditions. Single-specialty care often fails to address the interconnected nature of allergic diseases, leading to suboptimal outcomes.

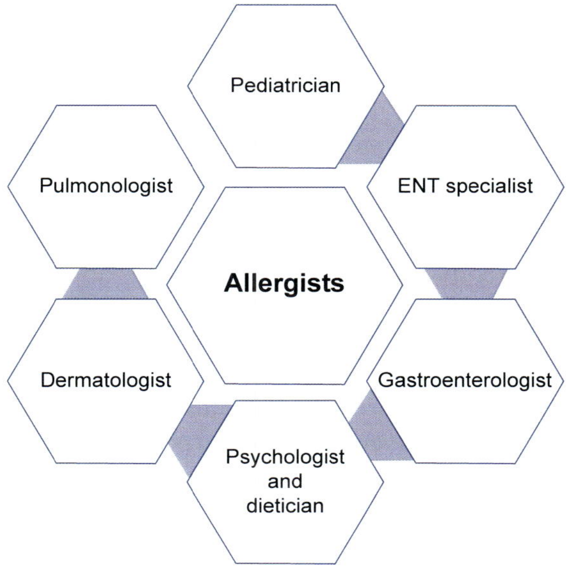

Fig. 1: Multidisciplinary collaboration.

A multidisciplinary approach ***(Fig. 1)****:*

- Enables comprehensive evaluation and management
- Reduces fragmentation of care
- Facilitates shared decision-making
- Ensures appropriate referrals and follow-up

Role of Various Specialists

Allergists/Clinical Immunologists

- They are the main experts and central coordinators for the diagnosis and treatment of allergies.
- They perform and explain tests like skin prick tests, blood tests for immunoglobulin E (IgE), component-resolved diagnostics (CRD), and drug challenge tests.

- They treat patients with difficult asthma using fewer steroids and advanced medicines like biologics [such as anti-IgE or anti-IL-5 (interleukin 5)].
- They create personalized treatment plans using immunotherapy—either by injection (SCIT) or drops/tablets under the tongue (SLIT).
- They also manage serious conditions like anaphylaxis, mast cell disorders, and primary immune system problems.

Pediatricians

- Pediatricians are often the first point of contact for children showing early signs of allergic disease, such as eczema, recurrent wheeze, or food intolerance.
- They are skilled at identifying red flags for IgE-mediated allergies, monitoring growth in food-allergic children, and recognizing progression along the allergic march.
- Provide critical input in childhood vaccination and infection control in atopic children
- Key in family counseling and long-term monitoring

Pulmonologists

- Pulmonologists specialize in the management of asthma, a condition that frequently coexists with allergic rhinitis and atopic dermatitis.
- They use advanced diagnostic tools such as spirometry, bronchodilator reversibility testing, fractional exhaled nitric oxide (FeNO), and bronchial provocation testing to assess and monitor respiratory function in allergic patients.

Gastroenterologists

- Specialize in managing gastrointestinal (GI) allergies like eosinophilic esophagitis, which often coexists with food allergy
- *Utilize advanced diagnostics:* Endoscopic biopsies

Dermatologists

- Dermatologists manage a wide range of skin allergies, including urticaria, angioedema, contact dermatitis, and atopic dermatitis.
- They utilize specialized diagnostic tools such as patch testing, dermatoscopy, and histopathology, especially for chronic or atypical skin conditions.
- They play a key role in identifying and diagnosing drug-induced skin reactions.

Ear–Nose–Throat Specialists

- Essential for diagnosing and managing upper airway allergies—chronic rhinosinusitis, nasal polyps, and allergic rhinitis
- Perform endoscopic assessments for patients with nasal symptoms unresponsive to medical therapy

Dietitians

- Assess nutritional risks in food-allergic children or elimination diets
- Create balanced, allergen-free diets
- Advise on unnecessary food restrictions
- Educate families about label reading, hidden allergens, and safe food introduction

Psychologists

- Address anxiety in children, adolescents, and adults, especially those with life-threatening allergies
- Help in behavioral therapies for atopic dermatitis, urticaria, or treatment adherence issues.
- Help in improving quality-of-life index in allergy patients

TRAINING AND EDUCATION

Current Landscape

Despite the high disease burden, allergy training remains underdeveloped in India:

- Allergy is not recognized as a distinct specialty by medical councils.

- Lack of structured training leads to misdiagnosis or empirical treatments.
- Very few centers offer hands-on training in allergy diagnostics or immunotherapy.

Postdoctoral Training Programs in Allergy and Clinical Immunology

To build a skilled workforce:

- A 3-year superspecialty programs like DM or DNB must be developed in tertiary hospitals or academic centers.
- Alternatively, 1- to 2-year full-time fellowship/postgraduate diploma programs must be developed.
- Curriculum should be competency-based, including:
    - Skin prick and patch testing
    - Spirometry and FeNO
    - Drug and food challenges
    - Immunotherapy preparation and monitoring
    - Emergency management of anaphylaxis
- Inclusion of modules on CRD, biologics, and environmental allergens

Continuing Medical Education and Skill-Building Workshops

- Regular continuing medical education (CME) programs to update general practitioners, pediatricians, and dermatologists on:
    - New guidelines [e.g., Global Initiative for Asthma (GINA), World Allergy Organization (WAO), European Academy of Allergy and Clinical Immunology (EAACI)]
    - Emerging diagnostic tools
    - Rational pharmacotherapy
    - Emergency management of anaphylaxis
    - Referral pathways
- Regional and national societies [e.g., IAP Pediatric Allergy and Applied Immunology (PAAI), Indian College of Allergy, Asthma and Applied Immunology (ICAAI), etc.] should facilitate *interactive workshops*, case presentations, and panel discussions.

Online Certification Courses

At present, few courses are already in place-like Diploma in Pediatric Allergy and Asthma (DPAA) and Diploma in Allergy and Asthma (DAA) at WAO Centers of Excellence, IAP Pediatric Allergy and Asthma Course (IAP-PAAC), and Advance Asthma Certificate Course, etc.

- To develop many more 6–12 months' modular courses through:
    - Government health universities
    - Online education portals (e.g., dIAP, IMA eLearning, NPTEL)
    - Certification in "Basic Allergy Practice" or "Pediatric Allergy Care" for primary care providers
    - Use of virtual laboratories, simulation tools, and case-based e-learning to supplement practical learning

Training of Allied Health Professionals

- Nurses must be trained in:
    - Skin test preparation
    - Immunotherapy administration
    - Monitoring during food and drug challenges
- Dietitians should be included in structured allergy care education modules.

ESTABLISHING SPECIALIZED ALLERGY CENTERS

Vision for Allergy Centers of Excellence

Specialized centers are necessary to offer comprehensive, evidence-based, and multidisciplinary care, while also serving as regional hubs for research, education, and policy development. Recently, Sir Ganga Ram Hospital at New Delhi, Christian Medical College at Vellore and DY Patil

Hospital and School of Medicine at Navi Mumbai have been designated as "Centre of Excellence" by WAO. We need more such reference centers, at least one in each state.

Structural Components

Outpatient and Diagnostic Services

- Weekly dedicated allergy clinics
- *Diagnostic infrastructure:*
  - Skin prick and patch testing setups
  - Spirometry and FeNO
  - Enzyme-linked immunosorbent assay (ELISA) and ImmunoCAP for IgE testing
  - Nasal provocation testing and peak flow monitoring
- Provision for oral food/drug challenges under intensive care unit (ICU) supervision.

Immunotherapy Unit

- Preparation of standardized allergen extracts (with licensing and quality control)
- Facility for SCIT and SLIT
- Protocols for updosing, maintenance, and long-term follow-up
- Monitoring adverse reactions and rescue protocols

Inpatient and Emergency Services

- Beds for anaphylaxis observation, severe eczema flares, or drug hypersensitivity reactions
- ICU access for complex cases undergoing diagnostic testing or biologic infusions

Research and Clinical Trials

- Study regional allergen prevalence (e.g., pollens, mites, food allergens).
- Develop Indian-specific CRD panels.
- Conduct trials on cost-effective immunotherapy, biosimilars, and novel biologics.
- Collaborate with universities and pharma companies.

BOX 1: Tech-based innovations for allergy care.

Mobile Apps:
- Daily symptom tracking
- Reminder alerts for immunotherapy
- Identifying local pollen/allergen levels

SMS campaigns:
- Educating parents about food allergies
- Promoting World Allergy Week

QR-coded emergency cards:
- Anaphylaxis patients carry these for instant ER guidance

Education and Awareness Wing

- Develop IEC (information, education, and communication) materials (posters, videos, handouts) in local languages.
- Host "asthma schools", caregiver training workshops, and school health programs.
- Digital outreach via apps, webinars, and SMS reminders.
- Public engagement and technology use **(Box 1)**

National and Regional Network Integration

- Link tertiary allergy centers with district hospitals and primary health centers (PHCs) through telemedicine and referral systems.
- Build shared electronic health records (EHRs) for allergy tracking.
- Align with national programs like Ayushman Bharat for policy support and funding.
- Promote public-private partnerships for expanding reach, affordability, and innovation.

SUMMARY

The chapter provides a comprehensive roadmap for establishing a national ACN in India to address the growing burden of allergic diseases. It highlights the pressing challenges—including economic, regulatory, educational, and infrastructural gaps—that hinder quality allergy care. The chapter proposes a three-pronged strategy:

(1) A multidisciplinary team-based approach involving specialists across pediatrics, pulmonology, dermatology, ENT, dietetics, psychology, and immunology; (2) Structured training programs, fellowships, and certification courses to build skilled human resources; and (3) the development of specialized allergy centers of excellence equipped with diagnostics, immunotherapy units, emergency care, and research facilities. The chapter emphasizes integration with national health programs, telemedicine, and digital tools to scale access and impact.

Key Learning Points

- *Multidisciplinary collaboration is essential:* Allergic diseases often span multiple organ systems. Collaborative care involving allergists, pediatricians, pulmonologists, dermatologists, ENT specialists, dietitians, and psychologists ensures comprehensive, patient-centered allergy management.
- *Training and education are foundational pillars:* India lacks formal recognition of allergy as a medical specialty. Structured training programs, fellowships, and CME initiatives are critical to empower generalists and specialists with diagnostic and therapeutic skills.
- *Specialized allergy centers must be developed:* Centers of Excellence must offer outpatient and inpatient care, immunotherapy, diagnostics, research, and education. These hubs should be established in each state and integrated through a national network.
- *Technology and public engagement can catalyze progress:* Use of telemedicine, mobile Apps, EHRs, and online certification courses can expand reach and improve continuity of care. Awareness campaigns and school programs can boost community-level impact.
- *Policy support and multisectoral investment are crucial:* Realizing the vision of an effective ACN requires alignment with public health policies, academic initiatives, and support from governmental and private stakeholders.

SUGGESTED READING

1. Barker S, Daniels L, Chang YS, Chikovani T, DunnGalvin A, Gerdts JD, et al. Allergy education and training for physicians. World Allergy Organ J. 2021;14(10):100589.
2. Krishna MT, Mahesh PA, Vedanthan P, Moitra S, Mehta V, Christopher DJ. An appraisal of allergic disorders in India and an urgent call for action. World Allergy Organ J. 2020;13(7):100446.
3. Krishna MT, Singh AB, Gaur SN, Mahesh PA. Research priorities and strategies to improve asthma and allergy care in India. Clin Exp Allergy. 2022;52(3):367-9.
4. Mahesh PA, Moitra S, Mabalirajan U, Garg M, Malamardi S, Vedanthan PK, et al. Allergic diseases in India: Prevalence, risk factors and current challenges. Clin Exp Allergy. 2023;53(3):276-94.
5. Matricardi PM, Dramburg S, Alvarez-Perea A, Antolín-Amérigo D, Apfelbacher C, Atanaskovic-Markovic M, et al. The role of mobile health technologies in allergy care: An EAACI position paper. Allergy. 2020;75(2):259-72.
6. Oppenheimer J, Bender B, Sousa-Pinto B, Portnoy J. Use of Technology to Improve Adherence in Allergy/Immunology. J Allergy Clin Immunol Pract. 2024;12(12):3225-33.
7. Vassilopoulou E, Skypala I, Feketea G, Gawlik R, Dunn Galvin A, Meyer R, et al. A multi-disciplinary approach to the diagnosis and management of allergic diseases: An EAACI Task Force. Pediatr Allergy Immunol. 2022;33(1):e13692.

Index

Page numbers followed by *b* refer to box, *f* refer to figure, *fc* refer to flowchart, and *t* refer to table.

S

T

U

V

W

X

Z